Comprehensive Manuals of Surgical Specialties

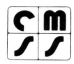

Richard H. Egdahl, editor

Claude E. Welch   Leslie W. Ottinger   John P. Welch

Manual of Lower Gastrointestinal Surgery

Includes 138 color illustrations and 77 illustrations in black and white

Springer-Verlag
New York   Heidelberg   Berlin

Comprehensive Manuals of Surgical Specialties

SERIES EDITOR

Richard H. Egdahl, M.D., Ph.D., Professor of Surgery, Boston University Medical Center, Boston, Massachusetts 02118

AUTHORS

Claude E. Welch, M.D., D.Sc., F.A.C.S., Clinical Professor of Surgery Emeritus at Harvard Medical School; Senior Surgeon, Massachusetts General Hospital, Warren Building, 275 Charles Street, Boston, Massachusetts 02114

Leslie W. Ottinger, M.D., F.A.C.S., Harvard University Associate Professor of Surgery at the Massachusetts General Hospital; Visiting Surgeon, Massachusetts General Hospital, Warren Building, 275 Charles Street, Boston, Massachusetts 02114

John P. Welch, M.D., F.A.C.S., Adjunct Assistant Professor of Surgery at Dartmouth Medical School; Assistant Professor of Surgery, University of Connecticut, 85 Jefferson Street, Hartford, Connecticut 06106

MEDICAL ILLUSTRATORS

Edith Tagrin, Chief, Medical Art Unit, Massachusetts General Hospital, Boston, Massachusetts 02118

Robert J. Galla, Medical Art Unit, Massachusetts General Hospital, Boston, Massachusetts 02118

Library of Congress Cataloging in Publication Data

Welch, Claude E.
   Manual of lower gastrointestinal surgery.

   (Comprehensive manuals of surgical specialties)
   Includes bibliographical references and index.
   1. Colon (Anatomy)—Surgery. 2. Rectum—
Surgery. I. Ottinger, Leslie W., joint author.
II. Welch, John Paton, 1942- joint author.
III. Title.
RD544.W44   617'.5547   79-9534

Printed in the United States of America.

9 8 7 6 5 4 3 2 1

ISBN 0-387-90205-8 Springer-Verlag New York Heidelberg Berlin
ISBN 3-540-90205-8 Springer-Verlag Berlin Heidelberg New York

I hav finally kum to the konklusion,
that a good reliable sett ov bowels
iz wurth more tu a man, than enny
quantity ov brains.

Josh Billings
(early American aphorism)

Editor's Note

Comprehensive Manuals of Surgical Specialties is a series of surgical manuals designed to present current operative techniques and to explore various aspects of diagnosis and treatment. The series features a unique format with emphasis on large, detailed, full-color illustrations, schematic charts and photographs to demonstrate integral steps in surgical procedures.

Each manual focuses on a specific region or topic and describes surgical anatomy, physiology, pathology, diagnosis and operative treatment. Operative techniques and stratagems for dealing with surgically correctable disorders are described in detail. Illustrations are primarily depicted from the surgeon's viewpoint to enhance clarity and comprehension.

Other volumes in preparation:

Manual of Vascular Surgery
Manual of Cardiac Surgery
Manual of Liver Surgery
Manual of Soft Tissue Tumor Surgery
Manual of Orthopaedic Surgery
Manual of Upper Gastrointestinal Surgery
Manual of Plastic Surgery
Manual of Ambulatory Surgery

Richard H. Egdahl

Preface

The surgeon who desires an atlas of techniques covering operations on the colon and rectum almost surely prefers a concise volume rather than an encyclopedic compilation of the innumerable procedures that have been described in the literature. This book includes the operations that have proved to be useful and have survived the test of time. They now are in general use in the Massachusetts General Hospital.

Space limitations have necessitated exclusion of detailed illustrations of a number of infrequently performed procedures, such as pelvic exenteration for cancer of the rectum. In such instances bibliographic references have been provided for ready reference. The bibliography emphasizes recent contributions because they are easily available to the reader.

Critical comments by the authors concerning certain technical procedures may be due to personal bias and certainly do not imply that the alternative methods are undesirable. Furthermore, the brevity of discussion of anatomy, physiology, and pathology and the neglect of details of medical therapy of numerous colorectal diseases must be attributed to the fact that this volume is directed primarily toward the practicing surgeon.

Thanks are due to the artists Mrs. Edith Tagrin and Mr. Robert Galla, and to Miss Evelyn Hall for help in the preparation of the manuscript.

Claude E. Welch, M.D.
Leslie W. Ottinger, M.D.
John P. Welch, M.D.

Contents

Introduction

This volume is devoted primarily to a description of operative procedures on the colon and rectum. For this reason various diseases, including their symptoms and alternatives to surgical therapy, will be discussed only briefly. The treatment of many of these diseases by medical measures clearly will not receive the emphasis that it should in practice.

At first glance it might appear that operations on the large bowel are relatively simple in theory, involving only removal of a lesion, and then, when appropriate, reconstruction of intestinal continuity. However, all surgeons who have worked in this area will recognize the numerous variations that are required upon these simple themes. The frequency of complications encountered either at the time of operation or afterward make this type of surgery difficult and dangerous. In this volume the authors will emphasize the techniques that they have found to be satisfactory, safe, and effective. Other methods will also be described and, when appropriate, the reasons one is preferred over another will be given.

This volume covers primarily diseases in adults. Infants and children have special problems, such as imperforate anus, colonic atresia, complicated fistulas between the urogenital tract and the rectum, Hirschsprung's disease, and idiopathic ileocolic intussusception. Inasmuch as they will be covered in a separate volume, they will not be discussed here except as they are encountered in adults.

Since the primary concern in this book is with technical procedures, it is appropriate to delineate historical trends and to list names of some of the great pioneers; many operations still bear their names.

The history of colorectal surgery may be divided into several epochs. The first was the preanesthetic era, which lasted until 1850. The next century saw the great expansion of abdominal surgery and the definition of diseases that could be treated appropriately by such techniques. The past three decades since World War II may be called the modern era and have seen a dramatic reduction in mortality, not due primarily to better surgical skills, but to great improvements in ancillary care.

In the preanesthetic era colorectal surgery was confined chiefly to the treatment of traumatic injuries and anal diseases. One major event was the famous fistula-in-ano of Louis XIV.[21(p.393)] The successful cure by the royal surgeon, Felix, elicited a remarkable display of generosity from the monarch that included the rehabilitation of French surgery and led to the foundation of the French Academy of Surgery in 1731.

Nevertheless, colorectal surgery essentially was restricted to the treatment of hemorrhoids, fissures-in-ano, and fistulas for many years after that. For example, hemorrhoidectomy 150 years ago was a very grim procedure. The second patient admitted to the Massachusetts General Hospital suffered from hemorrhoids. According to the surgical records, four strong men held the patient in a knee–chest position while the surgeon, of course without the benefit of any anesthesia, grasped the huge, protruding hemorrhoids in clamps and excised them. The pain from the procedure was compounded by the copper sulfate enemas that were given regularly on succeeding days until healing finally resulted.

St. Mark's Hospital for Fistulas and Other Diseases of the Rectum was opened in London in 1835. It has been the most important center for the study of colorectal diseases for the past 150 years.

After the advent of anesthesia and antisepsis, the second period of colonic surgery was characterized by explorations of various diseases that could be conquered by surgery. Meanwhile, however, many old methods of treatment were retained. Until 1900, for example, the optimum treatment of a fissure-in-ano consisted of division of the sphincters and the posterior wall of the rectum upward for a distance of several inches. Prior to this date a few surgeons had investigated the possibility of the use of colonic stomas for the relief of intestinal obstruction due to cancer of the rectum. Reybard, in 1823, had carried out a successful resection and anastomosis of the sigmoid colon.[54] Travers, in 1812, had laid the basis for successful intestinal suture.[61] Cancer of the lower rectum, since it was essentially an external cancer, was also amenable to therapy. Lisfranc first successfully removed one in 1826[33]; the first extraperitoneal excision of cancer of the rectum done in the Massachusetts General Hospital was performed by John Warren in 1842.

With the advent of anesthesia and antisepsis curative operations for cancer of the colon became feasible. The first successful right colectomy was done by Maydl in 1883[38] and a transsacral approach for cancer of the rectum was first used by Kraske in 1885.[30] However, because of the proved dangers of intraperitoneal anastomosis, three surgeons in the last few years of the 19th century—Mikulicz,[42] Bloch,[9] and Paul[48]—independently but almost simultaneously described and popularized the use of a diverting colostomy with delayed anastomosis after the excision of a cancer of the colon. The earliest description of this operation, however, according to Maingot, was by Bryant in 1883.[12]

Other diseases that proved curable by surgery included appendicitis, which was first identified in 1886 by Fitz.[19] Soon afterward appendectomy became one of the most common abdominal operations. Diverticulitis was essentially an unknown disease in 1900; fistulas from the colon to the bladder were observed occasionally but the presence of diverticulitis was not suspected. Although in 1907 W.J. Mayo et al.[40] described a few cases in which resection of the colon had been necessary for diverticulitis, this disease attained very little prominence until the modern era.

In 1908 Miles described his combined abdominoperineal resection for cancer of the rectum; the principles of a one-stage operation that combined excision of the tumor with a wide removal of mesentery and lymphatics marked him as a pioneer in cancer surgery.[43] The contributions that were made by him in St. Mark's Hospital were continued by numerous surgeons thereafter, including Lockhart-Mummery, Abel, and Parks. Dukes' classification of rectal cancer was developed in that institution in 1932,[17] and important histologic work has since been carried on by Bussey and by Morson. Sphincter-saving operations for cancer of the rectum were developed by Quenu in 1897[50] and Hochenegg in 1897.[27] They were revived later by Babcock,[4] followed by Bacon. Hartmann described his operative procedure in 1923.[25] The low anterior resection was developed by Dixon in 1939,[15] and D'Allaines described his perineal anastomosis in 1946.[14]

Idiopathic ulcerative colitis was a rare disease essentially untreated by surgery until the decade following 1930 when pioneers such as McKittrick and Miller promoted surgical treatment of the disease.[41] Crohn's disease was first described by Crohn et al. in 1932.[13] The modern techniques for the treatment of idiopathic ulcerative colitis that are based upon total proctocolectomy developed much later; one of the early papers championing this operation was published by Miller et al. in 1949.[44]

The modern era of colorectal surgery began during World War II. During the war Ogilvie developed the principle of colostomy for the treatment of colon wounds[47]; this procedure saved many lives in those difficult circumstances. World War II led to the development of a huge number of reasonably well-trained surgeons who were scattered widely across the United States; hence the techniques of colorectal surgery were disseminated extremely rapidly. Antibiotics, improved anesthesia, the science of accurate replacement of electrolytes, plasma, and blood, hyperalimentation, and the treatment of specific organ failure have led to a dramatic reduction in the mortality of various operative procedures. The names of some surgeons and operations such as Wangensteen's "second look"[64] and Turnbull's "no touch technique"[63] have stimulated investigation into the validity of such procedures. Chemotherapy and radiation therapy have been developed as aids in the treatment of cancer.[1,18] The development of the flexible colonoscope and the increasing conviction that adenomas are the usual precursors of cancer have made the 1970s the decade of the polyp.[67]

The American Proctologic Society was organized at the turn of the century and the first president, Joseph Matthews, served in the years 1899–1900. The name was later changed to the American Society of Colon and Rectal Surgeons. The Society for Surgery of the Colon, founded by Drs. Robert Turell, Warren Cole, and John Waugh in 1960, became the Society for Surgery of the Alimentary Tract 3 years later. Drawing strong support from general surgeons, the American Board of Colon and Rectal Surgery was established in 1949. The first issue of the periodical *Diseases of the Colon and Rectum* appeared in 1958.

The succeeding pages will demonstrate the modern techniques developed by surgeons for colorectal diseases. Some of the most important historical landmarks are listed in Table 1.1. Many of the older contributions were described in unavailable publications. In this table the generally accepted dates are given.

The Reference Section of this chapter is divided into two portions. The first is a list of important general references that may be consulted for further information; the second includes references to the technical historical development of colorectal surgery.

References

General References

These monographs or textbooks contain information on many aspects of colorectal lesions.

Bacon H.E. (1949) Anus–rectum–sigmoid colon, 3rd edn, Vols 1 and 2. Lippincott, Philadelphia

TABLE 1.1.   Some Historical Landmarks of Colorectal Surgery

1686	Felix	Cure of Louis XIV's fistula-in-ano[21(p393)]
1710	Littré	Concept of colostomy
1776	Pillore	First cecostomy[49]
1812	Travers	Inverting intestinal suture[61]
1823	Reybard	Successful resection and anastomosis of cancer of the sigmoid[54]
1826	Lembert	Develops his suture[31]
1826	Lisfranc	First successful excision, cancer of the rectum[33]
1829	Amussat	First elective colostomy[2]
1835		St. Mark's Hospital, London, opens its doors
1842	Long	First use of ether anesthesia[21(p505)]
1846	Morton	First public demonstration of ether (at Massachusetts General Hospital)[21(p505)]
1846	Semmelweiss	Introduction of surgeons to clean hands[21(p435)]
1869	Lister	Use of methods of antisepsis[21(p588)]
1879	Czerny	Abdominoperineal resection of cancer of the rectum[36]
1882	Bryant	First exteriorization and resection cancer of the colon[12]
1883	Maydl	First right colectomy for cancer[38]
1885	Kraske	Transsacral approach to rectal cancer[30]
1886	Fitz	Description of appendicitis[19]
1889	Hochenegg	Pull-through resection for cancer[27]
1892	Murphy	Button method of anastomosis[46]
1892	Bloch	Exteriorization resection[9]
1893	Mikulicz	Exteriorization resection[42]
1895	Kelly	First modern sigmoidoscope[62]
1895	Paul	Exteriorization resection[48]
1897	Quenu	Anorectal resection with preservation of sphincter[50]
1899		Founding of the American Proctologic Society
1900	Landsteiner	Description of four primary blood groups[58(p146)]
1901	Matas	Intratracheal anesthesia[37]
1904	Friedrich	Modern right colectomy[20]
1906	Bloodgood	Two-team technique for cancer of the rectum[10]
1906	Mayo	Two-team technique for cancer of the rectum[39]
1907	Mayo	Resection for diverticulitis[40]
1908	Miles	Abdominoperineal resection[43]
1911	Kausch	First use of intravenous glucose for nutrition[28]
1912	Hartwell, Hoguet	Use of intravenous normal saline[26]
1913	Strauss et al.	Electrocoagulation of cancer of the rectum[59]
1921	Levin	Gastroduodenal tube[32]
1923	Hartmann	Turn-in of rectal stump[25]
1928	Fleming	Discovery of penicillin[58(p235)]
1930	Rankin	Obstructive resection for cancer of the colon[51]
1931	Wangensteen, Paine	Constant suction of Levin tube[65]
1932	Babcock	Pull-through operation[4]
1932	Domagk	Introduction of Prontosil as an antibiotic[58(p214)]

Birenbaum W. (1975) The anorectum. In: Dunphy J.E., Way L.W. (eds) Current surgical diagnosis and treatment, 2nd edn. Lange, Los Altos, Calif, p 642

Birenbaum W., Schrock T.R. (1975) Large intestine. In: Dunphy J.E., Way L.W. (eds) Current surgical diagnosis and treatment, 2nd edn. Lange, Los Altos, Calif, p 606

Bockus H.L. (ed) (1976) Gastroenterology, 3rd edn, Vol 2. Saunders, Philadelphia

Garrison F.H. (1929) An introduction to the history of medicine. Saunders, Philadelphia

Goligher, J.C. (1975) Surgery of the anus, rectum and colon, 3rd edn. Macmillan, London, New York

Hardy J.D. (ed) (1972) Rhoads textbook of surgery. Principles and practice, 5th edn. Lippincott, Philadelphia

Maingot R. (1979) Abdominal operations, 7th edn, Vols 1 and 2. Appleton-Century-Crofts, New York

TABLE 1.1 (*Continued*)

1932	Crohn et al.	Description of Crohn's disease[13]
1932	Dukes	Classification of cancer of the rectum[17]
1935	McKittrick, Miller	Operations for ulcerative colitis[41]
1938	Gilchrist, David	Metastatic patterns of cancer of the colorectum[22]
1939	Dixon	Low anterior resection for cancer[15]
1939	Lloyd-Davies	Two-team resection for cancer of the rectum[34]
1942	Churchill	Establishment of blood banks for the U.S. Army[7]
1942	Griffith, Johnson	Use of curare in anesthesia[23]
1944	Ogilvie	Exteriorization of wounds of the colon[47]
1946	D'Allaines	Perineal anastomosis for cancer of the rectum[14]
1949	Swenson	New operation for Hirschsprung's disease[60]
1949	Wangensteen	Concept of second-look[64]
1949		Founding of American Board of Colon and Rectal Surgery
1949	Miller et al.	One-stage proctocolectomy for ulcerative colitis[44]
1951	Bierman et al.	Selective arteriography[8]
1951	Skukys	Development of nonflammable fluorine compounds as anesthetics[52]
1952	Barnes	Original concept of no-touch technique for cancer of the colon[5]
1952	Brooke	New type of ileostomy[11]
1952	Moore, Ball	Metabolic response to surgery[45]
1952	Grinnell, Hiatt	High ligation, inferior mesenteric artery[24]
1952	Yancey et al.	Pull-through operation with retention of rectal sphincters for polypoid disease[68]
1953	Severinghaus, Bradley	Practical use of blood gases[56]
1957	Duschinsky et al.	Discovery of 5-FU[18]
1958	Ault	Radical left colectomy for cancer[3]
1959	Wells	Development of Ivalon sling for rectal prolapse[66]
1960		Founding of the Society for Surgery of the Alimentary tract
1961	Soave	Pull-through operation with retention of rectal sphincters for Hirschsprung's disease[57]
1963	Barron	Rubber band technique for hemorrhoids[6]
1966	Ravitch, Rivarola	Introduction of staplers in the United States[53]
1967	Ripstein	Concept of subtotal colectomy for cancer of the colon[55]
1967	Madden, Kandalaft	Reintroduction of electrocoagulation for cancer of the rectum[35]
1967	Turnbull	Popularization of no-touch technique for cancer of the colon[63]
1968	Dudrick et al.	Introduction of hyperalimentation[16]
1969	Kock	Continent ileostomy[29]
1970	Allen, Fletcher	Heavy preoperative radiation for cancer of the rectum[1]
1971	Wolff, Shinya	Development of colonoscopic polypectomy[67]

Ottinger L.W. (1974) Fundamentals of colon surgery. Little, Brown, Boston

Proceedings of the 1977 Workshop on Large Bowel Cancer, National Large Bowel Cancer Project, Houston, Texas, Jan 21–23, 1977. Cancer, 40 [Suppl]: 2405 (1977)

Sabiston D.C. Jr. (ed) (1977) Davis-Christopher textbook of surgery. The biological basis of modern surgical practice, 11th edn. Saunders, Philadelphia

Schwartz S.I., et al (eds) (1979) Principles of surgery, 3rd edn. McGraw-Hill, Hightstown, New Jersey

Turell R. (ed) (1969) Diseases of the colon and rectum, 2nd edn, Vols 1 and 2. Saunders, Philadelphia

Wangensteen O.H. (1955) Intestinal obstructions, 3rd edn. Thomas, Springfield, Ill

Wangensteen O.H., Wangensteen S.D. (1978) The rise of surgery. University of Minnesota Press, Minneapolis

Welch C.E. (1958) Intestinal obstruction. Year Book, Chicago
Welch C.E., Hedberg S.E. (1975) Polypoid lesions of the gastrointestinal tract, 2nd edn. Saunders, Philadelphia

Historical References

1. Allen C.V., Fletcher W.S. (1970) Observations on preoperative irradiation of rectosigmoid carcinoma. Am J Roentgenol Radium Ther Nucl Med 108: 136
2. Amussat J.Z. (1841) Deuxième mémoire sur la possibilité d'établir un anus artificiel dans les régions lombaires gauche et droite sans ouvrir le péritoine. Gaz. d. hôp, Paris. (See Wangensteen and Wangensteen, The rise of surgery, pp 120, 612)
3. Ault G.W. (1974) A technique of cancer isolation and extended dissection for cancer of the distal colon and rectum. In: Maingot R. (ed) Abdominal operations, 6th edn, Vol 2. Appleton-Century-Crofts, New York, p 2010
4. Babcock W.W. (1932) Carcinoma of rectum. One-stage simplified proctosigmoidectomy with formation of perineal anus. Surg Clin North Am 12: 1397
5. Barnes J.P. (1952) Physiologic resection of right colon. Surg Gynecol Obstet 94: 722
6. Barron J. (1963) Office ligation of internal hemorrhoids. Am J Surg 105: 563
7. Beecher H.K. (1955) Resuscitation of men severely wounded in battle. In: Surgery in World War II: Vol 2, General surgery. Department of the Army, Washington, D.C., p 24
8. Bierman H.R., et al (1951) Intra-abdominal catheterization of viscera in man. Am J Roentgenol 66: 555
9. Bloch O. (1894) Case of extra-abdominal excision of entire descending colon and of parts of transverse colon for cancer. Hosp-Tid Kbh 4: 1053
10. Bloodgood J.C. (1906) Surgery of carcinoma of upper portion of rectum and sigmoid: Combined sacral and abdominal operations. Surg Gynecol Obstet 3: 284
11. Brooke B.N. (1952) Management of an ileostomy including its complications. Lancet 2: 102
12. Bryant T. (1883) A successful case of lumbar colectomy. Med Chir Trans 65: 131
13. Crohn B.B., Ginzburg L., Oppenheimer G.D. (1932) Regional enteritis. JAMA 99: 1323
14. D'Allaines F. (1946) Traitement chirurgical du cancer du rectum. Éditions Médicales Flammarion, Paris
15. Dixon C.F. (1939) Surgical removal of lesions occurring in the sigmoid and rectosigmoid. Am J Surg 46: 12
16. Dudrick S.J., Wilmore D.W., Vars H.M., Rhoads J.E. (1968) Long-term total parenteral nutrition with growth, development, and positive nitrogen balance. Surgery 64: 134
17. Dukes C.E. (1932) The classification of cancer of the rectum. J Pathol Bacteriol 35: 323
18. Duschinsky R., Pleven E., Heidelberger C. (1957) The synthesis of 5-fluoropyrimidines. J Am Chem Soc 79: 4559
19. Fitz R.H. (1886) Perforating inflammation of the vermiform appendix; with special reference to its early diagnosis and treatment. Trans Assoc Am Physicians 1: 107
20. Friedrich P.L. (1904) Prinzipelles zur operati ven Behandlung der Ileocoaltumoren, gleichzietig ein Bietrag zur Symptomatik und Behandlung der Invaginatio in Colon Transversum. Arch Int Chir 2: 231
21. Garrison F.H. (1929) An introduction to the history of medicine. Saunders, Philadelphia
22. Gilchrist R.K., David V.C. (1938) Lymphatic spread of carcinoma of the rectum. Ann Surg 108: 621
23. Griffith H.R., Johnson G.E. (1942) The use of curare in general anesthesia. Anesthesiology 3: 418

24. Grinnell R.S., Hiatt R.B. (1952) Ligation of inferior mesenteric artery at aorta in resections for carcinoma of sigmoid and rectum. Surg Gynecol Obstet 94: 526

25. Hartmann H. (1931) Chirurgie du rectum. Masson et Cie, Paris

26. Hartwell J.A., Hoguet J.P. (1912) Experimental intestinal obstruction in dogs with special reference to cause of death and treatment by large amounts of normal saline solution. JAMA 59: 82

27. Hochenegg J. (1897) Zur Therapie des Rectum Carcinoms. Wien Klin Wochenschr

28. Kausch W. (1911) Über intravenöse und subkutane Ernährung mit Traubenzucker. Dtsch Med Wochenschr, p 89

29. Kock N.G. (1969) Intra-abdominal "reservoir" in patients with permanent ileostomy. Arch Surg 99: 223

30. Kraske P. (1885) Zur Exstirpation hochsitzenden Mastdarmkrebse. Verh Dtsch Sch Ges Chir 14: 464

31. Lembert A. (1826) Mémoire sur l'enteroraphie avec la description d'un procédé nouveau pour pratiquer cette opération chirurgicale, répetoire general d'anatomie et de physiologie et de cliniqe. Chirurgicale 2: 100

32. Levin A.L. (1921) New gastroduodenal catheter. JAMA 76: 1007

33. Lisfranc J.L. (1826) Mémoire de l'excision de la partie inferieure du rectum devenue carcinomateuse. Rev Med Fr 2: 380

34. Lloyd-Davies O.V. (1939) Lithotomy–Trendelenburg position for resection of rectum and lower pelvic colon. Lancet 2: 74

35. Madden J.L., Kandalaft S. (1971) Electrocoagulation in the treatment of cancer of the rectum: A continuing study. Ann Surg 174: 530

36. Maingot R. (1974) Abdominal operations, 6th edn, Vols 1 and 2. Appleton-Century-Crofts, New York, p 2044

37. Matas R. (1901) Artificial respiration by direct intralaryngeal intubation with a modified O'Dwyer tube and a new graduated air-pump in its applications to medical and surgical practice. Trans Am Surg Assoc 19: 392

38. Maydl C. (1883) Ein Beitrag zur Darmchirurgie. Wiener Med Presse, Vienna (Monogr 14); abstracted in Zentralb Chir 10: 487

39. Mayo C.H. (1906) Cancer of sigmoid and rectum. Surg Gynecol Obstet 3: 236

40. Mayo W.J., Wilson L.B., Giffin H.Z. (1907) Acquired diverticulitis of the colon and its surgical treatment. Twenty-Eighth Meeting of the American Surgical Association, Washington, D.C., May 7–9; see Transactions of the American Surgical Association, Taylor Publishing Co., Dallas, Texas.

41. McKittrick L.S., Miller R.H. (1935) Idiopathic ulcerative colitis; review of 149 cases with particular reference to value of, and indications for surgical treatment. Ann Surg 102: 656

42. Mikulicz J. (1903) Chirurgische Erfahrungen über das Darmcarcinom. Arch Klin Chir 69: 28

43. Miles W.E. (1908) A method of performing abdomino-perineal excision for carcinoma of the rectum and of the terminal portion of the pelvic colon. Lancet 2: 1812

44. Miller C.G., Gardiner C. McG., Ripstein C.B. (1949) Primary resection of the colon in ulcerative colitis. J Can Med Assoc 60: 584

45. Moore F.D., Ball M.R. (1952) Metabolic response to surgery. Thomas, Springfield, Ill

46. Murphy J.B. (1892) Cholecysto-intestinal, gastro-intestinal, entero-intestinal anastomosis, and approximation without sutures. Med Rec 42: 665

47. Ogilvie W.H. (1944) Abdominal wounds in the Western Desert. Surg Gynecol Obstet 78: 225

48. Paul F.T. (1895) Colectomy. Liverpool Med Chir J 15: 374

49. Pillore de Rouen: Quoted in Ref. 2, pp 85-88

50. Quenu J.A.E.E. (1897) Bull Soc Chir Paris 23: 163

51. Rankin F.W. (1930) Resection and obstruction of the colon (obstructive resection). Surg Gynecol Obstet 50: 591

52. Raventos J. (1956) Action of fluothane: A new volatile anesthetic agent. Br J Pharmacol 11: 394

53. Ravitch M.M., Rivarola A. (1966) Enteroanastomosis with an automatic stapling instrument. Surgery 59: 270
54. Reybard J.F. (1844) Mémoire sur une tumeur cancéreuse affectant, l'S iliaque du colon: Ablation de la tumeur et de l'intestin. Bull Acad Natl Med (Paris) 9: 1031
55. Ripstein C.B. (1967) Radical colectomy for carcinoma of the colon. Dis Colon Rectum 10: 40
56. Severinghaus J.W., Bradley A.F. (1958) Electrodes for blood pO$_2$ and pCO$_2$ determination. J Appl Physiol 13: 515
57. Soave F. (1964) Hirschsprung's disease: New surgical technique. Arch Dis Child 39: 166
58. Sourkes T.L. (1966) Nobel Prize winners in medicine and physiology 1901–1965. Abelard-Schuman, New York
59. Strauss A.A., Strauss S.F., Crawford R.A., et al (1935) Surgical diathermy of carcinoma of the rectum; its clinical end results. JAMA 104: 1480
60. Swenson O. (1950) A new surgical treatment for Hirschsprung's disease. Surgery 28: 371
61. Travers B. (1812) An inquiry into the process of nature in repairing injuries of the intestines, illustrating the treatment of penetrating wounds, and strangulated hernia. Longmans, Green, London
62. Turell R. (1969) Diseases of the colon and anorectum, 2nd edn, Vol 1. Saunders, Philadelphia, p 188
63. Turnbull R.B. Jr. (1970) Cancer of the colon: The five- and ten-year survival rates following resection utilizing the isolation technique. Ann R Coll Surg Engl 46: 243
64. Wangensteen O.H. (1949) Cancer of the colon and rectum. Wis Med J 48: 591
65. Wangensteen O.H., Paine J.R. (1933) Treatment of acute intestinal obstruction by suction with tube. JAMA 101: 1532
66. Wells C. (1959) New operation for rectal prolapse. Proc R Soc Med 52: 602
67. Wolff W.I., Shinya H. (1971) Colonofiberoscopy. JAMA 217: 1509
68. Yancey A.G., et al (1952) A modification of the Swenson technique for congenital megacolon. J Natl Med Assoc 44: 356

Anatomy and Physiology of the Colon and Rectum

2

Anatomy of the Colon and Rectum

Colon

Divisions The colon is divided into sections that include the cecum, ascending colon, hepatic flexure, transverse colon, splenic flexure, descending colon, sigmoid, and rectum. While there is universal agreement about the major sections of the colon, the nomenclature of the lower portion of the large bowel has been a subject of some disagreement. Gilchrist's designation will be used in this book. He divides the rectum into two portions. The lowermost is the extraperitoneal rectum that lies entirely below the peritoneal floor and averages about 8 cm in length. The upper portion of the rectum is the intraperitoneal rectum; it is also about 8 cm in length and extends upward to the sigmoid, which is marked by the transition to a definite mesentery. In this method of nomenclature the old designation "rectosigmoid" is eliminated and replaced by the term "intraperitoneal rectum."

Blood Supply The right colon is supplied by the superior mesenteric artery via the ileocolic and right colic arteries (Fig. 2.1). The right colic artery is an inconstant vessel and may arise either directly from the superior mesenteric or from the ileocolic or middle colic vessels. The transverse colon is supplied by the midcolic artery; there are two main divisions—one running to the right and one running to the left. In many instances the two divisions of the midcolic are replaced by double colic arteries. The inferior mesenteric artery supplies the left side of the colon and the intraperitoneal rectum. The left colic branch originates about 3 cm below the origin of the inferior mesenteric and usually runs obliquely to the splenic flexure. There are two to six sigmoid branches that run to the sigmoid. The inferior mesenteric artery, renamed the superior hemorrhoidal as it crosses the left common iliac artery, runs to the rectum and divides into right and left branches.

In addition to these major vessels there is a small vessel that runs close to the colon around the whole circumference. This is known as the marginal artery of Drummond. It is not a large artery. Whether or not it can be depended upon to provide enough blood supply for the colon if the major arteries have been interrupted is questionable. Furthermore, it may

9

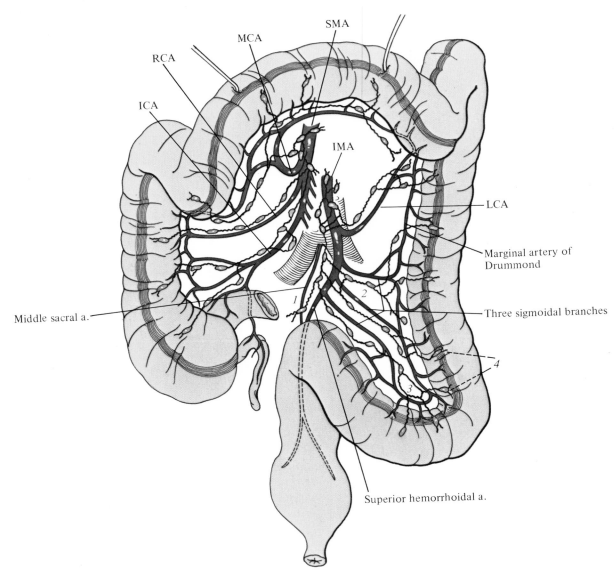

Fig. 2.1. Arterial supply and lymph nodes of the colon. The superior mesenteric vein lies to the right of the superior mesenteric artery and the inferior mesenteric vein to the left of the inferior mesenteric artery. ICA, ileocolic artery; RCA, right colic artery; MCA, middle colic artery; SMA, superior mesenteric artery; IMA, inferior mesenteric artery; LCA, left colic artery; 1, principal nodes; 2, intermediate nodes; 3, paracolic nodes; 4, epicolic nodes.

be absent in certain areas, particularly just proximal to the splenic flexure, near the lower sigmoid, or in the region of the proximal ascending colon. Consequently, any excision of the colon that involves division of the major vessels and depends upon the artery of Drummond for integrity of an anastomosis must be regarded with some suspicion. The surgeon must be certain of an adequate blood supply in all such cases.

Finally, there is a small artery (the middle sacral) that arises from the posterior surface of the aorta and runs downward on the anterior surface of the sacrum to the rectum.

The veins, in general, correspond to the arteries. Those accompanying the superior mesenteric distribution run very close to the arteries and to the right of the superior mesenteric artery. On the left side of the colon the inferior mesenteric vein lies to the left of the artery and departs from the artery at the site of the origin of the inferior mesenteric artery; it then runs upward behind the pancreas to drain into the splenic or, occasionally, the superior mesenteric vein.

Lymphatics The lymph nodes of the colon are divided into several groups. The epicolic nodes usually are very small and are found immediately on the surface of the colon. Those on the next level are known as the paracolic nodes and lie along the marginal artery. The intermediate nodes lie near the main branches of the mesenteric arteries. The principal nodes are localized near the superior or inferior mesenteric vessels or along the aorta.[1] Metastatic disease usually progresses regularly from one set of nodes to another, but we have had instances in which the intermediate groups of nodes have been skipped and metastasis from a lesion of the colon has been noted only in the principal nodes.

Nerves The nerves of the colon include the sympathetic and the parasympathetic fibers. The vagus supplies the right colon but has little or no function; after truncal vagotomy for duodenal ulcer there is little change in intestinal activity except for occasional unexplained diarrhea. The sacral parasympathetic outflow supplies the lower sigmoid colon and rectum. The sympathetic nerves supply the small intestine and colon. Sympathectomy from D-10 to L-3, as practiced in the past for the control of hypertension, abolished the sensation of distention.

Rectum

Divisions The anatomy of the rectum is much more complex. The outermost opening of the bowel is marked by the anal verge (Fig. 2.2). Progressing upward is the anal canal, which usually is about 2.5 cm in length; the lower three-quarters are lined by squamous epithelium.

The upper end of the anal canal opens into the lowermost portion of the rectum. Mucous membrane begins just below the upper end of the canal. This spot (the dentate or pectinate line) is marked by the presence of crypts that open upward and tend to catch fecal material. They may be the site of the original inflammation that leads to either complications of hemorrhoids or perianal abscesses or fistulas. Anal intermuscular glands are found between the sphincters, and they drain through narrow channels into the crypts.

Muscles The intrinsic muscles of the rectum (Fig. 2.3) include the external sphincter, which begins subcutaneously, extends upward for about 4 cm, and lies external to the internal sphincter. It is a voluntary circular muscle. Beginning just above the external sphincter, and lying between it and the mucosa is the involuntary internal sphincter which is about 1 cm in width. With advancing age or inflammation the lower portion of the internal sphincter may become fibrosed. This may lead to symptomatic hemorrhoids or produce a tight band (the pectinate band) that may require dilatation or section for relief.

The levator ani muscles surround the rectum and form the so-called levator sling. They run from the lateral margin of the ischium to the pubis and around the rectum and serve to maintain the pelvic floor as well as to support the bowel. The puborectalis is an important division of the levator ani muscle. It originates from the pubis and forms a sling posteriorly about the rectum. This section of the levators may become quite relaxed and incompetent, particularly in patients with prolapse of the rectum.

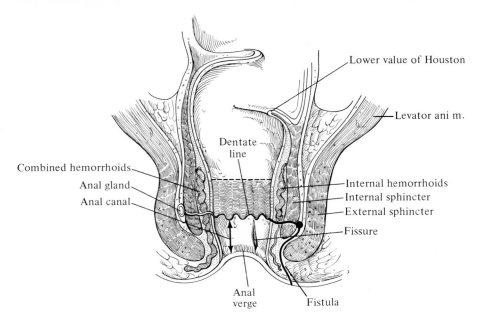

Fig. 2.2. Anatomy of the rectum and location of some common types of anal pathology.

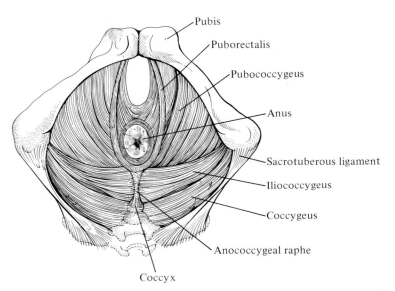

Fig. 2.3. Muscles of the perineum.

Blood Supply   Three sets of arteries supply the rectum (Fig. 2.4). The blood supply of the rectum is primarily through the superior hemorrhoidal artery. The corresponding vein becomes the inferior mesenteric at a higher level. The middle hemorrhoidal arteries, which lie in the lateral ligaments on either side, vary in number from zero to three and are branches of the internal iliac arteries. The inferior hemorrhoidal artery arises from the internal iliac via the internal pudendal. The middle and inferior hemorrhoidal veins empty into the internal iliac veins. Blood from the middle and inferior hemorrhoidal arteries will support viability of the lower 10 cm of the rectum after section of the superior hemorrhoidal.

There is also an important intrinsic blood supply of the lower rectum and the anal canal. This consists of the three hemorrhoidal vessels that are

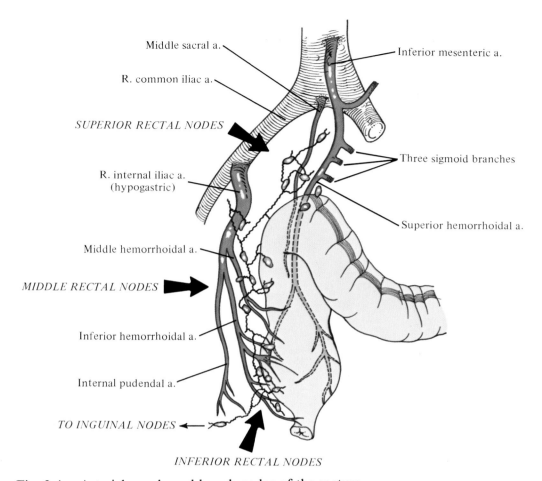

Middle sacral a.

R. common iliac a.

SUPERIOR RECTAL NODES

R. internal iliac a.
(hypogastric)

Middle hemorrhoidal a.

MIDDLE RECTAL NODES

Inferior hemorrhoidal a.

Internal pudendal a.

TO INGUINAL NODES

INFERIOR RECTAL NODES

Inferior mesenteric a.

Three sigmoid branches

Superior hemorrhoidal a.

Fig. 2.4.   Arterial supply and lymph nodes of the rectum.

located (when the patient is in the lithotomy position) at 4, 7, and 11 o'clock. These intrinsic hemorrhoidal vessels have been the site of considerable investigation. It has been proved by Thulesius and Gjöres that the hemorrhoidal veins contain an unusually high oxygen saturation,[6] indicating the presence of arteriovenous communications in the lower rectum. These tissues, therefore, are very similar to the erectile tissues noted in the genital tract, and it is presumed that the presence of this unusual amount of blood may aid in the maintenance of continence.[5]

Lymphatics   Lymphatic flow progresses upward in vessels closely related to the superior hemorrhoidal artery and vein. Lateral flow occurs along the middle hemorrhoidal vessels. From the anal canal, the flow can be lateral along the inferior pudendal and internal iliac artery and vein or to the inguinal lymph nodes in the groin.

Research by Gilchrist and others has shown that cancer of the rectum always spreads upward unless the nodes have been blocked completely by tumor; in this case metastases can occur either laterally or to the groin nodes.[1] Clinically, it is rare to find involvement of the iliac nodes with a cancer of the rectum. Groin nodes may be involved with either squamous cell carcinoma or adenocarcinoma originating in the anal canal.

Nerves   The rectum is supplied by the sympathetic and parasympathetic nerves. Somatic nerves supply the perianal area. The sympathetic supply

13

of the rectum, bladder, and sexual organs is via the presacral nerves and hypogastric plexus. They descend to the lower lateral sides of the pelvis, where they join with the parasympathetic nerves—the nervi erigentes—that come from the sacral canal. From the pelvic plexuses the nerves are distributed to the rectum, bladder, and sexual organs. Dissection of the presacral nerves can prevent forward ejaculation in the male. Destruction of the nervi erigentes can destroy the power of erection and orgasm in the male and can interfere with bladder function.

The sensory nerves in the perianal area carry exquisite pain sensations; therefore, any inflammation or irritation in this area causes extreme discomfort for the patient. These pain fibers are also present within the anal canal. However, there are none in the rectal mucous membrane, so that ordinary surgical procedures, such as biopsy, injection of hemorrhoids, electrodesiccation, etc., are tolerated without any sensation of pain. There are, however, other nerves in the anal canal. For example, it is recognized that the mucosa of the very lower part of the rectum is very important in the maintenance of a reflex arc that allows the individual to differentiate between gas and fecal discharge. When this very sensitve lowermost portion of the rectal mucosa is excised and sigmoid mucosa is brought down to the anus for anastomosis, this delicate reflex arc is broken and loss of continence occurs. After a period of retraining continence may be regained, particularly in children, but recovery in an adult is a very slow procedure and may never occur.

The rectum just above the dentate line is sensitive to distention and thus a desire for evacuation is produced when feces or a tumor is present. Nerves controlling this sensation are located in the myenteric plexus, which is found in the muscular wall of the rectum. Absence of nerves in the myenteric plexus occurs congenitally in patients with Hirschsprung's disease. These children have an extremely spastic anal sphincter and require extirpation of this abnormally innervated bowel in order to secure proper function.

The exact location of the anal orifice in the perineum has been of recent interest. Hendren has suggested that an anus located far anteriorly may lead to constipation because in the erect position pressure can drive the anterior rectal wall against the posterior and produce a functional obstruction.[2] This concept also is of importance in the descending perineum syndrome (q.v.).

Physiology of the Colorectum

It is impossible to include a full discussion of the physiology of the large bowel in this text even though the amount of information is trivial compared with that known about the upper gastrointestinal tract. There are several points, however, that are of interest to the surgeon.

The normal colon can absorb water, glucose, and some electrolytes. According to Rodgers et al., the colon, when perfused with a 0.9% saline solution, can absorb 2400 ml water, 400 mm sodium, and 560 mm chloride in 24 hr.[4] The absorption takes place almost entirely in the right colon, but after extensive colectomy there is compensation and the left colon can also increase its ability to absorb water. Diarrhea can occur and be severe after resection of the right colon for this reason alone.

The terminal ileum is the site of absorption of bile salts, cholesterol, and vitamin B_{12}. Wide resections of the terminal ileum should therefore be avoided if possible; obviously, however, a resection for cancer should not be compromised by this consideration. The loss of absorption of cholesterol can, as a matter of fact, be an advantage to certain patients. The institution of pernicious anemia from wide resections of the terminal ileum perhaps should be considered but has not been reported. The lack of absorption of bile salts is an important feature. Many colons are quite sensitive to the action of bile salts, which are known laxatives. Consequently, after a resection of the terminal ileum there may be increased diarrhea for this reason as well. Various absorptive substances such as cholestyramine (Questran) may absorb such bile salts and help in the treatment of diarrhea after colectomy.

It is difficult to ascribe any importance to loss of the ileocecal valve. It apparently never acts to obstruct the passage of intestinal contents from above downward unless foreign bodies such as gallstones or undigested food debris collect in the terminal ileum and obstruct it. It is also imcompetent in approximately 50% of all cases insofar as retrograde propulsion is concerned. Thus, in about one-half of patients with obstructive lesions of the colon there is ready reflux back into the small bowel and decompression of the colon in this fashion. If this valve is competent and will not allow decompression of the colon, a closed loop obstruction may be produced between the ileocecal valve and the obstructing lesion. Thus the ileocecal valve seems to be of much less physiologic importance than the pylorus.

The colon acts chiefly as a reservoir for feces. Consequently, the greater the length of bowel that is resected the more likely the patient is to have more frequent bowel movements. Resection of the left colon or sigmoid often changes the time clock, so that a patient with bowels that formerly were quite regular may find that they become irregular and movements appear with no definite schedule after a partial colectomy.

The physiology of defecation is very complicated and patients may adapt to entirely different patterns after surgical operations. Normally a slow, powerful peristaltic wave passes in a regular fashion down the colon at the time of defecation. It seems, according to Painter and Truelove's theory, that the replacement of this action by segmental contractions could be the origin of diverticular disease.[3] After a sigmoid colostomy in many instances the colon can be trained to work at a regular time without the use of irrigations, although in the United States irrigations at 2-day intervals are usually employed. After a period of adjustment many patients will need to wear only minimal or no protection whatsoever over the stoma.

The mechanism of defecation is initiated by pressure on the mucous membrane of the rectum located just above the dentate line. This pressure may be caused by feces, a tumor, or redundant mucosa. There are reflex colon contractions and defecation occurs. Ordinarily, peristaltic contraction of the colon begins in the right colon and extends distally; the left colon tends to straighten and shorten as the peristaltic wave progresses. If the bowel is empty the contractions continue but the symptom of tenesmus is produced. Direct irritation of the same area by such agents as glycerin suppositories may produce the same result.

The rectum may be the site of absorption of various medicines. Cortisone, local anesthetics, aminophylline, aspirin, alcohol, and electrolytes are all absorbed here, indicating the wide capabilities of this mucosa to absorb certain substances very rapidly. Opium suppositories, a favorite remedy for hemorrhoidal disease in the past, exert their effect only through the absorption of morphine and its general effect. It should be noted that much of the absorption in the rectum occurs into the systemic circulation via the inferior and middle hemorrhoidal veins, so that only the blood that returns via the portal circulation through the superior mesenteric veins allows many of these substances to be detoxified by the liver.

The anal sphincter is an extremely important organ in modern society. Undoubtedly it has great social advantages, but there may also be some disadvantages. For example, one of the complaints that is heard most frequently in offices these days is that of "gas." It will be noted that in many of these patients the inflation of the colon with air at the time of sigmoidoscopy will reproduce these complaints exactly. It is also interesting to note the almost total absence of any complaints of retained "gas" after either a sigmoid colostomy or an ileostomy has been done and the underlying disease has been removed. This observation leads to the clinical impression that colon distention can be a very important component of these common complaints.

Extent of Resection for Cancer

Since the extent of resection depends on the anatomic distribution of blood vessels and lymphatics, the standard operations for cancer can be shown diagrammatically (Fig. 2.5).

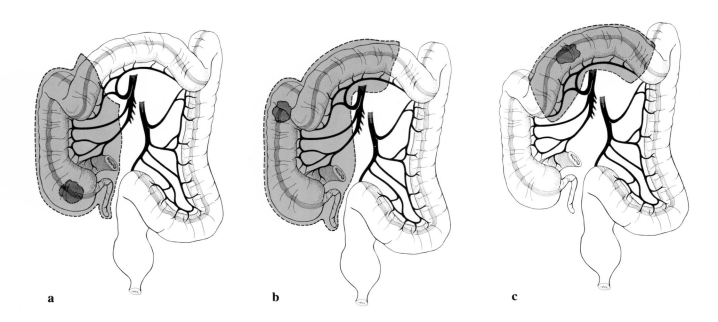

a   b   c

Fig. 2.5a–j. Extent of resection for cancers of the colorectum and the levels at which major blood vessels are interrupted. a. Cecum and lower ascending colon (right colectomy). b. Upper ascending colon and hepatic flexure (right and transverse colectomy). c. Transverse colon (transverse colectomy). d. Splenic flexure (limited resection, splenic flexure). e. Decending colon and upper sigmoid (limited resection left colon). f. Lower sigmoid and descending colon (sigmoid colectomy). g. Left colectomy (for any cancer of left colon). h. Subtotal colectomy. i. Cancer of the intraperitoneal rectum (low anterior resection). j. Extraperitoneal rectum (combined abdominoperineal resection).

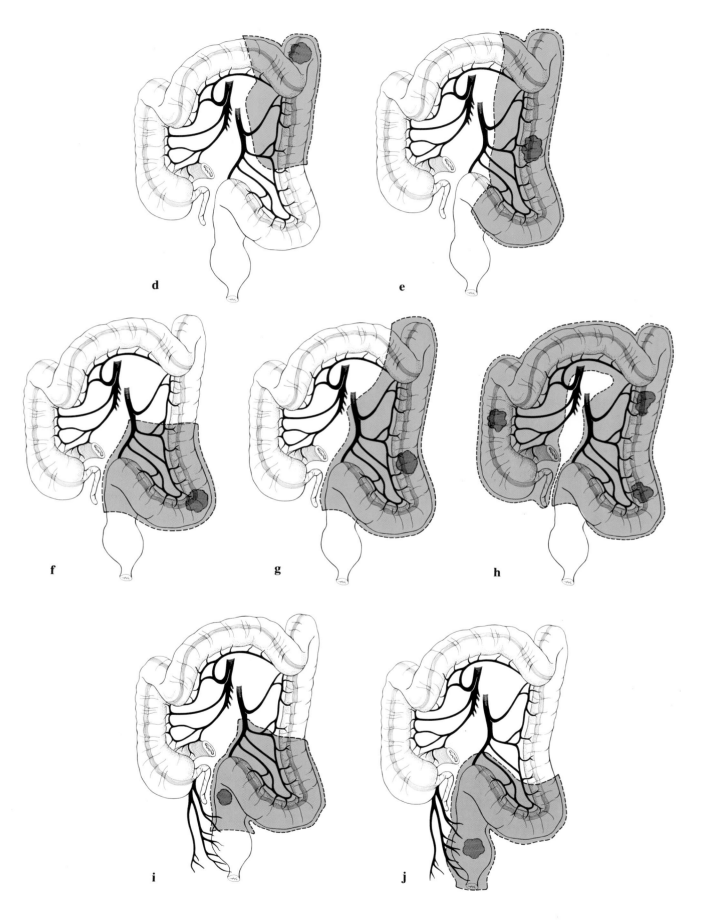

d

e

f

g

h

i

j

References

1. Gilchrist R.K., David V.C. (1938) Lymphatic spread of carcinoma of the rectum. Ann Surg 108: 621
2. Hendren W.H. (1978) Constipation caused by anterior location of the anus and its surgical correction. J Pediat Surg 13: 505
3. Painter N.S., Truelove S.C. (1964) Intraluminal pressure pattern in diverticulosis of the colon. Gut 5: 365
4. Rodgers J.B., Barnard H.R., Balint J.A. (1976) Colonic infusion in the management of the short bowel syndrome. Gastroenterology 70: 186
5. Stelzner F. (1976) Die Anorectalen Fisteln, 2nd edn (English translation). Springer, New York
6. Thulesius O., Gjöres J.R. (1973) Arterio-venous anastomoses in the anal region with reference to the pathogenesis and treatment of hemorrhoids. Acta Chir Scand 139: 476

General Principles of Surgery of the Colorectum

3

Symptoms and Diagnosis of Colonic Disease

The symptoms of colonic disease include rectal bleeding, abnormal bowel habits, changes in bowel habits, lower abdominal cramps, gas, nausea and vomiting, tenesmus, anemia, fever, abdominal pain, distention, and even extra-abdominal symptoms that may accompany ulcerative colitis. Rectal disease, in addition, may be accompanied by local pain, irritation, protrusion, and itching. It is important to note, however, that serious colonic disease may exist without any symptoms. This is particularly true of adenomatous polyps and early cancer.

For this reason screening techniques have been suggested to identify malignant disease before it reaches the stage of overt symptomatology.[18,24] Whether or not such measures as routine guaiac testing of stools will eventually turn out to be worthwhile is a moot question. Some studies have indicated it is valuable, but others have found it of little value.[22,24] Many polyps do not bleed, and if polypoid disease is to be regarded as highly important in the development of later cancer, as we believe it must, other diagnostic techniques must be considered. Pearl has called attention to the fact that patients who have red color blindness may fail to recognize bleeding from a body orifice; this possibility should be investigated.[35]

The diagnosis of colorectal disease is made primarily upon the history and physical examination. Careful vaginal and rectal examinations are essential, although it is surprising to note how many times they have been omitted or done in the wrong way.

A barium enema is usually the next diagnostic method employed after sigmoidoscopy. In combination with an air contrast study this will demonstrate the great majority of lesions of the bowel except for small polyps. Undoubtedly it is not satisfactory for the demonstration of polyps less than 1 cm in diameter, but for all practical purposes none of these lesions are malignant. In Lahiry and Hedberg's series only 1 of 897 polypoid lesions less than 1 cm in diameter contained cancer.[28]

Endoscopy Techniques

Sigmoidoscopy

Sigmoidoscopy is performed in the office. Often it is preferable to sigmoidoscope the patient before he is given an enema in order that the character of the bowel movements may be noted. This is particularly true if he has complained of small amounts of bright red rectal bleeding and the source is probably the anal ring; in these instances the stool above the anal ring will be guaiac negative. Then the patient is given a Fleet enema and re-examined with both the anoscope and the sigmoidoscope. The most comfortable position for the patient is the left lateral one. This procedure is essentially painless except when the upper portion of the rectum is reached. The examination is preferably carried out to a depth of 25 cm. However, if it is impossible to pass the angle at the upper end of the rectum, no forcible attempt is made because there is a danger of perforation. If a lesion has been demonstrated above this level by barium enema, or if symptoms suggest such a lesion, it is far better to use a colonoscope than to attempt to pass the rigid scope up to that area. Even when the procedure is done with the patient under general anesthesia there is a distinct possibility of perforation with the rigid scope if any force is used in the examination.

Digital examination must precede endoscopy. At times very low-lying polypoid lesions of the rectum that are easily palpable with the finger may be passed over by the endoscope.

Colonoscopy

After the barium enema the advisability of colonoscopy must be considered if the diagnosis has not been satisfactorily attained by other methods. Since colonoscopy is time consuming, expensive, and more dangerous in unskilled hands than the barium enema, the examinations are usually performed in the order stated here. It should be noted that the danger of perforation is also present with barium enemas and that the introduction of barium into the peritoneal cavity is followed by a very severe granulomatous reaction that can lead to many late complications unless the operation is carried out very rapidly and every bit of barium is removed from the peritoneal cavity. There has been some evidence that sterile barium introduced into the peritoneal cavity is essentially harmless. However, there is no question that when it is introduced through the colon, clean though it may be, infection is carried with it and consequently the intraperitoneal presence of such an enema is a very serious matter. Barium has also penetrated through a perforation into a mesenteric and then the portal vein; nine such cases were found by Juler et al.[27]

The colonoscope may reveal large lesions that were overlooked by barium enemas. However, it is not always possible to force the colonoscope into the right colon. The two methods of diagnosis are complementary. In a prospective study, Hogan et al. found that 94% of all polypoid lesions were detected by colonoscopy compared with 67% by barium enema.[25]

The key to the success of colonoscopy is the adequate preparation of the colon. This involves a 3-day preparation by the patient.

It is necessary to give the patient light sedation.[42] This can be accomplished by intravenous diazepam and, in case spasm of the bowel is encountered, simultaneous intravenous injection of glucagon. The technical problems include the advance and withdrawal of the scope, the requirement for rotary motions, the simultaneous injection of air, and the application of suction. All of these maneuvers are facilitated greatly by Hedberg's apparatus, which allows manipulation with both hands. A second viewing scope and a television monitor also make it possible for the entire procedure to be visualized by any observer. The scope is alternately advanced and retracted. Progress may be impossible if there have been marked adhesions in the pelvis from diverticulitis. The surgeon must also be aware of the dangers of endoscopy in the presence of active ulcerative colitis as the possibility of perforation is excessive. Inflation of the bowel preferably should be carried out with carbon dioxide. Inflation with room air or with nitrogen could lead to a toxic megacolon in patients with severe inflammatory disease.

Passage through a large sigmoid loop is aided by the so-called "alpha maneuver," in which the whole sigmoid must be twisted on its axis together with the inlying colonoscope.

As the splenic flexure is passed the transverse colon is identified by its almost triangular shape. Further passage into the ascending colon can be noted and the end of the examination is reached when the ileocecal valve is observed. At times the scope can be passed in a retrograde fashion through the valve into the terminal ileum.

There have been surprisingly few complications referable to colonoscopy. Most of them have been associated with concomitant polypectomy. Bleeding is the most common; this is nearly always self-limited but may be controlled by pitressin injections through a mesenteric arterial catheter, so that laparotomy rarely is necessary. Perforations have occurred, and if there is a perforation from the colonoscope, immediate laparotomy is indicated. Fortunately, other complications are extremely rare. If the desiccating unit is to be employed, it is very important that the colon be thoroughly flushed with a nonflammable gas since if there is methane or hydrogen present an operative explosion may occur. In some instances even the skilled operator will find it impossible to pass the colonoscope to the cecum; it is essential that the approximate area of observation be recorded in the record.

The flexible 60-cm colonoscope has been introduced recently. It provides greater diagnostic and therapeutic capabilities than the sigmoidoscope and is easier to use but not as effective as the longer colonoscope.

Preoperative Preparation and Anesthesia

The colon must be prepared very carefully for any of the more sophisticated procedures noted above. If, for example, colonoscopy is to be carried out, a 3-day preparation is employed. The details of the preparation include a liquid diet, laxatives, and enemas. The same preparation should be employed by the radiologist, particularly if he is looking for polyps. The usual preparation for barium enema includes castor oil the night before x-ray and an enema on the morning of the procedure, but the 3-day procedure again is advocated when small lesions are expected.

The preparation of the patient as well as the colon for operative procedures is extremely important. It will not always be possible to do this since many cases will have to be operated on as emergencies. We have followed the following principles of preparation for elective operation on the colon: The patient should remain on a low-residue diet for 3 days.[23] Mechanical preparation is by far the most important. Nichols et al. administered erythromycin by mouth and found that mechanical cleansing led to increased amounts of erythromycin in the fecal discharge and a higher level in the serum than when cleansing was not employed.[32,33] Laxatives such as magnesium citrate (8 oz) are given on the third and the second day prior to operation. Enemas are given on each day. Antibiotics are given according to the schedule described in the section.

Prior to operations on the colon the surgeon should be certain that the hemoglobin level and electrolytes are normal and that there are no abnormal clotting factors. A chest plate and electrocardiogram should be taken routinely in all patients over 45 years of age. Anemia is not uncommon with many diseases of the colon and must be corrected by transfusions. Severe malnutrition in patients with ulcerative colitis or Crohn's disease may require hyperalimentation.[12,14] Electrolytes are usually within the normal range except in extremely ill patients. Villous adenomas may be associated with hypokalemia and hypoproteinemia. Albumin levels also may be seriously diminished in patients with ulcerative colitis. Obviously, if the surgeon has time for appropriate preoperative preparation it is wise to attempt to correct any of these abnormalities prior to operation; in emergencies, however, it may be necessary to operate before all abnormal features can be corrected.

Blood should be available for transfusion if a resection is contemplated. Transfusions will almost always be necessary for patients who have combined abdominoperineal resections of the colon, although in the good-risk patient they will rarely be necessary for segmental or subtotal resections of the colon.

The anesthesia that is employed is usually a combination that includes intratracheal anesthesia, muscle relaxants, and pentothal. In a few poor-risk patients who have chronic pulmonary disease, epidural spinal anesthesia has been used and the blocks have been continued for a period of 24 hr afterward until the period of severe pain has passed.

Special warning should be given to the anesthesiologist if any of the antibiotics that cause respiratory depression, such as neomycin or kanamycin, are used for irrigation of the peritoneal cavity. These antibiotics are particularly dangerous in the presence of muscle-relaxing drugs and respiratory support may have to be continued for a long period of time after the operative procedure.

Antibiotic Therapy

Antibiotics are used for the treatment of many diseases of the colon. The major indications are for (1) therapy, e.g., in the treatment of acute inflammation, localized perforations, or local or generalized peritonitis due to diverticulitis, or (2) prophylaxis, involving oral antibiotic preparation of the colon prior to operation.[3,4,6,8,9,41]

The problems in all instances are exceedingly complex; no complete agreement has been reached. Many studies of colon flora have concentrated on the aerobic flora, whereas the anaerobic flora constitute at least 100 times as many bacteria by weight. Invasive infections therefore can occur from a large variety of organisms that can range from low-grade *Staphylococcus* to highly invasive *Clostridium* or *Bacteroides*. The most effective antibiotics against anaerobes widely used at present are chloramphenicol and clindamycin; metronidazole (Flagyl) is also effective against anaerobes, particularly of the *B. aerogenes* type.[5] However, clindamycin is not effective against many clostridia.

The side effects of many of these drugs also must be taken into consideration. For example, the penicillins and occasionally the cephalosporins may produce anaphylactic reactions. Chloramphenicol, though excellent for many gram-negative infectious agents including the anaerobes, occasionally will produce bone marrow depression. The aminoglycosides in some instances produce renal damage; clindamycin and lincomycin have also been associated with pseudomembranous colitis. Metronidazole has not been approved by the FDA for the purpose of control of anaerobes.

The surgeon therefore must choose an antibiotic that is perhaps not quite as effective but may be safer; but if the situation is extremely grave he may be required to use the most powerful antibiotics despite the possibility of side reactions.

It is impossible to cover in this text all of the aspects of antibiotic therapy or to recount the arguments that have been used for and against various programs. The following list includes the antibiotics usually employed at Massachusetts General Hospital:

I. Elective resections of the colon
    A. Preoperative preparation
        Neomycin (1 g) plus erythromycin base (1 g) p.o. at 1, 3, and 11 p.m. on day prior to operation
    B. At time of operative procedure
        Cephaloridine (1 g) i.m. 1–6 hr prior to operation
        Sodium cephalothin (1 g) i.v. during operation
    C. Postoperative
        None—except for persistent peritonitis or other complications
II. Emergency operations for perforated colon and peritonitis, before, during, and after operation
    A. Clindamycin (300 mg i.v. q 6 hr) plus gentamicin (1 mg/kg i.v. q 8 hr) or
    B. Chloramphenicol (500 mg i.v. q. 6 hr) plus gentamicin (1 mg/kg i.v. q. 8 hr)
III. Acute diverticulitis without peritonitis
    A. Tetracycline (250 mg p.o. q. 6 hr) (mild cases) or
    B. Sodium cephalothin (500 mg i.v. q. 6 hr) (more severe cases)

A recent survey of a number of surgeons showed that the majority favor oral neomycin–erythromycin on the day before surgery, in addition to vigorous mechanical preparation, as a preoperative measure. Several use parenteral antibiotics prior to or during operation. The majority use nothing afterward in uncomplicated cases. Individual preferences are shown in Table 3.1.

Anastomotic Techniques

Numerous anastomotic techniques are employed in the surgery of the colon and rectum. The principles underlying all of them include the production of a lumen that is wide enough to function normally, lack of tension, good blood supply, and lack of contamination at the time of the operation. In most instances special attention must be paid to the closure of the gap in the mesentery that is produced when two sections of the bowel are anastomosed. The desirability of drainage or proximal decompression will depend upon individual circumstances. The most important complication of anastomoses—leakage—can be affected profoundly by the technique used, as well as by other factors[26,38] (see Chapter 24).

TABLE 3.1. Antibiotics for Elective Surgery of the Colon

Surgeon[a]	Preparation	Immediately Preoperative	During Operation	Postoperative
Altemeier, W.A.	None	2 hr preop.; penicillin 1 million units i.v. tetracycline 0.5 g i.v.	Continue same dose of penicillin and tetracycline in each 1000 cc i.v. fluid for 48 hr	
Beahrs, O.H.	Neomycin 1 g Tetracycline 250 mg p.o. 4× daily for 2 days	None	None	Cephalothin 1 g, q. 6 hr i.v. for 3 days
Burke, J.F.	None	Cephaloridine 1 g i.m. on call to O.R.	Cephaloridine 1 g i.m. at end of case	None
Cohn, L., Jr.	Kanamycin 1 g p.o. q. hr × 4, then every 6 hr, for 3 days	None	None	None
Condon, R.E.	Neomycin 1 g Erythromycin base 1 g at 1, 2, and 10 p.m. day before	None	None	None
Dunphy, J.E.	Neomycin 1 g Erythromycin base 1 g p.o. t.i.d. day before	None	None	None
Gallagher, D.M.	Neomycin 1 g Erythromycin base 1 g p.o. 4 × starting 24 hr preop.	Ampicillin 2 g i.v. in all poor risks	Continue ampicillin i.v. in 50% of cases	Continue ampicillin 2 g i.v. q. 8 hr for 3 days
Goligher, J.C.	Phthalylsulfathiazole 2 g q. 4 hr for 4 days Neomycin 1 g q. 4 hr last 2 days Metronidazole 200 mg q 4 hr for 4 days	Lincomycin 600 mg i.m. Gentamicin 80 mg i.m.	None	Lincomycin 600 mg Gentamicin 80 mg i.m. q. 8 hr for 2–4 days
Hanley, P.H.	Neomycin 1 g Erythromycin base 1 g p.o. at 1, 2, and 11 p.m. day before	Cephazolin sodium 1 g i.v. at 12 and 6 a.m.	None	Cephazolin sodium 1 g i.v. q. 6 hr for 48 hr
Polk, H.C., Jr.	None	Cephaloridine 1 g i.m. on call to O.R.	Cephaloridine 1 g i.m. 5–6 hr after preop. dose	None
Remington, J.H.	Phthalylsulfathiazole 2 g 4 × daily for 3 days Neomycin 1 g Erythromycin base 1 g at 1, 2, and 11 p.m. day before	Cephazolin sodium 1 g i.m. 1 hr before	Ampicillin 1 g in wound before closing	None, except for low anterior anastomoses sodium cephalothin 1 g i.v. 4 × daily for 4 days
Turnbull, R.B.	Neomycin 1 g Erythromycin base 1 g p.o. at 1, 2, and 11 p.m. day before	None	Cephalosporins i.v.	Cephalosporins i.v. for 7 days in selected cases

[a] The data for W. A. Altemeier appear in Hardy JD (ed) (1977) Rhoads textbook of surgery, Lippincott, Philadelphia, p. 1254. The rest of the data are all from personal communications, January 1978.

Anastomoses may be classified as end-to-end, end-to-side, or side-to-side. Undoubtedly the most physiologic is the end-to-end anastomosis. However, in some instances in which the lumen of the bowel may be extremely small, as in some ileotransverse colonic anastomoses, this is impractical and either an end-to-side or a side-to-side anastomosis must be chosen. A side-to-end sigmoidoproctostomy is sometimes indicated after a low anterior resection not only for this reason but also because of the configuration of the sigmoid mesocolon. Side-to-side anastomoses in the colon are used rarely to bypass an obstructing irremovable carcinoma of the right colon or the splenic flexure.

Anastomoses also may be classified as open or closed depending upon whether or not the lumen of the bowel is exposed during the course of the procedure. The closed anastomosis, typified by the Parker-Kerr basting stitch technique, was a favorite many years ago but has been almost entirely replaced by the open anastomoses. The latter have the advantages that a more accurate suture may be made and that no bleeding vessels are left at the anastomotic line. The closed technique has been reported by some surgeons to lower the incidence of suture-line implantation of tumor cells. It should be noted, however, that where implantation occurs most frequently, namely in very low anterior resections and anastomoses, it is impractical to use a closed technique because of the relative inaccessibility of the rectal stump.

Anastomoses may be made with the mucous membrane inverted, so that healing occurs from serosal surfaces, or everted, so that the mucous membrane is extruded outside the anastomotic line.[17] Inverting anastomoses have stood the test of time. Despite some enthusiastic reports favoring everting sutures, they have been found experimentally in dogs to owe their integrity to intact omentum; Goligher also found a prohibitive incidence of leakage.[20] Everting sutures have been abandoned by most surgeons.[16,19,20,21]

End-to-End Anastomosis

This is the most common type of anastomosis used after resection of the colon. Since it is the prototype of all intestinal anastomoses it will be described in detail.

In Figure 3.1 it is assumed that the section of the colon containing the pathologic process has been isolated between Allen clamps, the bowel divided with the actual cautery, and the specimen removed. The bowel is now ready for anastomosis. The cautery is used rather than the Bovie unit because the slow heat of the cautery tends to reduce the amount of bleeding at the suture line. It is not necessary to excise the section of bowel that has been included in the clamp or traumatized by the cautery.

A two-layer technique is preferred. In exceptional instances, such as in children or in adults with extremely narrow colons, a one-layer silk anastomosis may be employed. The usual two-layer technique requires an outer layer of interrupted nonabsorbable sutures and an inner layer of catgut. It is possible that in the future a synthetic suture will replace catgut, which is susceptible to rapid proteolytic digestion throughout the gastrointestinal tract.[7,29] Deveney and Way have presented evidence that poly (glycolic acid) sutures (Dexon or Vicryl) may be superior to catgut.[11] Unless the lumen of the colon is very large, both layers are made of interrupted sutures in order to prevent any purse-string effect.

The outer posterior layer of 000 silk is placed first, beginning at the end farther from the surgeon (Fig. 3.1a). Interrupted Lembert or Cushing sutures, depending upon the size of the bowel, are placed along the whole length of the divided segments. Then as the first suture is tied the clamps are removed. In the well-prepared bowel this should involve no contamination whatsoever. The posterior row of sutures is then tied and the lumen of the bowel segments is exposed. The anterior surface of each segment is then clasped with an Allis clamp, demonstrating the open lumen. Each lumen is occluded with a pledget of gelfoam. For the sake of clarity, the Allis clamps and gelfoam will not be shown in the illustrations.

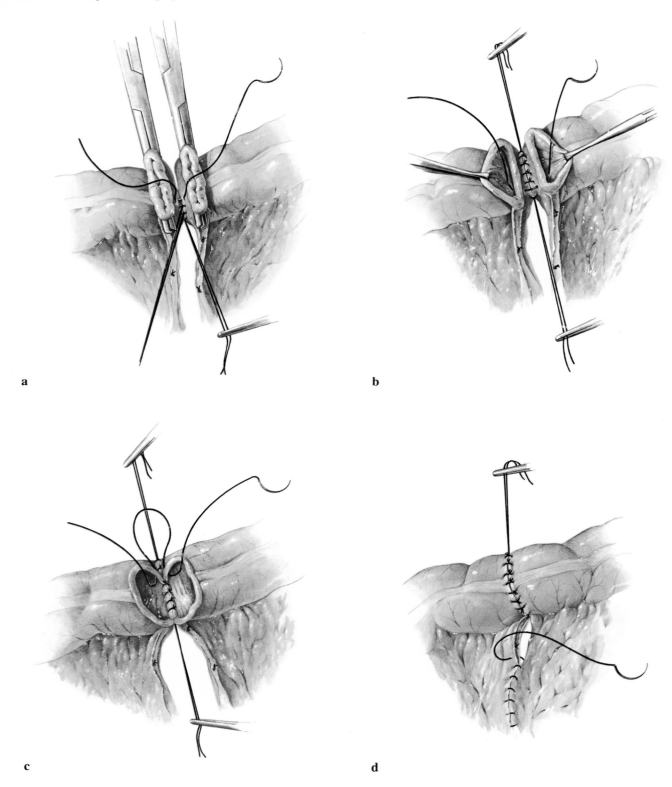

a

b

c

d

Fig. 3.1a–d. End-to-end anastomosis. Two-layer technique. a. Insertion of outer layer of interrupted 000 silk. b. The posterior outer row has been completed. The inner posterior row of interrupted 000 catgut or poly(glycolic acid) sutures is begun. c. The inner posterior row has been completed. The anterior inner row is now begun using inverting interrupted sutures. The last one or two sutures will be of the Lembert type. d. The outer anterior row has been completed, again of interrupted 000 silk. The mesenteric trap is closed with a running suture of catgut.

The second row of sutures, which is a posterior inner layer of interrupted 000 absorbable suture, begins at the far angle and continues around anteriorly (Fig. 3.1b). Sutures in the anterior inner row are placed so that the knots are tied within the lumen of the bowel except for the last one or two sutures, which are of the Lembert type (Fig. 3.1c). The final row of sutures is the outer anterior row, which again is of 000 silk (Fig. 3.1d). The surgeon then tests the lumen of the bowel to be certain that it is open by invaginating a finger through the anastomosis. The upper gelfoam plug can likewise be pushed through the anastomosis to assure patency.

End-to-Side Anastomosis

The end-to-side anastomosis is used most commonly after a resection of the right colon when the lumen of the ileum is small compared with the lumen of the transverse colon (see the section on Right Colectomy for Cancer in Chapter 6).

Side-to-End Anastomosis

A side-to-end anastomosis is used most commonly after low anterior resections for diverticulitis or cancer in which the left colon will lie comfortably in the base of the pelvis in a somewhat curved direction but will be kinked if an end-to-end anastomosis is attempted. This anastomosis is also particularly valuable if the lumen of the descending colon is much smaller than that of the rectum to which it is to be sutured. It will be described in Chapter 9 in the section on Low Anterior Resection.

Side-to-Side Anastomosis

A side-to-side anastomosis involves the apposition of two segments of bowel that circumvent the pathologic lesion that is deemed to be irremovable. It will be described in Chapter 6 in the section on Right Colectomy for Cancer.

Parker-Kerr Aseptic Anastomosis

The Parker-Kerr anastomosis is described because of its historical interest.[34] It is one of the "aseptic" methods of anastomosis of the colon. Historically, it was preceded by an anastomosis carried out over two clamps, followed by withdrawal of the clamps and final closure of the bowel—a method that provided relatively little contamination.

The essential feature of the Parker-Kerr method is that after the bowel has been resected the Allen clamp at either end is replaced by a basting suture of lubricated 00 catgut that is run over and over the clamp; the clamp is then removed and the basting stitch is tightened. This basting suture keeps the end of the bowel closed while the anastomosis is done. The anastomosis may be done in either one or two layers. As soon as it is complete the basting stitch is pulled out and a finger is passed through the anastomosis to assure patency.

This procedure furnished a nice technical method but it does have some disadvantages: The basting stitch may break as it is being withdrawn or it may be sutured in place so that it is impossible to remove. The inner surface of the bowel is not observed; thus the bowel may be occluded by sutures that pass from one side of the bowel to another across the lumen. Finally, there may be bleeding from the mucosal line that is not detected but would be found if the anastomosis were done in an open fashion.

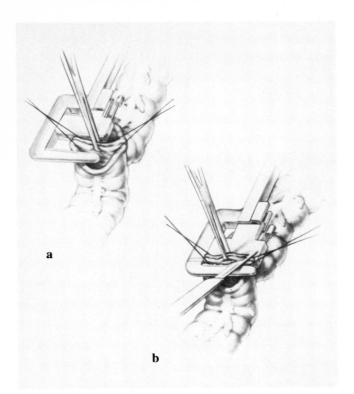

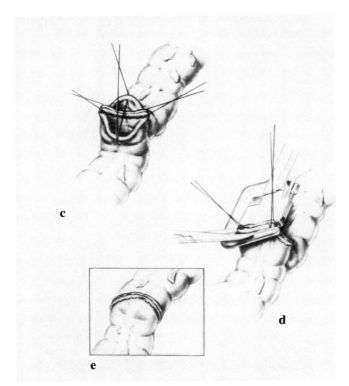

Fig. 3.2a–e. Anastomosis with stapler, triangulation technique. a. The colon has been resected and the two posterior margins are brought together. A clamp (either TA-55 or TA-30, depending on the diameter of the bowel) is placed at the midpoint to approximate the tissue edges. Ensure that all tissue edges are incorporated within the jaws. b. The pin is pushed firmly into place before the staples are fired. After the walls are stapled together, excess mucosa is trimmed away. c. The anterior surface of the bowel is divided into halves by a guy ligature. The third traction suture bisects both lips. d. The stapler is applied first on the right side, then on the left. e. The completed anastomosis has one posterior inverted and two anterior everted staple lines. (From Ravitch, M. M.: *Ann. Surg.* **175:**815, 1972.)

Anastomosis with the Stapler

Ravitch has been responsible for the popularization of staplers in this country. He modified Russian instruments that had been developed previously. It is possible to use the stapler for nearly all of the anastomotic procedures on the colon.[36,39] An instrument for low anterior anastomosis is discussed in Chapter 9.

Two methods of anastomosing the colon have been described. If the colon is freely mobile, an end-to-end anastomosis may be performed using the principle of triangulation (Fig. 3.2). After the resection has been completed, the posterior lips of the bowel are approximated and held in place with traction sutures (Fig. 3.2a). The TA-55 or TA-30 instrument is then applied and the two posterior walls are stapled together. Excess mucosa is trimmed away (Fig. 3.2b). In the second stage the anterior lips are bisected and traction sutures are applied (Fig. 3.2c and d). Either the TA-55 or TA-30 then can be used to close the anterior wall in two layers. It will be noted that this type of anastomosis has mucosa everted on the anterior row (Fig. 3.2e).

Another type of anastomosis, called the "functional" end-to-end anastomosis, brings the two loops of resected colon together in a side-to-side fashion (Fig. 3.3a). Each end of the bowel is then closed except for a small

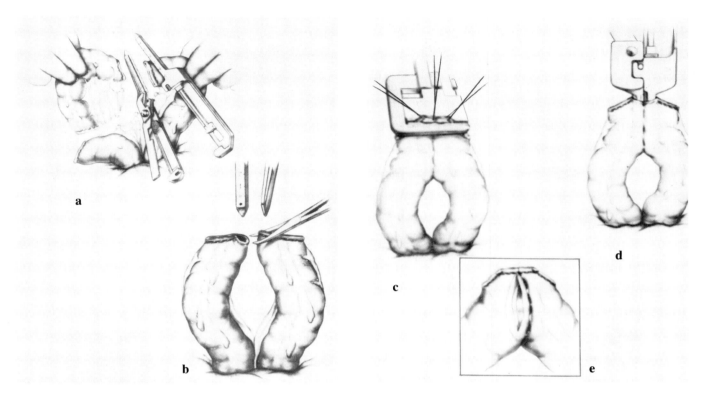

Fig. 3.3a–e. Anastomosis with the stapler, "functional" end-to-end technique. a. The two ends of the bowel have been closed by the TA-55 or TA-90. b. The two limbs are apposed side by side. The GIA stapler is inserted through the margin of each limb; both forks must be inserted fully to ensure maximal stomal size. c. The stapler is fired and the anastomosis is made by advancing the knife. d. The GIA is then withdrawn and the opening is closed either with the stapler or by suture. e. Note that this type of anastomosis produces essentially a side-to-side anastomosis. It also has one layer of everted mucosa in the anastomosis. (From Ravitch, M. M.: *Ann. Surg.* **175:**815, 1972.)

opening in the medial portion through which the two arms of the GIA stapler will be inserted. After it is inserted the instrument is closed and the blade cuts the new lumen between the staple lines (Fig. 3.3b and c). Finally, the GIA stapler is withdrawn and the opening that is left is closed with the TA-30 or TA-55 (Fig. 3.3d and e).

Although some surgeons are enthusiastic about the use of the stapler in colon surgery, a number of problems have developed: In many instances it is wise to invert the everting anastomosis if this can be done without obstruction of the lumen. The staples may not fire accurately enough to close all blood vessels so that bleeding from the suture line may be a problem. For this reason a careful inspection of the anastomosis should be made to be certain that there are no bleeders left. Late stenosis, stomal obstruction, perforation, and fistulization have all been reported.[13,15]

Proximal Decompression

Proximal decompression has been urged by many surgeons as a concomitant measure after resection of the left colon or after low anterior anastomoses. At one time such procedures were essentially routine; however, they may be hazardous. For example, the complications following closure of a colostomy are almost as numerous although admittedly not quite as serious as those of a primary resection and anastomosis of the colon. We now use Levin tube nasogastric suction for a period of 3–5 days, removing it when the patient passes gas by the rectum. In certain instances a gastrostomy catheter may be employed instead. However, a concomitant cecostomy is very rarely done. A concomitant transverse colostomy accompanying low anterior resection is considered advisable if the anastomosis is not entirely satisfactory in the surgeon's judgment, such as when there is some slight amount of uncontrolled bleeding or when there has been excessive contamination (see Chapter 15).

Some surgeons have passed a rectal tube through the anus and through a low anastomotic line to provide a type of decompression.[40] We have not used this method.

Drainage

For the usual resection and anastomosis of the colon no drainage is employed. There is no question that the old method of leading a drain down to an anastomosis invited leakage[1,2,30,31]; this has been proved clinically and in animal experiments. Therefore, drainage is employed only in special circumstances. For example, there may be a persistent ooze of blood after the splenic flexure has been mobilized; the colorectal anastomosis is placed low in the pelvis and a Penrose drain is placed in a subcostal area in the bed of the left colon to evacuate blood.[1] Such a drain can be removed after 48 hr. Occasionally such a situation also occurs after resection of the right colon.

The most important indication for the use of drainage, however, occurs when a low anterior resection and anastomosis has been performed.[10,37] If the rectum has been mobilized widely from the sacrum, the anastomosis usually lies anteriorly, and a space if left in the rectrorectal region that immediately fills with blood or serum. At times it may be possible to fill the space with omentum; usually, however, this method will not be possible. We prefer to insert a Shirley sump sucker that exits either through the lower angle of the wound or through a separate stab wound and keep it on suction for at least 48 hr (Fig. 3.4). If at this time the drainage has stopped, it may be removed. This technique is more satisfactory than the insertion of a stuffed Penrose drain, which has to drain uphill against gravity. Some surgeons prefer to insert a stuffed Penrose drain through the perineum into the retrorectal space. Unfortunately, if a fistula forms at this site it is very difficult to handle and we prefer drainage from above.

The use of drains in patients with localized abscesses, e.g., diverticulitis or appendicitis, is essential. Necrotic tissue in a localized area is another indication. In the presence of generalized peritonitis without a local abscess, the majority of surgeons advise against drains since they function only for a few hours. We have not employed continual peritoneal irrigation for sepsis; we use only parenteral antibiotics.

Incisions and Suture Material

The type of incision employed will be specified in the descriptions of individual operations. In general terms, midline or paramedian incisions allow excellent access to all sections of the peritoneal cavity. In obese patients resections involving the splenic flexure are easier through an upper transverse incision. Transverse incisions are excellent in the upper abdomen; however, if they are made close to the pubis, very troublesome postoperative hernias may develop. Incisions should not be made near the site of prospective stomas.

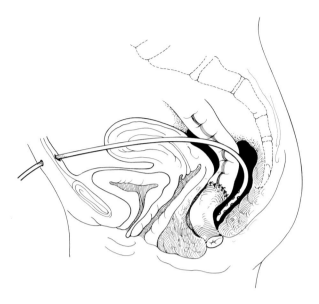

Fig. 3.4. Method of drainage by sump tube after a low anterior resection and anastomosis. The sump is placed posterior to the anastomosis and brought out through a stab wound in the lower abdomen.

For closure of incisions the surgeon has a choice of absorbable versus nonabsorbable sutures. There is no question that the nonabsorbable are far stronger in the early postoperative course. On the other hand, there is always the hazard that nonabsorbable sutures may have to be removed at a later date. Catgut has been the favorite absorbable suture, but this may very well be replaced by one of the synthetics in the near future. The usual closure has been continuous catgut in the peritoneum, interrupted 0 chromic catgut in the fascia, stay sutures of Mersilene, and silk sutures in the skin.

If nonabsorbable sutures are used, two options are 0 polyolifin (Prolene) applied as a continuous suture, or No. 30 interrupted wire sutures. Both silk and catgut have been used in the abdominal incisions, but in our experience they are more likely to be extruded than either polyolifin or wire.

Delayed primary closure has been employed by many surgeons, particularly after the closure of colonic stomas. At the time of the original operation stay sutures are placed, and the peritoneum and fascia are closed. The subcutaneous tissue and skin are packed lightly with a sponge. Four days later, with the aid of intravenous meperidine hydrochloride or diazepam, the sponge is removed and the sutures tied. This method has reduced the rate of postoperative infection in the closure of stomas or badly contaminated wounds; however, it is not necessary to use it in the usual colon resection.

References

1. Abramson D.J. (1976) Charles Bingham Penrose and the Penrose drain. Surg Gynecol Obstet 143: 285
2. Agrama H.M., Blackwood J.M., Brown C.S., et al (1976) Functional longevity of intraperitoneal drains. An experimental evaluation. Am J Surg 132: 418
3. Altemeier W.A., Thieme T., in discussion, Beahrs O.H., Hoehn J.G., Dear-

ing W.H. (1969) Surgery of the colon: Management and complications. Arch Surg 98: 485

4. Beahrs O.H., Hoehn J.G., Dearing W.H. (1969) Surgery of the colon: Management and complications. Arch Surg 98: 480
5. Brass C., Richards G.K., Ruedy J., et al (1978) The effect of metronidazole on the incidence of postoperative wound infection in elective colon surgery. Am J Surg 135: 91
6. Burdon J.G.W., Morris P.J., Hunt P., et al (1977) Trial of cephalothin sodium in colon surgery to prevent wound infection. Arch Surg 112: 1169
7. Clark C.G., Wyllie J.H., Haggie S.J., et al (1977) Comparison of catgut and polyglycolic acid sutures in colonic anastomoses. World J Surg 1: 501
8. Clarke J.S., Condon R.E., Bartlett J.G., et al (1977) Preoperative oral antibiotics reduce septic complications of colon operations: Results of prospective, randomized, double-blind clinical study. Ann Surg 186: 251
9. Cohn I. Jr. (1970) Intestinal antisepsis. Surg Gynecol Obstet 130: 1006
10. Collins C.D., Talbot C.H. (1969) Pelvic drainage after anterior resection of the rectum. Arch Surg 99: 391
11. Deveney K.E., Way L.W. (1977) Effect of different absorbable sutures on healing of gastrointestinal anastomoses. Am J Surg 133: 86
12. Dudrick S.J., Wilmore D.W., Vars H.M., Rhoads J.E. (1968) Long-term total parenteral nutrition with growth, development, and positive nitrogen balance. Surgery 64: 134
13. Elliott T.E., Albertazzi V.J., Danto L.A. (1977) Stenosis after stapler anastomosis. Am J Surg 133: 750
14. Fischer J.F. (1976) Total parenteral nutrition. Little, Brown, Boston
15. Fischer M.G. (1976) Bleeding from stapler anastomosis. Am J Surg 131: 745
16. Getzen L.C. (1969) Intestinal suturing. Part I: The development of intestinal sutures. Curr Probl Surg (Aug) 6: 1
17. Getzen L.C. (1969) Intestinal suturing. Part II: Inverting and everting intestinal sutures. Curr Probl Surg (Sept) 6: 1
18. Gilbert F.I. Jr., Cherry J.W., Downing D.E., et al (1974) Allied health personnel in cancer detection: Utilization of proctosigmoidoscopic technicians in detecting abnormalities of the lower bowel. Cancer 33: 1725
19. Gilchrist R.K., David V.C. (1938) Lymphatic spread of carcinoma of the rectum. Ann Surg 108: 621
20. Goligher J.C. (1976) Visceral and parietal suture in abdominal surgery. Am J Surg 131: 130
21. Goligher J.C., Graham N.G., De Dombal F.T. (1970) Anastomotic dehiscence after anterior resection of rectum and sigmoid. Br J Surg 57: 109
22. Goodman M.J. (1977) Mass screening for colorectal cancer—A negative report. JAMA 237: 2380
23. Gurry J.F., Ellis-Pegler R.B. (1976) An elemental diet as preoperative preparation of the colon. Br J Surg 63: 969
24. Hastings J.B. (1974) Mass screening for colorectal cancer. Am J Surg 127: 228
25. Hogan W.J., Stewart E.T., Geenen J.E., et al (1977) A prospective comparison of the accuracy of colonoscopy vs air–barium contrast exam for detection of colonic polypoid lesions. Gastrointest Endosc 23(4): 230
26. Jiborn H., Ahonen J., Zederfeldt B. (1978) Healing of experimental colonic anastomoses. The effect of suture technic on collagen concentration in the colonic wall. Am J Surg 135: 333
27. Juler G.L., Dietrick W.R., Eisenman J.I. (1976) Intramesenteric perforation of sigmoid diverticulitis with nonfatal venous intravasation. Am J Surg 132: 653
28. Lahiry S.K., Hedberg S.E. (1978) Fiberoptic colonoscopy and polypectomy. Complications and management. Meeting of the American Society for Gastrointestinal Endoscopy, Las Vegas, May 4
29. Laufman H., Rubel T. (1977) Synthetic absorbable sutures. Surg Gynecol Obstet 145: 597

30. Magee C., Rodeheaver G.T., Golden G.T., et al (1976) Potentiation of wound infection by surgical drains. Am J Surg 131: 547

31. Manz C.W., LaTendresse C., Sako Y. (1970) The detrimental effects of drains on colonic anastomoses: An experimental study. Dis Colon Rectum 13: 17

32. Nichols R.L., Condon R.E. (1971) Preoperative preparation of the colon. Surg Gynecol Obstet 132: 323

33. Nichols R.L., Condon R.E., DiSanto A.R. (1977) Preoperative bowel preparation. Arch Surg 112: 1493

34. Parker E.M., Kerr H.W. (1908) Intestinal anastomosis without open incisions by means of basting stitches. Bull Johns Hopkins Hosp 19: 132

35. Pearl S.S. (1978) Letter to the editor. CA 28: 238

36. Ravitch M.M., Steichen F.M. (1972) Technics of staple suturing in the gastrointestinal tract. Ann Surg 175: 815

37. Schaupp W.C. (1969) Drainage of low anterior anastomoses. Am J Surg 118: 627

38. Schrock T.R., Deveney C.W., Dunphy J.E. (1973) Factors contributing to leakage of colonic anastomoses. Ann Surg 177: 513

39. Steichen F.M. (1977) The creation of autologous substitute organs with stapling instruments. Am J Surg 134: 659

40. Stewart W.R.C., Samson R.B. (1968) Rectal tube decompression of left-colon anastomosis. Dis Colon Rectum 11: 452

41. Washington J.A. II, Dearing W.H., Judd E.S., et al (1974) Effect of preoperative antibiotic regimen on development of infection after intestinal surgery; prospective randomized, double-blind study. Ann Surg 180: 567

42. Welch C.E., Hedberg S.E. (1975) Polypoid lesions of the gastrointestinal tract, 2nd edn. Saunders, Philadelphia

4 Congenital Lesions

Almost all congenital lesions are manifested in infancy[3]; however, a few are encountered for the first time in adults.[2,4,7] Errors of rotation, paraduodenal hernias, and congenital diverticula are examples (see Chapter 10).

Errors of Rotation

Errors of rotation of the colon may lead to intestinal obstruction by a variety of mechanisms. Normal rotation, according to Dotts' classic description, takes place in three stages after the sixth week of fetal life.[1]

Stages of Development
The first stage occurs when the midgut (i.e., that section supplied by the superior mesenteric artery) lies in the umbilical cord. At this time the future small intestine lies to the right of the vitelline duct and artery, and the future distal ileum and colon lie to the left. If the gut returns to the peritoneal cavity in this fashion, nonrotation of the midgut is found. There may be fixation of some portions of the gut by adhesions, or there may be no attachment of the midgut either posteriorly or laterally. Such patients therefore are subject to volvulus of the entire midgut. However, the error may exist in the absence of any symptoms and may not be discovered until barium enema studies in adult life show that nonrotation is present (Fig. 4.1). It has been estimated that this condition is found once in every 20,000 barium enema examinations in the adult.

During the second stage of rotation the cecum rotates 270° in a counterclockwise direction anterior to the superior mesenteric artery. This change normally occurs during the 10th and 11th weeks of fetal life as the midgut is returning to the abdominal cavity. Normally the cecum will ascend from the left lower quadrant to the left upper quadrant, then move to the right upper and then to the right lower. If rotation stops when the cecum is in the right upper quadrant, the cecum may become fixed by dense adhesions that run from the liver across the duodenum. This is the error of malrotation. Clinically, either a high duodenal obstruction or volvulus of the midgut loop may be associated with this abnormality.

34

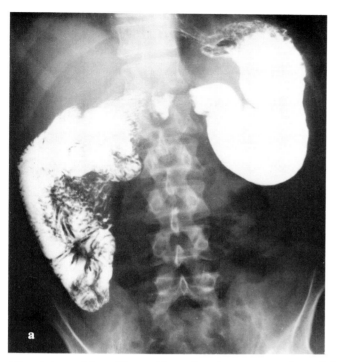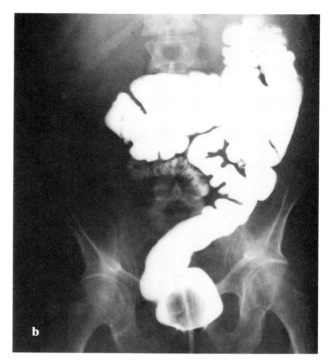

Fig. 4.1a and b.   X-ray films showing nonrotation of the intestine. a. Upper gastrointestinal series shows all small bowel in the right side of the abdomen. b. Barium enema.

The third stage of rotation occurs as the cecum descends and becomes fixed to the lateral peritoneum in the right lower quadrant. If this fixation does not occur the cecum may remain free and may be involved in volvulus either in childhood or in adult life.

The rare but serious error of reversed rotation occurs when the cecum rotates only 90° but in a clockwise direction. The duodenum then remains anterior to the superior mesenteric vessels and the transverse colon stays behind. The result is that the transverse colon may be compressed in a very small tunnel between the superior mesenteric artery and the aorta. This leads to obstruction. In addition, volvulus of the right colon and distal small intestine may occur or obstruction of the small intestine may result from adhesions. A preoperative diagnosis can be made by barium enema that shows the abnormal portion and constriction of the midtransverse colon.

Operative Procedures

Since in nonrotation of the colon (Fig. 4.2) the midgut usually is not completely attached to the posterior abdominal wall, volvulus of the cecum or distal ileum may occur. Depending upon the viability of the bowel, either detorsion and fixation of the cecum or resection and anastomosis of infarcted bowel will be necessary.

Malrotation (Fig. 4.3) is treated surgically by lysis of any adhesions that are obstructing the duodenum and replacement of the colon in a position of nonrotation (Ladd's operation) or by correction of volvulus. This type of obstruction is much more common in infancy than it is in later life.

Torsion of the cecum (Fig. 4.4) is caused by failure of fixation to the abdominal wall. It may be repaired by cecal fixation by suture, by cecostomy, or by resection and anastomosis; the last method is necessary if there is any vascular impairment (see Chapter 12).

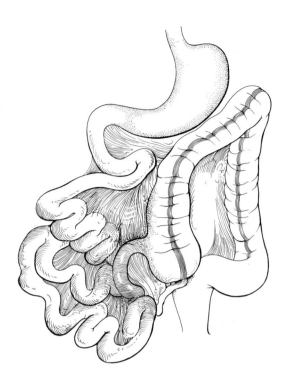

Fig. 4.2. Nonrotation. The small bowel lies entirely to the right side of the midline and the colon lies to the left.

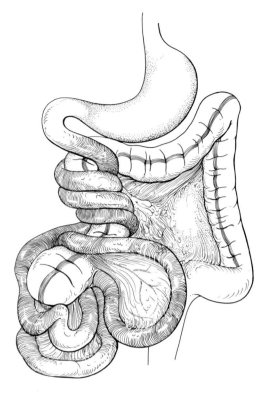

Fig. 4.3. Malrotation with volvulus. The entire small bowel and right colon have a common mesentery that is not fixed to the posterior abdominal wall. Volvulus is a common occurrence.

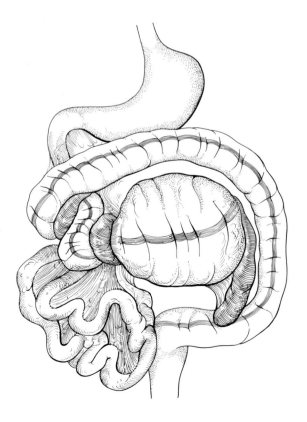

Fig. 4.4. Nonfixation of the cecum with torsion of the cecum. This is often instigated by adhesions near the midascending colon; torsion of the short portion of the ascending colon and the terminal ileum produces excessive distention of the cecum and gangrene.

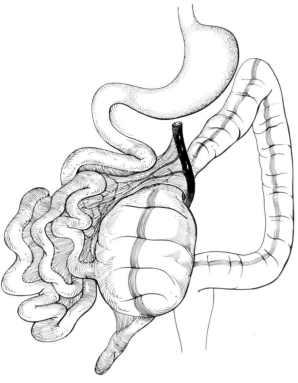

Fig. 4.5. Reversed rotation. The right colon has rotated posterior to the superior mesenteric artery and vein and obstruction results because this tunnel is very tight.

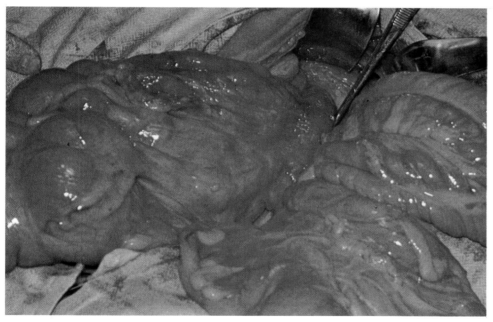

Fig. 4.6. Operative specimen of reversed rotation of the colon. The right colon is greatly distended due to obstruction in the tunnel behind the superior mesenteric artery. The left colon is of normal size. A subtotal colectomy and an ileosigmoid anastomosis cured the condition.

Reversed rotation (Figs. 4.5 and 4.6) requires a resection of the right, transverse, and descending colon with an ileosigmoidal or ileorectal anastomosis. The main technical difficulty occurs when the midcolic vessels are very short. It is necessary to free the transverse colon from its position between the superior mesenteric artery and the aorta; great care must be taken to preserve the vascular supply of the small intestine.

Paraduodenal Hernias

Right or left paraduodenal hernias are rare. Small intestine herniates into one or the other fossa and may produce a very confusing sight at laparotomy.

When the peritoneal cavity is entered the ascending colon and terminal ileum can be identified. However, the more proximal ileum seems to disappear behind a thin shield of tissue containing blood vessels; this is actually the mesentery of the descending colon. If it is necessary to free the small intestine, the blood supply of the distal colon may be compromised and an appropriate resection may be necessary.

Hirschsprung's Disease

Hirschsprung's disease is usually diagnosed very shortly after birth; however, a few cases elude diagnosis and treatment until adolescence or even adult life.[4-6] These patients tend to have greatly distended abdomens and repeated episodes of fecal obstruction, diarrhea, or enterocolitis. The underlying defect is the absence of intramural ganglion cells in the distal wall of the rectum. The aganglionosis extends for a variable distance upward, and in severe cases it involves the entire colon or even the entire alimentary tract. Only the patients who have had relatively short involvement will survive to adult life in the absence of surgical correction. Diagnosis usually has been made on the basis of a full-thickness rectal biopsy. Greatly increased acetylcholine esterase activity in the mucosa and muscularis mucosa in the distal rectum secured by a suction biopsy is also diagnostic of Hirschsprung's disease. In normal individuals anorectal manometry shows that rectal distention causes relaxation of the internal anal sphincter, but in Hirschsprung's disease contraction of the sphincter occurs.

The usual methods of treatment consist either of the Swenson operation, the Duhamel procedure, or the Soave procedure. A preliminary colostomy is necessary in adults; this may be a very difficult procedure because of the extreme distention of the colon. At the time of the definitive operation all rectum and colon that is devoid of ganglia on frozen section must be resected. The Swenson procedure involves a pull-through operation in which the incision is made about 1.5 cm above the dentate line anteriorly and at the level of the dentate line posteriorly so that an end-to-end anastomosis is effected between the ganglionic colon and essentially at the dentate line. The Soave procedure differs in that the internal and external sphincters of the rectum are left in place and the colon is drawn down through them. Both of these procedures are discussed in more detail in Chapter 9.

For a full discussion of the present status of Hirschsprung's disease the reader is referred to the comprehensive report by Sieber.[5]

References

1. Dott N.M. (1923) Anomalies of intestinal rotation: Their embryology and surgical aspects with report of five cases. Br J Surg 11: 251
2. Findley C.W. Jr., Humphreys G.H. II (1956) Collective review: Congenital anomalies of intestinal rotation in adults. Surg Gynecol Obstet (Intl Abstr Surg) 103: 417
3. Gross R.E. (1953) The surgery of infancy and childhood. Saunders, Philadelphia
4. Metzger P.P., Alvear D.T., Arnold G.C., et al (1978) Hirschsprung's disease in adults: Report of a case and review of the literature. Dis Colon Rectum 21: 113
5. Sieber W.K. (1978) Hirschsprung's disease. Curr Probl Surg (June) 15: 1
6. Todd I.P. (1977) Adult Hirschsprung's disease. Br J Surg 64: 311
7. Wang C.A., Welch C.E. (1963) Anomalies of intestinal rotation in adolescents and adults. Surgery 54: 839

Polypoid Lesions of the Colon

5

At the present time, unless the surgeon does his own endoscopy, the management of polypoid diseases of the colon must remain a joint responsibility of the radiologist, endoscopist, and surgeon. Generally a single pedunculated polyp or a few similar polyps scattered in separate sections of the colon are removed by colonoscopic polypectomy. Small sessile polyps may also be treated in this fashion. Patients with large sessile polyps, familial or multiple polyposis, and cancer developing in a polyp are candidates for operation. In some instances a single polyp is for some reason inaccessible to the colonoscope and removal by surgical means is necessary.

In these days watchful waiting in the treatment of polypoid lesions is unnecessary except in unusual instances. All doubt about the diagnosis can be resolved by colonoscopy. Even juvenile polyps that formerly were treated expectantly because of the frequency of self-amputation now should be treated by colonoscopic polypectomy. Multiple inflammatory polyps secondary to ulcerative colitis remain an exception because they tend to recur.

The operations that are employed for polypoid diseases of the colon include colotomy and polypectomy, segmental resection and anastomosis of the colon, subtotal colectomy, total proctocolectomy, and removal through the sigmoidoscope or colonoscope.[16] Rectal polyps will be discussed in Chapter 7. The adenoma–cancer relationship has been established firmly enough to warrant the removal of even apparently benign polypoid lesions unless there are strong contraindications.[2,5–8,10,11]

Colotomy and Polypectomy

Colotomy and polypectomy is indicated for a colonic polyp that is apparently benign and cannot be removed by the colonoscope.

The abdomen is opened through an adequate incision and the polyp is located by palpation. This may prove to be a very difficult procedure and occasionally it may be necessary to open the colon and insert a sterile sigmoidoscope in both directions to locate the lesion. If the lesion is soft and pedunculated, the chances of malignancy are small and a polypectomy may be carried out. On the other hand, if the polypoid lesion is hard or large, soft, and sessile, a segmental colectomy is advised.

The procedure of colotomy and polypectomy consists of opening the bowel with a short longitudinal incision over the base of the polyp. The location of the base is identified by pulling the polyp as far as possible caudally and then cephalad so that the point of attachment of the pedicle is midway between the two (Fig. 5.1a). The colon is opened in a longitudinal direction (Fig. 5.1b). The polyp is elevated from the colon. Two catgut sutures are tied around the base of the polyp and the specimen is excised.

If the pathologist is very adept at frozen sections, the specimen is examined in this fashion. If the lesion is benign the colon is closed in either a transverse or vertical direction with two layers of sutures—an inner of interrupted absorbable such as 000 catgut and an outer of interrupted 000 silk.

There are three important complications of colotomy and polypectomy:

1. Inability to find the polyp: If the polyp cannot be found easily on palpation a sterile sigmoidoscope should be readily available for introduction into the colon through an incision made at a point where the polyp is believed to lie. Alternatively, a colonoscope can be inserted through the anus and the polyp can be identified.

2. Bleeding: The stalk of a pedunculated polyp often contains large blood vessels, and unless they are tied accurately the vessels may retract within the wall of the colon and rapidly produce an intramural hematoma. This may require a resection in order to stop the bleeding. Postoperative hemorrhage can occur from the vessels in the base of the pedicle. Prevention is much more likely if two catgut ties are placed on the base of the pedicle rather than one. However, when bleeding does follow, it is usually rather profuse and occurs within a few hours. The best method of therapy is relaparotomy. It may be necessary to resect a section of bowel at this time to secure adequate hemostasis. An alternative method of therapy consists of vasopressin injection via the corresponding mesenteric artery.

3. Carcinoma: The pathologist may determine on final sections a day or so later that the lesion is carcinoma. If the cancer invades the stalk the possibility of lymphatic metastasis is present and in a good-risk patient a bowel resection is advisable. Unless proof has been obtained on frozen section, this will require a second laparotomy within a few days.

Primary Resection and Anastomosis of the Colon or Rectum

Primary resection and anastomosis is advocated for large sessile polyps or for any polyp not removable by the colonoscope.[2,16,17] If the lesion is on the right side of the abdomen, a standard right colectomy is performed, including a removal of the lymph nodes along the ileocolic vessels. If the lesion is in the sigmoid we have usually been somewhat less radical than in the usual cancer operation. We have tended to remove a generous segment of mesentery, but have not removed the inferior mesenteric artery for pedunculated polyps if no enlarged nodes are encountered. The metastases from a cancer in a pedunculated polyp that we have discovered have been very close to the colon rather than deep in the mesenteric nodes. Large villous adenomas located in the low sigmoid and extending into the rectum at the level of the peritoneal floor require removal of the inferior mesenteric pedicle. If the lesion is soft, only 2−3 cm of normal rectal mucosa is

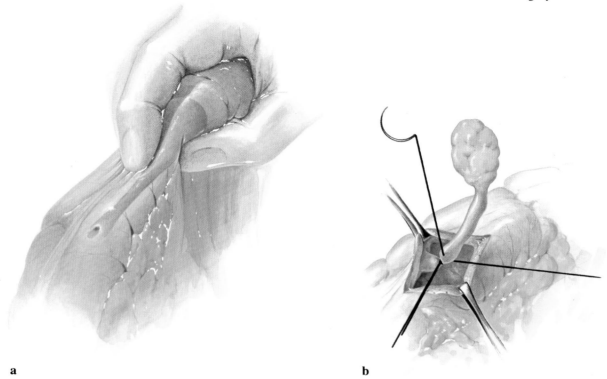

a   b

Fig. 5.1a and b. Colotomy and polypectomy. a. The location of the base of the polyp is determined by pulling the polyp upward and then downward. The midpoint represents the base. b. The colon is opened through a short vertical incision and the polyp is withdrawn. The base will be doubly ligated with catgut and the polyp will be excised. The incision will be closed in a transverse direction with an inner layer of interrupted catgut and an outer layer of interrupted silk.

removed. Anastomosis can be done either by the low anterior technique or by the D'Allaines procedure.[17]

Subtotal Colectomy

Subtotal colectomy is indicated for multiple polyposis of the colon. It is wise to resect the colon from the terminal ileum down to a point where the remainder can be observed accurately by sigmoidoscopy. The operation involves the principles described in Chapter 6.

This operation is indicated for patients with a large number of polyps.[3,4,10,13,16] The exact number is arbitrary and will depend on many other factors, such as the age and condition of the patient. It might be suggested that 10 or more polyps indicate a colectomy; if there are fewer polyps, endoscopic removal is usually elected. If there is any recurrence of polyps after removal of several at a previous date, a partial colectomy is desirable.

Surgery for Familial Polyposis

Familial polyposis develops in children and symptoms usually appear at about 12 years of age. Sigmoidoscopy at this time usually shows complete involvement of the colon and rectum with thousands of polyps. Patients with untreated disease develop cancer and generally are dead before age 40.

Surgery is indicated in the early teens. The preferred procedure at this time is a subtotal colectomy with an anastomosis of the ileum to the rectum at a site well within the view of the sigmoidoscope.

After the young person has recovered from this operation, there are several courses that are open. One is to continue a policy of watchful waiting. Sigmoidoscopy is carried out every 6 months and polyps are fulgurated as they appear. This is the method that is usually chosen. The polyps sometimes diminish in number in the rectal segment after subtotal colectomy, but in our experience new ones usually appear that require endoscopic removal by the snare through the sigmoidoscope.[3,4,11,13] This conservative approach is sanctioned by the results of the St. Mark's series; only 3 combined abdominoperineal resections have been required in this series of 73 patients.[11] Despite this optimistic report, it must be expected that resection of the rectum will be required at a second stage due to the development of another cancer. Very careful follow-up is necessary if this course is chosen. J. J. DeCosse (personal communication, 1978) has suggested that large doses of vitamin C p.o. may facilitate regression of polyps.

A second method of therapy is to remove the colon and rectum and form a permanent ileostomy as soon as the disease is discovered. This is the method that is certain to prevent any development of colorectal cancer, but it is carried out at the price of a permanent ileostomy. Factors that make such a course desirable include female sex, early development of polyps, and innumerable polyps in the rectum.

In recent years a third method, the Soave procedure for multiple and familial polyposis, has been used.[15] This may be done as either a primary or a secondary procedure following a subtotal colectomy and ileoproctostomy. This procedure is described in Chapter 9.

Soper (personal communication, 1977) has reported 12 cases treated in this fashion with good results in all of them. However, at times a protracted period was necessary before the patient recovered full continence. This operation has been used only a few times in Massachusetts General Hospital; the postoperative course in these older patients usually has been slow and complicated.

Endoscopic Removal of Colorectal Polyps

The principles of endoscopic removal of polypoid lesions of the colon and rectum are the same regardless of whether excision is carried out through the sigmoidoscope or the colonoscope: (1) the procedure must avoid perforation of the bowel; (2) there should be complete hemostasis; (3) the entire lesion should be removed for microscopic section if possible; (4) decision on further treatment must be made if the lesion shows malignant change; and (5) proper follow-up is necessary. The technical principles, however, are quite different depending upon whether the lesion is removed through the sigmoidoscope or the colonoscope; therefore these two methods will be discussed separately.

Removal of Rectal or Low Sigmoid Polyps Through the Sigmoidoscope

A large-bore sigmoidoscope that has lighting at the inner end of the scope is necessary. We prefer the Welch-Allyn scope that has a bore of approximately 3 cm. The bowel is prepared by enema. If the anal canal is very tight a preliminary intravenous injection of 50 mg meperidine hydrochloride

(Demerol) will ease the passage of the scope. However, manipulations other than those due to introduction of the scope should be relatively painless.

The lesion is identified. Stalked lesions are the most favorable for total removal. Sessile lesions ranging up to 4 cm in diameter can be destroyed by electrodesiccation, although the chances of recurrence are distinctly greater since many of them are villous adenomas.

In most instances the snare can then by passed around the polyp close to the base of the pedicle. This maneuver may be aided by the insertion of a suction tip applied to the end of the polyp that will draw it downward and allow more accurate application of the snare. The snare is then tightened, and with alternating bursts of coagulation and cutting current from the Bovie unit the entire lesion is removed. It is advisable to leave a short pedicle so that if further bleeding occurs there will be an opportunity for control by electrodesiccation that will not injure the wall of the bowel.

If there is some persistent bleeding from the base of the pedicle the area may be cauterized by electrodesiccation. Unless a plastic suction tube is inserted to remove the smoke and blood that is seeping from the open area, this electrodesiccation may be difficult and it may damage the wall of the bowel if it is done inaccurately. Other methods of hemostasis include the application of a small pledget soaked in epinephrine solution to the bleeding area with the biopsy forceps. After control has been obtained it is also possible to apply a silver nitrate stick on a long applicator to a small bleeding vessel. It should be emphasized that unless complete control is secured there may be profuse bleeding after the operation that will require secondary control. When the area is high, it may even require an anterior resection and anastomosis if the bleeding is excessive.

The danger of perforation of the bowel is always present. It is much more dangerous to excise polypoid lesions on the anterior or lateral walls than on the posterior wall. Furthermore, when the lesion is above the peritoneal floor, i.e., at a depth greater than 8 cm, the possibility of penetration into the peritoneal cavity must be considered. Unskilled cauterization has also led to perforation of the bladder.

The diagnosis of a perforation may be made immediately or it may be delayed for several days. If it occurs at the time of sigmoidoscopy or desiccation of a polyp, immediate laparotomy is indicated with closure of the perforation. Usually there has been wide enough contamination such that a transverse colostomy is necessary as well, but this option should depend upon the judgment of the surgeon.

Some polypoid lesions are extremely large and the pedicle cannot be visualized through the sigmoidoscope. In such instances we have attacked the polyp from the top and, with multiple biopsies as the desiccation progressed, destroyed the polyp from the head down toward the base. It is advantageous to be able to see the pedicle because histologic section of this area will be most important, particularly if there is any carcinoma in the tip of the polyp.

Sessile polyps also present a more difficult problem. It is necessary to destroy them with multiple biopsies and then electrodesiccation carried down essentially to the muscular wall. It is better to resort to repeated desiccations rather than to carry the original procedure so deeply that the bowel wall is penetrated. It should be noted that villous adenomas tend to extend from visible margins with great ease and a recurrence after apparently successful destruction of such a lesion is not unexpected.

The question then arises as to what should be done if carcinoma is discovered in the polyp.[12,14,19] It should be recalled that the old diagnosis of "carcinoma in situ" is not regarded as tenable by pathologists. In order for a true carcinoma to be present there must be invasion of the muscularis mucosa at some point in the polypoid lesion. Cellular atypia without invasion below the mucous membrane indicates a benign lesion that will not recur provided that it has been completely destroyed. If, however, there is definite carcinoma at the tip and it has penetrated into the body of the polyp below the muscularis mucosa, then a decision must be made as to whether or not a further operative procedure is necessary. We believe that if the pathologist is able to demonstrate an invasive carcinoma that has involved the muscle of the colon at the base of the polyp, and the lesion is located in the sigmoid or intraperitoneal rectum, resection and anastomosis is the therapy of choice.

If the lesion is in the extraperitoneal rectum, we believe that local removal of a small polyp with cancer in the tip is the preferable operation even though the optimal curative operation would be a Miles resection. The mortality rate of a combined abdominoperineal operation together with the presence of a permanent colostomy would make it advisable to be content with the lesser operation, but very close follow-up of the patient is necessary. In this instance the situation is somewhat different than it is if a lesion is discovered higher in the colon, where a resection and anastomosis can be carried out with less risk and without the problem of a permanent colostomy.

The follow-up examinations after removal of a rectal polyp include frequent enough observations to be certain that the polyp has been completely destroyed. Further examination by sigmoidoscopy is carried out at 6-month intervals for 3 years and at yearly intervals thereafter. It is probably also advisable to carry out a colonoscopy and a barium enema at least at 3-year intervals. A table of suggested follow-up examinations will be given later.

Colonoscopic Polypectomy

When the polypoid lesion must be removed through the colonoscope (Fig. 5.2), many of the same problems arise.[1,16,18] The pedunculated polyp is relatively easy to handle. Small sessile lesions can be successfully treated. We believe, however, that the large lesions over 3 cm in diameter are best treated by segmental resection of the colon because there is an increased danger of perforation if they are destroyed widely by electrodesiccation. At the time of the operative procedure the retrieval of the polyp is sometimes difficult. The polyp may be entrapped in the suction apparatus and withdrawn together with the scope. At times the polyp is lost and must be retrieved with an evacuation produced by an enema.

Bleeding is the most common complication. Polypoid lesions removed by colonoscope are therefore amputated at least 1 cm from the base of the stalk in order that an adequate pedicle may again be seen and desiccated if necessary (see Fig. 5.3). After control has apparently been obtained, however, there may be further bleeding a few hours later. In our experience this bleeding nearly always is minor and does not require any particular care. In other instances it has been controlled by selective anteriography and injection of pitressin. In very rare instances continuing rebleeding requires laparotomy and resection of the involved segment. In Lahiry and Hedberg's series of 2336 polypectomies the incidence of hemorrhage was 1.8%.[9] All hemorrhage either stopped spontaneously or was treated successfully by transfusion, recauterization, or angiography. Bleeding usually occurs early but can occur as late as 10 days.

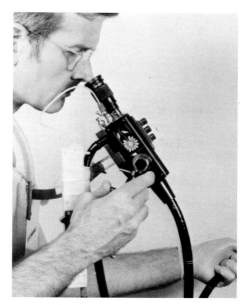

Fig. 5.2. The colonoscope in use demonstrating Hedberg's appliance for easy "solo" manipulation.

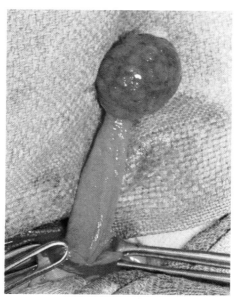

Fig. 5.3. Colonic polyp removed by colotomy and polypectomy. In contrast, the base of the stalk is left with colonoscopic polypectomy.

The second most important complication is perforation. The wall of the colon is exceedingly thin and deep electrocoagulation can lead to either immediate or delayed perforation. Frequently on the day after a colonoscopic polypectomy the abdomen is slightly tender over the site of the polyp removal. This has been referred to as the "coagulation syndrome," but actually represents a subacute perforation. Some endoscopists have regarded this as a fairly benign occurrence. However, if it is associated with more general abdominal tenderness and the presence of free air on an erect abdominal plate, laparotomy should be performed and repair carried out, usually by resection and anastomosis of the involved segment. A perforation with wide contamination requires a resection combined with a double-barreled colostomy and reconstruction at a later date. Fortunately, such episodes are exceedingly uncommon. In Lahiry and Hedberg's series the incidence of perforation was 0.5% and usually occurred after the removal of sessile polyps.[9]

If the pathologist makes the diagnosis of carcinoma, the question arises as to whether or not a laparotomy with resection of the involved segment should be undertaken (Table 5.1). Wolff and Shinya have advocated segmental resection if there is a highly anaplastic carcinoma, the line of resection is close to the carcinoma, or there is definite lymphatic invasion found in the stroma of the polyp.[19] We certainly agree with all these indications. However, the mortality of segmental resection of the colon for a polypoid lesion is only about 2% and cancer found only in the tip of a polyp does occasionally metastasize. Even though the carcinoma is confined to the distal portion of the stalk, the risk of recurrence or metastasis is probably greater than 1 in 50; on this basis a secondary resection is indicated in the good-risk patient.

Follow-up studies after polypectomy are based on the belief that if the colon can be freed of all polypoid lesions it is unlikely that any more of these lesions or invasive carcinomas will develop within a 3-year period. This opinion is based on the findings of Gilbertsen, who studied recur-

45

TABLE 5.1. Incidence of Cancer in Polyps Removed by Colonoscopy (Based on 101 Cancers in 2073 Polyps)

Diameter of Polyp (cm)	Adenomatous	Villo-glandular	Villous Adenoma	Cancer	Miscel.	Total No.	Percent
0–0.9	0/506	0/142	0/10	1	0/238	1/897	0.1
1–1.9	2/363	27/328	5/29	10	0/102	44/832	5.3
2–2.9	1/60	19/136	8/22	6	0/24	34/248	13.7
≥3	1/14	9/53	6/17	6	0/6	22/96	22.9
Total No.	4/943	55/659	19/78	23	0/370	101/2073	
Percent	0.4	8.5	24.4	100	0		4.9

Courtesy of Dr. S. E. Hedberg.

TABLE 5.2. Suggested Follow-Up Examinations after Polypectomy or Colectomy for Polypoid Disease or Cancer

	Benign Polyps	Cancer
History	q. 6 mo for 3 yr, then q. 1 yr	q. 6 mo for 5 yr, then q. 1 yr
Physical examination	q. 6 mo for 3 yr, then q. 1 yr	q. 6 mo for 5 yr, then q. 1 yr
Sigmoidoscopy	q. 6 mo for 3 yr, then q. 1 yr	q. 6 mo for 5 yr, then q. 1 yr
Stool guaiac	q. 6 mo for 3 yr, then q. 1 yr	q. 6 mo for 5 yr, then q. 1 yr
Complete blood count	q. 1 yr	q. 1 yr
Barium enema	q. 2 yr	q. 1 yr
Colonscopy (total)	q. 3 yr	q. 1 yr
Chest x-ray	—	q. 1 yr
Carcinoembryonic antigen	—	q. 6 mo for 3 yr
Liver scan	—	As indicated

rences after the removal of rectal polyps. We now advise a second colonoscopy 6 months after the polypectomy, and succeeding ones at 3-year intervals in the patient who is asymptomatic.[6,7,14]

The rate of recurrence of colon polyps has been studied by Henry et al.[7] They found that prior to the advent of colonoscopy the risk of developing a second polyp was approximately 30%. Most recurrences were found within 1 year after operation and they were more common with villous adenomas or multiple polyposis.

The frequency and extent of follow-up examinations are clearly a compromise between the necessity for the discovery of polyps and expense and patient acceptance. Our philosophy is summarized in Table 5.2.

The situation obviously is different if the polyp contained carcinoma and a simple polypectomy was carried out, or if the patient had carcinoma of the colon with concomitant polyps. More frequent examinations are then essential. Usually a sigmoidoscopy is done every 6 months and a barium enema once a year for 5 years; the optimal frequency of total colonoscopy has not been determined, but it probably should be done about once a year.

References

1. Abrams J.S. (1977) A hard look at colonoscopy. Am J Surg 133: 111
2. Bacon H.E., Eisenberg S.W. (1971) Papillary adenoma or villous tumor of the rectum and colon. Ann Surg 174: 1002
3. Bernstein W.C., in discussion, Schaupp W.C., Volpe P.A. (1972) Management of diffuse colonic polyposis. Am J Surg 124: 221

4. Dunphy J.E., in discussion, Schaupp W.C., Volpe P.A. (1972) Management of diffuse colonic polyposis. Am J Surg 124: 220

5. Fenoglio C.M., Lane N. (1975) The anatomic precursor of colorectal carcinoma. JAMA 231: 640

6. Gilbertsen V.A. (1974) Proctosigmoidoscopy and polypectomy in reducing the incidence of rectal cancer. Cancer 34 (suppl): 936

7. Henry L.G., Condon R.E., Schulte W.J., et al (1975) Risk of recurrence of colon polyps. Ann Surg 182: 511

8. Jackman R.J., Beahrs O.H. (1968) Tumors of the large bowel. Saunders, Philadelphia

9. Lahiry S.K., Hedberg S.E. (1978) Fiberoptic colonoscopy and polypectomy. Complications and management. Meeting of the American Society for Gastrointestinal Endoscopy, Las Vegas, May 4

10. Morson B. (1974) The polyp–cancer sequence in the large bowel. Proc R Soc Med 67: 451

11. Morson B.C., Bussey H.J.R. (1970) Predisposing causes of intestinal cancer. Curr Probl Surg (Feb) 7: 1

12. Okike N., Weiland L.H., Anderson M.J., et al (1977) Stromal invasion of cancer in pedunculated adenomatous colorectal polyps. Arch Surg 112: 527

13. Schaupp W.C., Volpe P.A. (1972) Management of diffuse colonic polyposis. Am J Surg 124: 218

14. Shatney C.H., Lober P.H., Gilbertsen V.A., et al (1974) The treatment of pedunculated adenomatous colorectal polyps with focal cancer. Surg Gynecol Obstet 139: 845

15. Soave F. (1964) Hirschsprung's disease: New surgical technique. Arch Dis Child 39: 116

16. Welch C.E., Hedberg S.E. (1975) Polypoid lesions of the gastrointestinal tract, 2nd edn. Saunders, Philadelphia

17. Welch J.P., Welch C.E. (1976) Villous adenomas of the colorectum. Am J Surg 131: 185

18. Wolff W.I., Shinya H. (1973) Polypectomy via the fiberoptic colonoscope. Removal of neoplasms beyond reach of the sigmoidoscope. N Engl J Med 288: 329

19. Wolff W.I., Shinya H. (1975) Definitive treatment of "malignant" polyps of the colon. Ann Surg 182: 516

6 Cancer of the Colon

In this chapter the standard operations for cancer of the colon will be discussed in detail. Inasmuch as there are many instances in which the diagnosis is not entirely certain at the time that surgery is performed, brief comments will also be made about some other indications for these standard operations. A detailed review of all aspects of colorectal cancer can be obtained from other reports and reviews.[6,8,17,18,25,30,32,33,36,40,43,46,50–53]

Right Colectomy

A right colectomy is carried out most frequently for cancer or extensive polypoid disease of the right colon. When the colon is resected for cancer, a wide resection of the mesentery is desirable. When the colectomy is done for benign lesions (Crohn's disease, diverticular disease, benign tumors, torsion of the cecum, angiodysplasia, or appendiceal disease), removal of wide areas of mesentery is unnecessary.

Cancer
When the cancer is located in the cecum or ascending colon the usual operation involves removal of approximately 15–20 cm of terminal ileum and all of the mesentery down close to the superior mesenteric vessels, and ligation of the ileocolic vessels, the right colic artery, and the right branch of the midcolic artery near their origins. When the lesion is as high as the hepatic flexure, less terminal ileum is excised but it is advisable to remove the entire midcolic artery as well as the ileocolic and right colic vessels. When the left branch of the midcolic artery has been excised it is necessary to be absolutely certain that there is adequate blood supply to allow an anastomosis of the terminal ileum to the distal transverse colon; otherwise the resection should be carried out to a much lower level and will probably end in the sigmoid.

The usual operation for cancer begins with one suture being tied around the lumen of the colon distal to the tumor and another around the terminal ileum close to the ileocecal valve (Fig. 6.1a). A tie is then placed around the major vessels that will be removed, midway between the colon and the superior mesenteric artery. The omentum is freed from the stom-

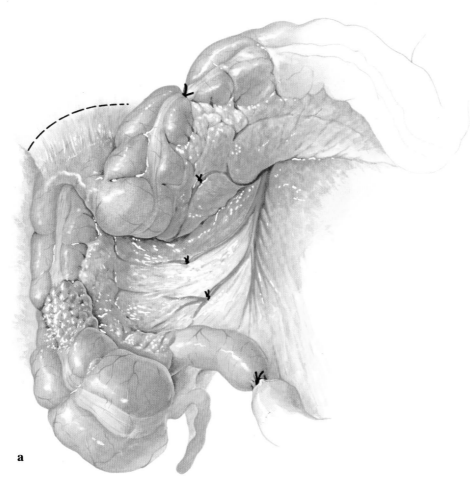

a

Fig. 6.1a–c. Right colectomy. a. The tumor is exposed. Ties have been placed around the terminal ileum and transverse colon and the major vessels have been interrupted approximately midway along their course to the colon from the superior mesenteric artery. The suspensory ligaments of the colon in the right upper quadrant will be divided and ligated (see broken black line).

ach and from the duodenum. Any adhesions about the terminal ileum are mobilized. The peritoneum is then identified at the point of attachment of the colon and an incision is made along this line. A dense ligament will be found near the hepatic flexure that binds the colon to the parietes or the lower portion of the right lobe of the liver; this ligament contains blood vessels that must be clamped and tied. If the tumor involves peritoneum or muscle, a wide resection of peritoneum or abdominal wall is required as well. When these attachments have been cut the colon is gradually turned forward (Fig. 6.1b). The duodenum is readily identified. A rather troublesome vein often runs just anterior to the duodenum and must be ligated. The whole mesentery may then be elevated. This maneuver reveals the right spermatic or ovarian vein, which is often divided at the time that the cecum is elevated from the lateral abdominal wall. Further dissection demonstrates the ureter. The ureter runs immediately beneath the peritoneum at the level of the bifurcation of the iliac arteries; hence with a large tumor of the cecum it is in danger unless it is guarded very carefully.

After the colon has been turned forward, Allen clamps are applied to the ileum and to the transverse colon at the projected site of division. A deep V of mesentery is removed (Fig. 6.1c). The ileocolic vessels are ligated with two sturdy ties of catgut about 1 cm from their origin. The right

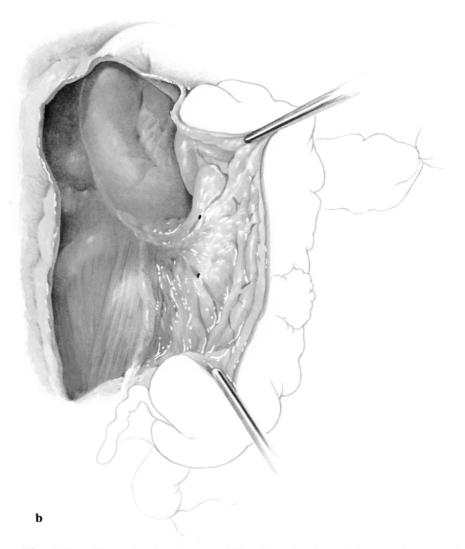

b

Fig. 6.1b.   The colon has been mobilized by division of the attachments along the lateral white line and is turned forward. The duodenum is exposed widely, and as the dissection is carried deeper on the mesentery the ureter is exposed. The spermatic or ovarian vein will cross behind the mesentery at a low level and will be divided.

colic artery is often missing or may arise from either the midcolic or ileocolic artery. If present, it is ligated separately. Either the right branch of the midcolic or all the midcolic vessels are then ligated in turn. The bowel is then divided with the actual cautery and the specimen is removed. It should be examined by the pathologist to confirm the original diagnosis. When cancer of the colon is accompanied by numerous polyps, a subtotal colectomy should be considered at this time.

The bowel is then prepared for anastomosis. It is advisable to close the large rent in the mesentery first. This step is begun near the point of ligation of the ileocolic vessels; the mesenteries of the transverse colon and the terminal ileum are then united by a continuous catgut suture. This is done before the anastomosis for two reasons. First, if a vessel is caught with this suture or if there is an undue amount of bleeding, it may be necessary to remove a further section of terminal ileum in order to secure adequate circulation for the anastomosis. Furthermore, with closure of this trap any rotation of terminal ileum is completely avoided.

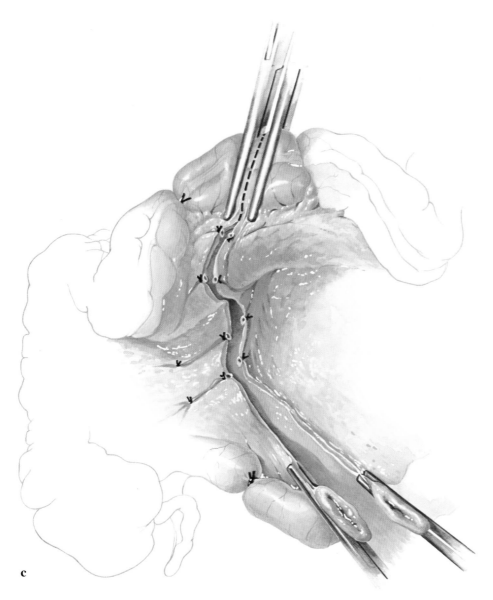

c

Fig. 6.1c. The mesentery is divided. The major vessels—the ileocolic, right colic, and right branch of the midcolic—will be divided just distal to their origins. The ileum has been divided and the transverse colon will be divided along the broken black line.

  If a no-touch technique is to be employed, this is the first stage of the procedure; thereafter the lateral attachments of the colon will be cut and the bowel will be delivered. See Fig. 6.2 for alternative methods of anastomosis.

  The anastomosis is then made, preferably by the end-to-end technique (Fig. 6.2a). If there is a marked discrepancy in the size of the lumina, this is not possible, and either an end-to-side or a side-to-side ileotransverse colostomy is desirable. The end-to-side and the side-to-side anastomoses will be described here. The usual end-to-end technique is described in Chapter 3 in the section on Anastomotic Techniques.

  For an end-to-side anastomosis the proximal end of the transverse colon must be closed with three layers of sutures; the inner two are of 000 absorbable suture and the outer is of 000 silk (Fig. 6.2b). The end-to-side

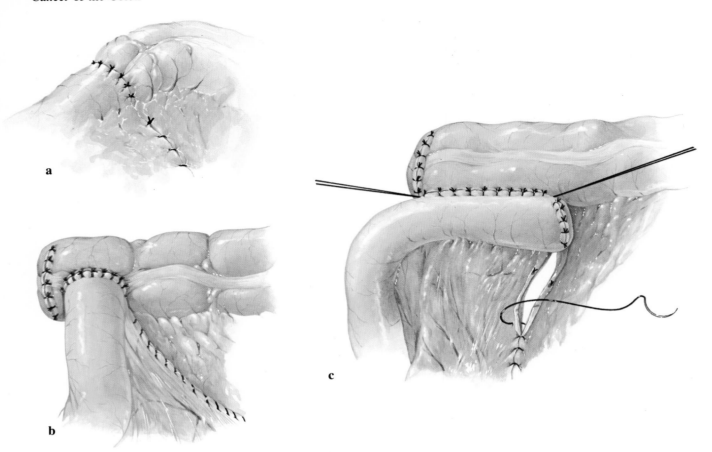

Fig. 6.2a–c. Methods of anastomosis in right colectomy. a. The operation is usually completed by an end-to-end anastomosis. b. Alternative method of anastomosis by end-to-side technique. If the lumen of the ileum is extremely small the end of the colon is inverted with three layers of sutures—the inner two of catgut, the outer of silk. A two-layer end-to-side ileocolic anastomosis is made as shown. All sutures in the ileocolic anastomosis are interrupted. c. Alternative method of anastomosis by side-to-side technique. Both ends of the ileum and colon are turned in and a side-to-side anastomosis is made in two layers with interrupted sutures.

anastomosis is then placed a short distance from this point. The anterior wall of the colon is elevated between Allis clamps and a row of interrupted 000 silk sutures is placed between the terminal ileum and the transverse colon. The clamp on the terminal ileum is then removed and a small plug of gelfoam is placed within the lumen of the ileum. A corresponding opening is then made through the wall of the colon and the lumen of the colon is again protected with gelfoam. The posterior inner row of interrupted 000 absorbable suture is then placed. Similar sutures are placed anteriorly so that the knots are tied within the lumen of the bowel, with the exception of the last one or two, which must be Lembert sutures. The outer anterior layer of interrupted 000 silk is then placed and tied.

For a side-to-side anastomosis a layer of interrupted silk sutures is placed (Fig. 6.2c). The lumen of the two segments is then opened and the posterior inner layer is made with interrupted or continuous absorbable suture. This is continued anteriorly, and finally the anterior outer layer of silk completes the anastomosis. Side-to-side anastomoses may be required in infants. However, distention of the blind end of the upper segment may occur years later and produce a blind loop syndrome; hence this is not a procedure favored by pediatric surgeons.

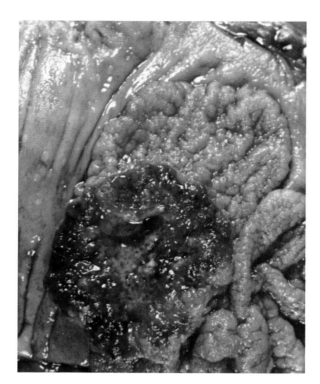

Fig. 6.3. Carcinoma of the colon developing in a villous adenoma.

If the colectomy involves wide removal of the transverse colon and the blood supply is not as adequate as desired in the region of the splenic flexure, it is necessary to mobilize the left colon to a lower level. It is very difficult to anastomose the descending colon and impossible to close the trap between the ileum and descending colon under any circumstances. Consequently, it is much wiser to carry the dissection down to the sigmoid and perform a subtotal colectomy than to be left with an unsatisfactory anastomosis or a wide trap that cannot be closed.

Diseases That Are Confused with Cancer of the Colon

In all sections of the colon, polypoid disease, Crohn's disease, diverticular disease, and some infectious diseases such as amebiosis and tuberculosis can be confused with cancer. In addition, in the right colon, appendiceal disease must be added.

Polypoid Disease

The cecum may be the site of large villous adenomas. In general terms a single, large villous adenoma is removed in the same fashion as a carcinoma of the colon because, although it may be soft and feel benign, evidence of microscopic cancer is frequently found (Fig. 6.3). Therefore, it is desirable to have a wide dissection of the mesenteric lymph nodes. If there are numerous polyps in the right colon, it is almost certain that the patient should have a subtotal colectomy at this time even though previous colonoscopy has shown little polypoid disease in the left colon; otherwise, chances are high that this patient will develop further polyps or cancer at a later date.

Crohn's Disease

There is no essential difference between the operation for this disease and that for cancer, except that there is no need to excise wide areas of mesentery or the mesenteric lymph nodes (see Chapter 11). Therefore, an anastomosis can be made at any appropriate point in the transverse colon. However, the gross appearance of the colon may be confusing; immediate examination by the pathologist is essential to exclude cancer.

Diverticular Disease

Diverticulitis of the right colon is relatively uncommon in the continental United States but is very common in Hawaii. Some of these patients require operations as emergency procedures because of perforation or abscess formation. In such instances the disease may very well be confused with appendicitis or a cancer of the colon with subacute perforation. A right colectomy following the technique described for cancer is employed.

Appendiceal Disease

A right colectomy may be required for certain diseases of the appendix (see Chapter 26). In some instances acute appendicitis may result in a localized perforation or a mass of almost ligneous character that involves the terminal ileum and right colon so widely that it is impossible to be certain that the disease is appendicitis at the time of operation. Under these circumstances it is far better to carry out an immediate right colectomy than to attempt to extricate an appendix from such a field because of the danger of sepsis, obstruction, or fistula formation. Cancer of the appendix, although very rare, also requires a right colectomy.

Mucoceles of the appendix often represent low-grade carcinomas and consideration here should be given to a primary right colectomy as the initial operation. If the appendix is sectioned through an area involved by disease, the possibility of later pseudomyxoma peritonei must be recognized. This disease also can occur primarily and is now believed to represent in many cases a form of cancer of the appendix.

Patients with large carcinoids of the appendix likewise are treated by right colectomy. Carcinoids over 2 cm in diameter, microscopic involvement of the lymphatics, and the line of resection of the tumor lying very close to the tumor itself are all indications for right colectomy.

Drainage

Drainage is seldom necessary after right colectomy, but if an abscess is encountered at the time of operation, drainage is indicated. Drainage also may be necessary if capillary bleeding is not completely controlled at the time of the anastomosis. The patient is maintained on Salem sump gastric suction for 3–5 days after the operation until peristaltic sounds have returned and gas has been passed by the rectum.

Transverse Colectomy

The surgeon has the choice of four procedures for the removal of carcinomas of the transverse colon. Resections must be based upon the exact location of the tumor and the mobility of the transverse colon as well as the age and the build of the patient.

For tumors in the proximal transverse colon we prefer to carry out a standard right colectomy with division of the ileocolic and midcolic vessels at the base (Fig. 6.4). The anastomosis can then be made between the terminal ileum and distal transverse colon, assuming that an adequate blood supply is furnished by the left colic artery. It is possible to close the mesenteric trap very adequately after this resection.

If the tumor is in the midtransverse colon and the patient is old and

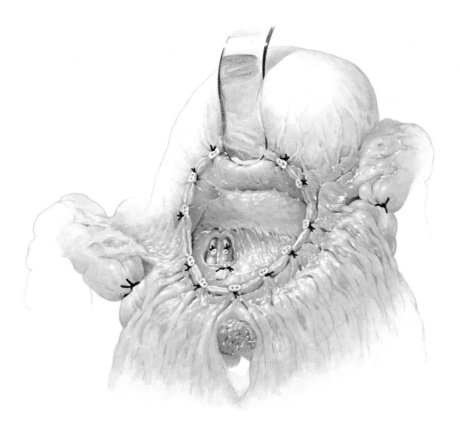

Fig. 6.4. Transverse colectomy. If the tumor is bulky the gastrocolic omentum and contiguous portion of the gastroepiploic vessels and nodes are removed en bloc with the transverse colon. In this picture ties have been placed around the colon proximally and distally. Mobilization of the stomach demonstrates the mid-colic artery and vein, which must be ligated close to their origins from their superior mesenteric vessels. To secure an anastomosis without tension the hepatic and splenic flexures may need to be freed. The resection may be extended by a right or a subtotal colectomy.

the colon is freely movable, a segmental resection may be carried out. The midcolic vessels are ligated near their sources and then the two ends of the transverse colon may be anastomosed across the midline. This operation does involve some hazard because it may be extremely difficult to close the trap behind the bowel, and if the anastomosis of the colon is left unsupported there are the usual dangers of herniation of the small intestine behind the anastomosis. In addition, a segmental resection is not as adequate a cancer operation as the wider resection. Consequently, this procedure is used rarely.

When the tumor is located in the distal portion of the transverse colon, the surgeon again has several options. In an older patient a segmental resection running from the midtransverse to the middescending colon may be feasible. The section of mesentery then removed is essentially that supplied by the left colic artery. A more adequate operation and the one that we recommend if the patient is a good risk is a subtotal colectomy with anastomosis of the ileum to the intraperitoneal rectum. Any anastomosis of the ileum to the descending colon is difficult due to the depth of the colon, the shortness of the mesentery, and the increased difficulty of closing the trap in this area. Technically it is much simpler to carry the dissection of the colon much lower and to perform the standard subtotal colectomy.

The no-touch technique is also applicable for tumors of the transverse colon (see the section on the no-touch technique).

Left Colectomy

A left colectomy provides a wide excision of the mesentery of the descending colon and sigmoid.[3,36,37] Since it involves the removal of the entire inferior mesenteric supply, the left colic artery must be sacrificed and the mesentery is removed from the distal transverse colon down to a point approximately 5 cm above the pelvic floor.

Ties are first placed around the bowel above and below the tumor (Fig. 6.5a). It may also be possible to place ties about the main vessels that run to the area of the tumor. These ties are not placed as low as the inferior mesenteric, but about halfway between it and the colon. This will interrupt most of the blood supply to the tumor-bearing area. Mobilization is then begun by dividing the attachments to the lateral peritoneum, beginning with the attachments at the sigmoid flexure. The left spermatic or ovarian vessels usually require ligation and division. The colon is turned to the right, and as the peritoneum is cut inferiorly the left ureter is identified and retracted. The colon can than be reflected toward the right immediately anterior to the ureter and the aorta (Fig. 6.5b). Any lymph nodes that are present in this area are removed along with the specimen. The inferior mesenteric pedicle is identified and the inferior mesenteric artery and vein are separately divided and ligated.

The distal transverse colon is then mobilized so that the splenic flexure is approached from both above and below. After the flexure is freed, attention is again turned to the lower portion of the dissection, where the sigmoid and intraperitoneal rectum will be mobilized. The peritoneum is incised on the right side and both ureters are again identified. The dissection is carried distally. The mesentery is divided and ligated at the level of the prospective division of the bowel at the lower level. The distal transverse colon (at a spot where blood supply is good and length of colon adequate) and rectum are then clamped with Allen clamps and divided with the cautery. An end-to-end anastomosis then is made.

The most difficult portion of the operation is the management of the large defect that is left after this wide excision. It is rarely possible to effect any closure of the mesenteric trap if the excision has been wide. Furthermore, if a trap such as this cannot be closed adequately, it is better to leave it wide open than to leave a small hole that might be more dangerous due to incarceration of a loop of small bowel. Furthermore, the closure of the trap may kink the jejunum at the ligament of Treitz and produce obstruction if it has been pulled too tightly. For these reasons we believe that the best way to handle this anastomosis is to leave the trap wide open. Usually the colon can be placed posteriorly after the anastomosis so that the small bowel will ride anteriorly.

Complications of the total left colectomy include damage to the ureter and problems with the trap and with anastomotic dehiscence. Careful protection of the ureter obviously is necessary. The problems with the trap have already been discussed. If the trap is left wide open, it is clear that there will not be much support for the anastomosis; consequently there is an increased chance of dehiscence. In order to prevent this it may be possible to buttress the anastomosis by closing a small portion of the rent in the mesentery that is adjacent to the bowel; this will give some additional sup-

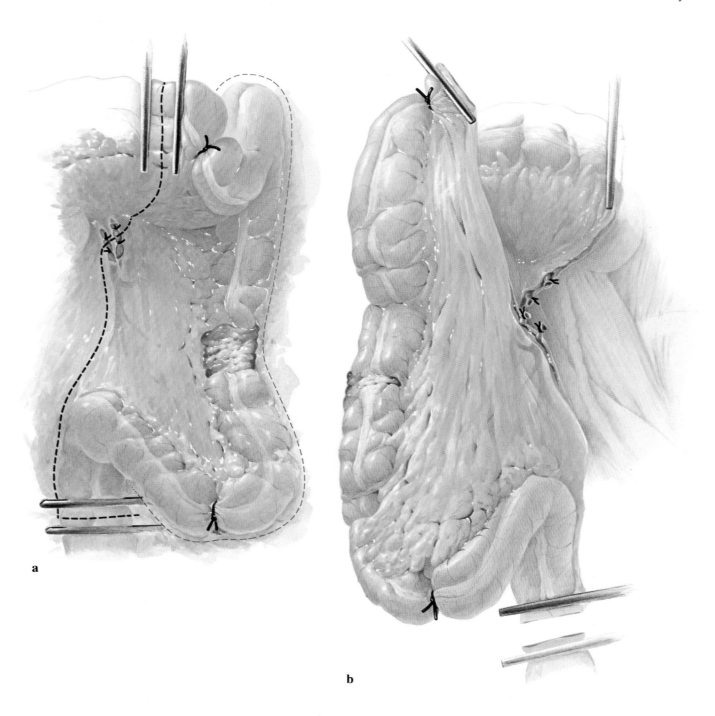

Fig. 6.5a and b. Left colectomy (no-touch technique). a. Clamps are placed on the transverse colon and intraperitoneal rectum and the bowel is divided with the cautery. The mesentery of the transverse colon is divided down to the inferior mesenteric artery and vein. Exposure of the vessels is aided by division of the peritoneum to the right of the peritoneal rectum. The inferior mesenteric artery will be divided close to the origin from the aorta and the inferior mesenteric vein at a slightly higher level. The broken black line indicates the incision line; this is followed by freeing the colon along the broken red line and by mobilization of the splenic flexure. b. As the colon is turned to the right, the lower pole of the left kidney and ureter are exposed.

Continuity will be restored by an end-to-end anastomosis (see Fig. 3.1).

port and may be valuable. It is clear that any tension on an anastomosis that is unsupported by a closed mesenteric trap is likely to cause trouble. Therefore, it is absolutely imperative that an adequate length of transverse colon be obtained during the dissection so that the anastomosis will lie without any tension whatsoever.

One warning should be given. In some patients the mesentery of the transverse colon is unusually short and it is absolutely impossible to draw the transverse colon down for an anastomosis in the pelvis. Hence, occasionally it may be necessary to resect the entire colon and perform an anastomosis of the ileum to the rectum.

Sigmoid Colectomy

Sigmoid colectomy is indicated for patients who have a lesion located in the sigmoid provided that a margin of at least 5 cm can be obtained below the tumor and there are no enlarged lymph nodes at the origin of the inferior mesenteric artery. If these are present, a more extensive operation in-

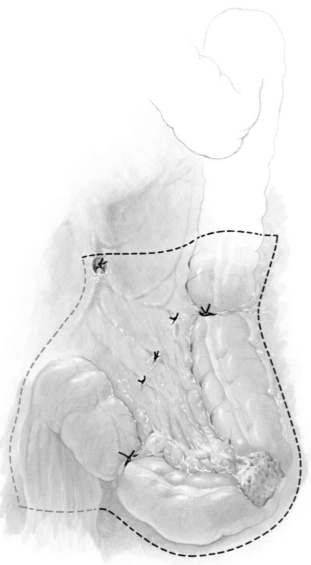

Fig. 6.6. Sigmoid colectomy. Fig. 6.6a. Ties are placed about the colon distal and proximal to the tumor. The line of division of the peritoneum is indicated by the broken black line. The inferior mesenteric vessels will be divided below the left colic branch. Exposure is secured by freeing the sigmoid laterally and turning it to the right. The right side of the mesentery is divided along the broken red lines.

a

cluding a total left colectomy should be considered as the procedure of choice.

In our experience,[50] as well as that of Busuttil et al.,[13] the cure rate following segmental resection is as high as that after total left colectomy. It also is applicable to poor-risk patients. The sigmoid may be removed either by the usual technique (Fig. 6.6) or, if the tumor is small, by the no-touch technique described later in this chapter.

In the usual technique ties are first placed around the colon above and below the tumor. Another suture is placed in the mesentery approximately halfway down to the inferior mesenteric artery in order to obliterate the vessels that directly feed the tumor. The sigmoid colon is then easily mobilized from the left side of the abdomen by dividing the peritoneum and carrying the dissection down in a retroperitoneal fashion. The ureter is identified and retracted. The dissection can be carried to as low a level as required, with a minimum of 5 cm and preferably more below the tumor. The peritoneum on the right side of the sigmoid mesentery is divided. The right ureter is usually far laterally, but it must be observed in case the tumor is bulky. The mesentery is elevated from the aorta and iliac vessels and dissection can be carried to the origin of the inferior mesenteric. At this point it is necessary to be certain that the ureter is not adherent, which it may be in occasional patients. The vessels are usually divided just distal to the left colic branch and ligated en bloc with two strong ties of catgut. If the patient if thin and there is relatively little fat, individual ligation of the inferior mesenteric artery and vein is preferable. A deep V in the mesentery is outlined to be removed together with the tumor. The mesentery is divided up to the sigmoid at the upper end of the dissection and Allen-Kocher clamps are applied. The dissection is carried distally on the pelvic vessels and on the sacrum down to the lower level of the dissection. Here the mesentery of the bowel is divided and ligated. The colon is di-

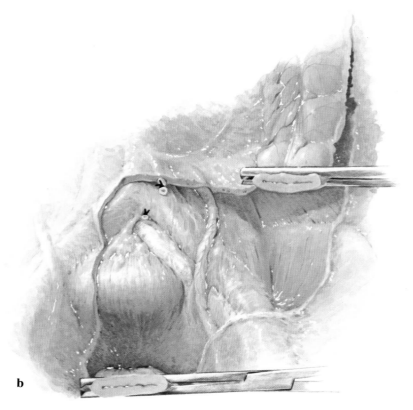

b

Fig. 6.6b. Exposure after excision of the sigmoid. The iliac arteries and veins and the sacrum are exposed. An end-to-end anastomosis is done. Mobilization of the splenic flexure may be required.

59

vided with the cautery between clamps. Good pulsations of the vessels should be present at the upper end of the dissection. Pulsating vessels are impossible to identify at the lower end as a general rule. The mesentery is closed to the peritoneum on the right side but the left side is left open. The details of the end-to-end anastomosis are described in Chapter 3 in the section on Anastomotic Techniques.

Frequently one or both ovaries are included with the resection in the female. The fact that there are ovarian metastases relatively frequently has led to the advocacy of bilateral oophorectomy in females with such cancers as a routine measure.[12.] We have done this frequently, particularly with bulky tumors (Fig. 6.7), but have no conclusive evidence that it improves longevity. Since it is not uncommon for these tumors to be adherent to adjacent organs, a portion of the bladder, small bowel, or ureter may require resection. If the bladder is opened it is usually closed with two layers of catgut and the patient is maintained with Foley catheter drainage. If there has been an exceedingly wide excision a suprapubic cystotomy tube is left in as well. An adjacent loop of small bowel may require resection along with the tumor, in which case continuity is restored by an end-to-end anastomosis. If the ureter is definitely adherent to the tumor, assuming that it is known that the opposite kidney is functioning, it is advisable to remove a section of ureter. The ureter may be tied proximally; in most instances the kidney will atrophy in a painless fashion, but at times a secondary infection may occur in the kidney and require a nephrectomy.

Anomalies of the urinary tract are frequent enough to warrant an intravenous pyelogram prior to the operation if the tumor is large. In unusual cases there may be a single pelvic kidney that will be very suggestive of an extension of the sigmoid tumor and the unsuspecting surgeon might remove the sole functioning kidney.

Approximately 30 cases have been reported in which cancers have developed at the site of a ureterosigmoid anastomosis; such cases require an ileal loop urinary conduit at the time of resection.[23,40]

Subtotal Colectomy

Subtotal colectomy is indicated for many colonic diseases, including carcinoma of the colon[35] (particularly when it is associated with other polypoid lesions), multiple polyposis, Crohn's disease, ulcerative colitis, and massive hemorrhage from the colon from an undetermined source. The operative procedures in all these instances are essentially similar, except for the fact that when one is dealing with definite carcinoma or extensive polypoid disease the resection of the mesentery needs to be wider than it would if the disease were due solely to inflammation.

A generous left paramedian incision is preferred. After general exploration the area of the bowel that is to be removed is identified. Usually the ileum is divided a short distance proximal to the ileocecal valve and the intraperitoneal rectum is divided at some level that is less than 25 cm from the anal verge so that the remaining rectum can later be kept under observation with the sigmoidoscope. If the lesion is a definite carcinoma the usual precautions of placing ties about the proximal and distal bowel are carried out and, if possible, vessels that lead to the tumor are ligated.

Aspiration of the contents of the colon by means of a sucker introduced through the terminal ileum in an area that will later by excised may

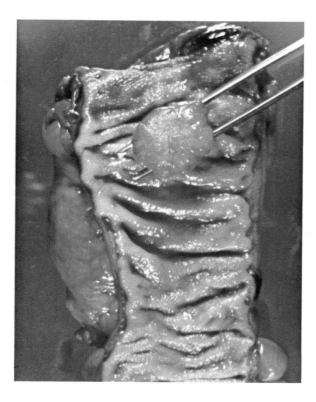

Fig. 6.7. Polypoid carcinoma of the sigmoid.

reduce the frequency of contamination if the procedure is done for an obstructing tumor, ulcerative colitis, or toxic megacolon. This deflation is carried out prior to any mobilization of the bowel.

Dissection usually begins in the transverse colon. If the lesion is malignant the omentum should be removed along with the colon. In the absence of cancer the omentum may be saved and can be employed later to help close the trap that will lie behind the stomach.

After mobilization of the transverse colon the right colon is usually the next easiest area to approach. The right colon is freed by division of the peritoneum at the white line and the colon is turned forward. The suspensory ligaments running from the liver or parietal peritoneum to the colon must be divided and ligated. As the colon is brought forward the spermatic vessels or the right ovarian vessels may be noted in the line of resection and may require division and ligation. If the dissection is carried to a very deep level the right ureter is also observed. The appendix is elevated with the colon as it is freed from the right gutter. The duodenum is identified. It is then possible to accurately divide and ligate the major vessels—the ileocolic, right colic, and midcolic arteries and veins—at a proper location.

Attention is then turned to the left side of the abdomen and dissection is begun in the area of the attachment of the sigmoid flexure. The sigmoid is then mobilized and resected to the right. Again ligation of the spermatic vein or the left ovarian vein may be necessary. The ureter is carefully observed and retracted. The splenic flexure is approached from both the distal transverse colon and the descending colon. This is the most difficult part of the resection; if the lesion is ulcerative colitis perforation is most likely to occur in this location. Division of the colosplenic ligament requires ligation of these vessels, which can be quite troublesome if they are allowed to bleed. After the colon is mobilized it will be possible to identify the left colic and sigmoid vessels individually.

A decision must then be made whether or not to remove the inferior mesenteric pedicle. If it is removed the dissection needs to be carried deeper in the pelvis to be certain that the blood supply from the middle hemorrhoidal vessels will be adequate at the anastomotic line. In many instances it can be left in place and the individual sigmoid vessels can be divided. However, if the lesion is malignant and arises anywhere in the left colon, it is necessary to remove the entire inferior mesenteric pedicle and to carry the dissection in the pelvis down to a point about 5–6 cm above the pouch of Douglas in order to be certain of a good blood supply.

The entire specimen is removed after division of the bowel at appropriate levels with the cautery between Allen clamps. The trap left between the mesentery of the terminal ileum and the intraperitoneal rectum is closed with a running catgut suture. The anastomosis is preferably of the end-to-end type. However, if there is any discrepancy in the size of the two lumina, a side-to-end ileoproctostomy is indicated.

Complications are common after subtotal colectomy. Some important ones are discussed below:

1. Intestinal obstruction: After such an extensive operation there are wide areas that have been deperitonealized, and therefore adhesions are much more common than after other operations. In addition, if the lower end of the lesser omental bursa remains open the bowel may herniate behind the stomach and perhaps from left to right behind the portal triad. Consequently, if omentum has been left in, as can be the case with ulcerative colitis, it can be sutured to the mesentery of the transverse colon to obliterate this potential trap. In some instances a peritonealization of either the right or left gutter can be carried out if it has not been necessary to excise wide areas of peritoneum.

A type of physiologic obstruction appears to exist in patients with these anastomoses. For example, the normal pressure within the small bowel is only about 10 cm H_2O. In the colon, in order to provide evacuation, a pressure of 30 cm H_2O or more is frequent. Consequently, there will be a period of adjustment before it is possible for the patient to have normal bowel movements, and decompression with a gastric sump tube for a period of several days will be necessary. Some surgeons have avoided this complication by inserting a long rectal tube through the anus and upward beyond the anastomosis.[42] We have not employed this method.

2. Anastomotic dehiscence: This anastomosis is more difficult than the usual anastomosis of colon to colon or small bowel to small bowel. There appears to be a tendency for kinking to occur above the anastomosis, leading to partial obstruction, and this may sometimes then be complicated by localized perforation.

In Massachusetts General Hospital the morbidity and mortality of subtotal colectomy for cancer has been distinctly higher than that of segmental resection of the colon. For example, in the latest series, the mortality of subtotal colectomy was 17%, right colectomy 6%, and anterior resection 2%.[50] It is mainly for this reason that the operation is not employed as frequently as has been advocated by some other surgeons. Another problem is that after subtotal colectomy in old patients the shortened bowel may lead to severe and incapacitating diarrhea. This is very difficult to control and may continue for a protracted period of time. If it becomes acute it may be fatal. We therefore are somewhat loath to advocate subtotal colectomy except for the specific indications that are mentioned earlier in this section.

No-Touch Technique

The principle of the no-touch technique is that the mobilization of the tumor-bearing portion of the colon is left until the last portion of the operation and follows the division of the regional vessels, lymphatics, and mesentery. The theory underlying it is that there will be a reduction in the metastases that might occur if the tumor were manipulated vigorously during the operation.

The advantages of this procedure have been emphasized by Turnbull.[44,45] His statistics indicate that it is superior to the usual method of mobilization. However, there are a number of features that render this conclusion somewhat speculative. For example, the larger the tumor the more difficult it is to employ the no-touch technique. Furthermore, Stearns, of Memorial Hospital, New York City, has shown, using standard techniques, that the end results were the same when the first step in the operation involved mobilization of the tumor-bearing segment. The one common feature of the two operations, and probably the most important, was the wide excision of the mesentery.

The no-touch technique is applicable to relatively small tumors of the right, transverse, descending, or sigmoid colon. It is impossible to interrupt all of the blood supply of the intraperitoneal rectum prior to mobilization of cancers in that location, nor is it possible to avoid vigorous manipulation of such tumors as they are being removed.

Right Colon

It is possible to isolate the entire section of bowel and blood supply before any mobilization of the colon from the right gutter is undertaken. This method has the obvious advantage, emphasized by Barnes[5] and later Turnbull,[45] of avoiding operative manipulation of the tumor. On the other hand, the possibilities of damage to the superior mesenteric vessels, duodenum, and ureter are increased, and great care must be taken if this type of dissection is to be used. We have employed it in tumors that are comparatively small and in patients in whom there is no question of the anatomy. However, if the patient is very obese or the dissection is particularly difficult, the accurate control of blood vessels, we believe, is more important than any theoretical considerations concerning the no-touch technique. The details of the technique are as follows:

The tumor is identified in the ascending colon. The terminal ileum is divided between Allen-Kocher clamps with the cautery. The transverse colon is then divided at an optimum point between Allen clamps with the cautery. The dissection is then carried through the posterior peritoneum. Care must be taken in elevating the mesentery of the colon from the posterior structures. The dissection is carried close to the superior mesenteric vein, which must be identified accurately and not damaged. At the lower portion of the dissection it is possible to damage the ureter if the dissection is carried to too deep a level. Furthermore, the duodenum lies in immediate apposition to the mesentery of the colon, so that it must be handled with great care. As the dissection proceeds the ileocolic vessels are identified and divided. The dissection is then carried upward. If there is a right colic vessel it is divided in the same fashion, and finally the right branch of the midcolic artery is divided and ligated.

The gastrocolic omentum is then divided and the colon is separated from the liver, the gallbladder, and the upper portion of the duodenum, to which it may be adherent. Finally, the right colon is elevated from its bed. If necessary, a section of peritoneum can now be excised around the tumor. The specimen is removed and the anastomosis completed.

Cancer of the Transverse Colon

The principles that are followed are exactly the same whether a segmental resection, right colectomy, or subtotal colectomy is to be performed. The essential features of the operation are first the division of the bowel proximal and distal to the tumor at an appropriate site for the anastomosis. The mesentery of the bowel is then exposed. If a subtotal colectomy is to be performed, this is most easily done by first elevating the right colon and then elevating the left colon from its bed. The blood vessels may then be ligated.

The midcolic vessels are located in a relatively difficult position to expose without some manipulation of the transverse colon. If possible, the gastrocolic omentum is divided and the dissection is carried down along the right margin of the lesser omental bursa so that the vessels can be identified at a low level. They are then divided and ligated a short distance above their emergence from the superior mesenteric artery and vein.

Carcinoma of the Sigmoid

Again the principles are almost exactly the same. If a segmental resection is to be performed, the descending colon well above the tumor is divided between Allen clamps with the cautery and the intraperitoneal rectum is divided an adequate distance below the tumor. The upper dissection is then carried out: the mesentery is divided down to the origin of the inferior mesenteric artery. At this stage in the dissection great care must be taken to avoid the left ureter, which may run very close to the mesentery of the sigmoid. The inferior mesenteric vessels are then divided and ligated. Usually this division is made just distal to the left colic branch. The mesentery of the sigmoid colon and intraperitoneal rectum may then be elevated. The peritoneum is divided on the right side, and the right ureter is identified. The peritoneum is then divided on the left side and close to the lower end of the dissection, again with identification of the ureter. The mesentery may then be elevated and divided at the lower end of the dissection. Attention is then finally turned to the freeing of the sigmoid tumor from the lateral peritoneum. The spermatic vessels often require ligation. The colon and mesentery are turned forward, again after identification of the ureter during this portion of the dissection. The entire specimen is removed (Fig. 6.7).

Mikulicz Procedure

The operation now usually known as the Mikulicz procedure was first developed by Bryant[10] and then described almost simultaneously by Paul,[31] Bloch,[9] and Mikulicz[29] in the latter part of the 19th century as a method of treating cancer of the colon that would not involve the dangers of an anastomosis placed within the peritoneal cavity. The procedure consisted of the withdrawal of the loop of colon containing the cancer and the suture of the two limbs of the colon together to form a rather long double tube that would extend several centimeters within the peritoneal cavity (Fig. 6.8). The whole loop was then exteriorized, a clamp was applied, and the bowel was removed. This formed a double colostomy. At a later date a special

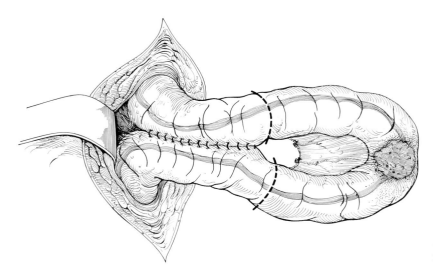

Fig. 6.8. Mikulicz procedure. A redundant sigmoid has been lifted out of the abdomen along with the tumor. The two limbs of colon are sutured together at the base so that the spur can later be crushed with a clamp. The wound will be closed and the colon amputated between clamps at the broken line. This operation is of historical interest only; it is totally inadequate for the removal of a carcinoma of the colon.

clamp could be introduced deeply into each limb and an anastomosis made by tightening of the clamp and consequent pressure necrosis of the adjacent walls of the colon. The remaining fistula was finally closed superficial to the peritoneum. The last variant of this method was Rankin's obstructive resection (1930).[34]

This procedure has now been entirely abandoned and is only of historical interest. There were many problems associated with it. It was not a good cancer operation because the mesentery was not removed as widely as it should be. The procedure itself was complicated, and the exact site of the clamp was never known, since it was applied blindly. Cutting of the spur proved to be dangerous at times because sutures unifying the two colonic limbs to form the spur would open for a distance and a loop of small bowel would become adherent; the clamp could then seize the small bowel and cause its necrosis, as well as necrosis of the walls of the colon. The dangers of intraperitoneal anastomosis have been reduced to a minimum in modern surgery, and after closure of a colonic stoma the colon is now replaced in an intraperitoneal position.

Hartmann Procedure

The Hartmann procedure consists of a resection of the sigmoid and intraperitoneal rectum for cancer and the formation of a proximal colostomy.[24] The important feature of the operation is the retention of the rectal stump, which is left in situ (Fig. 6.9). A similar procedure may be desirable for certain patients with ulcerative colitis or perforated diverticulitis.

This operation originally was employed for cancer in poor-risk patients. At least 5 cm of normal intraperitoneal rectum and the corresponding section of mesentery should be removed beyond the tumor. Unless there are proximal metastases that have blocked the entire lymphatic chain, theoretically there will be no metastases distal to the tumor. This operation, therefore, can be curative in poor-risk patients, but at the price of a permanent colostomy. With the increasing safety of anastomotic procedures, this operation has lost favor.

However, the operation is applicable in cases of perforated diverticulitis in which an anastomosis would be dangerous. The perforated sigmoid can be excised and if the distal bowel is too short to be brought out as a

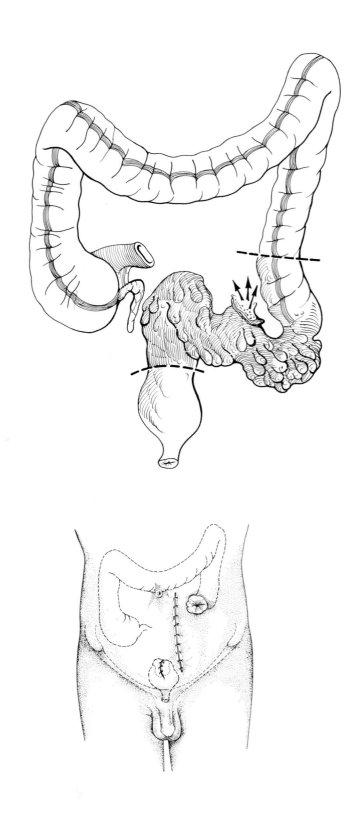

Fig. 6.9. Hartmann procedure (performed for perforated diverticulitis). The sigmoid and intraperitoneal rectum have been resected. The proximal colon is brought out as a colostomy. The distal end is turned in with three layers of sutures and preferably left within the peritoneal cavity.

stoma, it can be turned in by the Hartmann method. A similar situation may occur in some patients with ulcerative colitis or Crohn's disease in whom the rectal stump is left in place.

Despite these advantages the operation does have some drawbacks. For example, if it is used for ulcerative colitis, there may be bleeding from the retained rectal stump. If it is employed for cancer, too narrow a margin of large bowel distal to the tumor may be obtained. However, the most important complication peculiar to this operation is either a low-grade perforation of the stump and the formation of a pelvic abscess, or the formation of a pelvic abscess in the presence of a well-closed stump. Such abscesses are comparatively frequent. Infection about the closed stump may also occur if the peritoneum has been closed over it, and in these instances a retroperitoneal infection follows. Gongaware and Slanetz found, in 100 patients, that postoperative infections developed in 30% of those in whom the stump was left within the peritoneal cavity and 75% of those in whom it was placed below the peritoneum.[22] We are convinced that if the surgeon has the option of placing the stump either above or below the peritoneal floor, it should be placed above the peritoneal floor. If necessary, drains can be led to that area; even if fistulization occurs, it will be of no significance since spontaneous closure can be expected after a period of time since the rectum has been defunctionalized.

Palliative Operations

Palliative operations may be required for cancer of the colon that is judged to be incurable because of distal metastases or extensive local invasion.[41,43]

The most common condition that is found is carcinoma that is locally removable but is incurable because of multiple liver metastases. A palliative resection and anastomosis is of great value in such instances. It may eliminate the local symptoms of bleeding or obstruction and reduces the bulk of tumor that is present within the abdomen. It will allow the use of chemotherapy directed solely to the liver; a different therapeutic technique may be employed than when tumor is also present in other areas in the peritoneal cavity. One of the fluoropyrimidines has been used most often.[16]

Extensive fixation of the tumor may make it necessary to carry out a palliative entero- or colocolostomy around the tumor. This is not as satisfactory as a resection. If the lesion is in the right colon, for example, and the ileocecal valve is functional, a closed loop obstruction may occur between the ileocecal valve and the tumor, and the patient could therefore become quite uncomfortable from cramps. In these days such a palliative side-tracking operation is rarely done.

Classification and Prognosis of Carcinomas of the Colorectum

The prognosis of cancer of the colorectum depends to a major extent upon the depth of involvement by tumor and the spread to lymph nodes or other organs. Many systems of classification have been developed. One of the major problems is that it is impossible to determine the extent of the invasion on clinical examination of the patient prior to the removal of the tumor. Consequently, nearly all systems have been based upon the pathologist's examination of resected specimens, except in instances in which distant metastasis can be confirmed by preoperative examinations.

The earliest and most widely accepted classification is that developed by Dukes.[15] He classified such tumors as type A, B, or C. Group A tumors are localized to the rectum and do not show penetration beyond the serosal coat of the bowel. Group B tumors extend through the bowel wall into the fat. Group C includes those tumors that have invaded the perirectal tissues and spread to regional lymph nodes. This group is divided into two subcategories: in C-1 the nodes are localized close to the tumor; in C-2 they extend up to the line of division of the major artery (Table 6.1).

As Goligher[21] and Rubio et al.[38] emphasized, quite a different classification has been attributed to Dukes by many U.S. authors, e.g., Astler and Coller.[2] For example, A lesions have been defined as those that do not penetrate deep to the muscularis mucosae, B lesions as those that extend through the muscularis mucosae but are confined within the wall of the bowel, and C lesions as those that have progressed to the pericolic tissues and/or metastasized to lymph nodes. The import of such a classification would be that such A lesions would be regarded by most pathologists now as carcinoma in situ rather than as invasive carcinoma; Dukes did not include them in his category A. The B lesions, by the same definitions, would be exactly the same as Dukes' group A tumors.

It is apparent that if the system given by some of the U.S. authors is followed, the postoperative results will be much better than those reported by Dukes. For example, so-called A lesions will be 100% curable and so-called B lesions will have the same cure rate as Dukes' group A tumors.

Obviously, some carcinomas will not have grown through the wall of the colon but will have metastasized to regional lymph nodes. In either system these lesions should be placed in category C.

Because the variations in grading have added an element of confusion in the past, many institutions have merely described the tumors and not attempted to place them in different categories. The American Joint Committee for Cancer Staging and End Results, however, has recommended a new classification for carcinoma of the colon that is based upon the TMN classification.[7,28] T refers to the primary tumor, N to the regional lymph node involvement, and M to the distal metastases. The classification necessarily must be made retrospectively since it is impossible in many instances to classify the tumor accurately otherwise.

The carcinomas are also divided into five stages. Stage 0 represents carcinoma in situ. In stage IV, the most malignant, there is evidence of distal metastasis. In stage I the tumor is confined to the wall of the bowel with no metastasis, in stage II it extends beyond the bowel wall with no metastasis, and in stage III there is evidence of regional lymph node but no distal metastasis.

The comparison of statistics on therapy of cancer of the colorectum from different institutions is made difficult by many other factors. One of the major ones is that some reports are based on crude death rates, e.g., the Massachusetts General Hospital series, whereas others are based on adjusted death rates. In the latter case death due to other diseases would be excluded from the statistics and the cure rates would be correspondingly elevated. For example, if in a specific age group 25% would be expected to die in 5 years from all causes, an adjusted death rate would show significantly more cures than the crude death rate.

The sex and age of the patients at the time of admission to the hospital

TABLE 6.1. Systems of Classification of Polyps and Cancer

		MGH	Dukes'	Other	Joint Commission on Staging
1		a. Adenoma (simple tubular) b. Adenoma, villoglandular c. Adenoma, villous	a. Same b. Adenoma, papillary c. Same	Same	0
2		Adenoma	Adenoma	Carcinoma in situ A	0
3		a. Cancer arising in adenoma b. Polypoid cancer c. Infiltrating cancer (no metastasis)	A	B	I
4		Cancer invading mesentery (no metastasis)	B	C_1	II
5		a. Cancer arising in adenoma; epi- or paracolic lymph node metastasis b. Cancer, epi- or paracolic lymph node metastasis	C_1	C_1	III
6		a. + b. Cancer; distal lymph node metastasis	C_2	C_2	III

are also important.[1,47] Whereas some clinics show an average admission age of 62, the corresponding figure in the Massachusetts General Hospital series was 69; the crude death rate could be expected to be considerably higher in the Massachusetts General Hospital series because more deaths from other causes occur within 5 years from age 69 than from age 62.[4] The latest figures available from the Department of Health, Education and Welfare (personal communication from A.J. Asire, Statistician, End Results Section, Biometry Branch, April 7, 1978) indicate that in white males the survival probability 5 years later for those age 62 is 0.87, and for those age 69 it is 0.75; for white females the corresponding figures are 0.94 and 0.85.

Other factors that contribute to the prognosis include the presence or absence of acute obstruction or of perforation.[48,49] The overall survival figures will be smaller in institutions that have many patients admitted with such emergency problems. It may be concluded that the best statistics will be reported by clinics that treat cancer at a relatively early age and have few emergencies and a high number of females. Veterans hospitals, in which at present the average age of patients with cancer of the rectum is 69, will have poorer survival figures.

The crude 5-year survival rate of patients with cancer of the colorectum in the Massachusetts General Hospital is 54% after resection for cure; when adjusted for age it approaches 70%.[14,50]

Buckwalter and Kent have studied various factors that predict the likelihood of survival.[11] Their conclusions are as follows:

1. Tumor size: There is no definite correlation between the size of the tumor and survival rate.
2. Extent of penetration. This is a most important factor.
3. Annular lesions: These lesions seem to be more serious than others.
4. Obstruction: Most series of figures show poorer prognosis with this complication, though our figures provide more optimism.[48]
5. Proximal and distal margins. The evidence is conflicting. We believe that a margin of 5 cm should be the minimal margin of distal resection for tumors of the rectum and rectosigmoid if cure is to be expected. The level of peritoneal reflection is not important in the ultimate prognosis.[27]
6. Metastasis to lymph nodes: This is a very important factor.[19,20]
7. Number of metastases to lymph nodes: If more than five are involved, 5-year survival is less than 10%.
8. Location of involved lymph nodes: Following Dukes' classification, figures indicate a 5-year survival rate of 53% in patients with C_1 lesions and 22% in those with C_2. Patients with retrograde metastases have a uniformly fatal prognosis.
9. Venous invasion: This is questionable as a prognostic sign. This important conclusion is confirmed by recent studies by Khankhanian et al.[26]
10. Perineural invasion: This finding indicates a poor prognosis.
11. Tumor configuration: Polypoid tumors tend to grow slowly and metastasize late in comparison to those that are sessile or ulcerating.
12. Grading: Poorly differentiated tumors have a much poorer prognosis.
13. Margins: Tumors with sharp demarcation appear to have a much better prognosis.
14. Inflammatory infiltrate about the tumor: This finding indicates better host resistance.

The Massachusetts General Hospital figures for 1937–1970, covering delay from onset of symptoms to treatment, rate of resectability, and operative mortality, are given in Figure 6.10.[50]

References

1. Andersson Å., Bergdahl L. (1976) Carcinoma of the colon in children: A report of six new cases and a review of the literature. J Pediatr Surg 11: 967

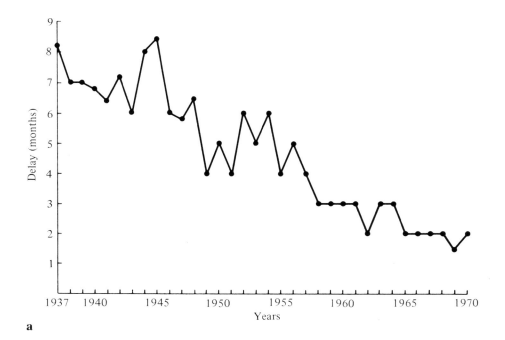

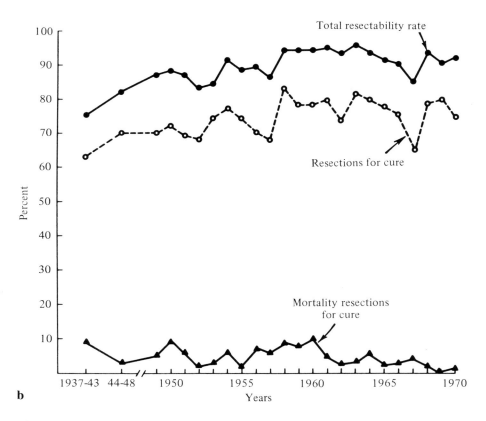

Fig. 6.10a and b. Massachusetts General Hospital statistics on surgery for cancer of the colon, 1937–1970. a. Delay from onset of symptoms to treatment. b. Resectability rate and operative mortality. (From Welch and Donaldson.[50])

2. Astler V.B., Coller F.A. (1954) The prognostic significance of direct extension of carcinoma of the colon and rectum. Ann Surg 139: 846
3. Ault G.W. (1974) A technique of cancer isolation and extended dissection for cancer of the distal colon and rectum. In: Maingot R. (ed) Abdominal operations, 6th edn, Vol 2. Appleton-Century-Crofts, New York, p 2010

4. Axtell L.M. (1963) Computing survival rates for chronic disease patients. JAMA 186: 1125
5. Barnes J.P. (1952) Physiologic resection of right colon. Surg Gynecol Obstet 94: 722
6. Beahrs O.H., Wilson S.M. (1975) Cancer of the colon and rectum: A review of the newer technics in diagnosis and treatment. Adv Surg 9: 235
7. Beart R.W. Jr., Van Heerden J.A., Beahrs O.H. (1978) Evolution in the pathologic staging of carcinoma of the colon. Surg Gynecol Obstet 146: 257
8. Berge T., Ekelund G., Mellner C., et al (1973) Carcinoma of the colon and rectum in a defined population. An epidemiological, clinical and postmortem investigation of colorectal carcinoma and coexisting benign polyps in Malmö, Sweden. Acta Chir Scand 1: [Suppl] 86
9. Bloch O. (1892) Om extra-abdominal behandling af cancer intestinalis (rectum derfra undtaget). Nord Med Ark 2 (1): 1, 2(8): 1
10. Bryant T. (1883) A successful case of lumbar colectomy. Med Chir Trans 65: 131
11. Buckwalter J.A. Jr., Kent T.H. (1973) Prognosis and surgical pathology of carcinoma of the colon. Surg Gynecol Obstet 136: 465
12. Burt C.A.V. (1960) Carcinoma of the ovaries secondary to cancer of the colon and rectum. Dis Colon Rectum 3: 352
13. Busuttil R.W., Foglia R.P., Longmire W.P. Jr. (1977) Treatment of carcinoma of the sigmoid colon and upper rectum. A comparison of local segmental resection and left hemicolectomy. Arch Surg 112: 920
14. Donaldson G.A., Welch J.P. (1974) Management of cancer of the colon. Surg Clin North Am 54: 713
15. Dukes C.E. (1932) The classification of cancer of the rectum. J Pathol Bacteriol 35: 323
16. Duschinsky R., Pleven E., Heidelberger C. (1957) The synthesis of 5-fluoropyrimidines. J Am Chem Soc 79: 4559
17. Egdahl R.H., Mannick J.A., Williams L.F. Jr. (1972) Core textbook of surgery. Grune & Stratton, New York, p 113
18. First National Conference on Cancer of the Colon and Rectum. Cancer 28: 1 (1971)
19. Gabriel W.B., Dukes C., Bussey H.J.R., et al (1935) Lymphatic spread in cancer of the rectum. Br J Surg 23: 395
20. Gilchrist R.K., David V.C. (1938) Lymphatic spread of carcinoma of the rectum. Ann Surg 108: 621
21. Goligher J.C. (1976) The Dukes' A, B and C categorization of the extent of spread of carcinomas of the rectum. Surg Gynecol Obstet 143: 793
22. Gongaware R.D., Slanetz C.A. Jr. (1973) Hartmann procedure for carcinoma of the sigmoid and rectum. Ann Surg 178: 28
23. Haney M.J., McGarity W.C. (1971) Ureterosigmoidostomy and neoplasms of the colon: Report of a case and review of the literature. Arch Surg 103: 69
24. Hartmann H. (1931) Chirurgie du rectum. Masson et Cie, Paris
25. Jackman R.J., Beahrs O.H. (1968) Tumors of the large bowel. Saunders, Philadelphia
26. Khankhanian N., Mavligit G.M., Russell W.O., et al (1977) Prognostic significance of vascular invasion in colorectal cancer of Dukes' B class. Cancer 39: 1195
27. Kirklin J.W., Dockerty M.B., Waugh J.M. (1949) The role of the peritoneal reflection in the prognosis of carcinoma of the rectum and sigmoid colon. Surg Gynecol Obstet 88: 326
28. Manual for staging of cancer 1978. American Joint Committee for Cancer Staging and End-Results Reporting, Chicago
29. Mikulicz J. (1903) Chirurgische erfahrungen über das darmcarcinom. Arch Klin Chir 69: 28
30. Mzabi R., Himal H.S., Demers R., et al (1976) A multiparametric computer analysis of carcinoma of the colon. Surg Gynecol Obstet 143: 959
31. Paul F.T. (1895) Colectomy. Liverpool Med Chir J 15: 374

32. Polk H.C. Jr., Ahmad W., Knutson C. (1973) Carcinoma of the colon and rectum. Curr Probl Surg (Jan) 10: 1

33. Proceedings of the 1977 Workshop on Large Bowel Cancer. National Large Bowel Cancer Project. Cancer 40 [Suppl]: 2405 (1977)

34. Rankin F.W. (1930) Resection and obstruction of the colon (obstructive resection). Surg Gynecol Obstet 50: 591

35. Ripstein C.B. (1967) Radical colectomy for carcinoma of the colon. Dis Colon Rectum 10: 40

36. Rosi P.A. (1969) Selection of operations for carcinomas of the colon. In: Turell R. (ed) Diseases of the colon and rectum, 2nd edn, Vol 1. Saunders, Philadelphia, p 478

37. Rosi P.A., Cahill W.J., Carey J. (1962) A ten year study of hemicolectomy in the treatment of carcinoma of the left half of the colon. Surg Gynecol Obstet 114: 15

38. Rubio C.A., Emås S., Nylander G. (1977) A critical reappraisal of Dukes' classification. Surg Gynecol Obstet 145: 682

39. Snyder D.N., Heston J.F., Meigs J.W., et al (1977) Changes in site distribution of colorectal carcinoma in Connecticut, 1940–1973. Am J Dig Dis 22: 791

40. Sooriyaarachchi G.S., Johnson R.O., Carbone P.P. (1977) Neoplasms of the large bowel following ureterosigmoidostomy. Arch Surg 112: 1174

41. Stein J.J. (1974) Comments on carcinoma of the colon and rectum. Cancer 34: 799

42. Stewart W.R.C., Samson R.B. (1968) Rectal tube decompression of left-colon anastomosis. Dis Colon Rectum 11: 452

43. Takaki H.S., Ujiki G.T., Shields T.S. (1977) Palliative resections in the treatment of primary colorectal cancer. Am J Surg 133: 548

44. Turnbull R.B. Jr. (1970) Cancer of the colon: The five- and ten-year survival rates following resection utilizing the isolation technique. Ann R Coll Surg Engl 46: 243

45. Turnbull R.B. Jr. (1975) The no-touch isolation technique of resection. JAMA 231: 1181

46. Wallack M.K., Brown A.S., Rosato E.F. (1976) The treatment of cancer of the large intestine. Surg Gynecol Obstet 142: 97

47. Walton W.W. Jr., Hagihara P.F., Griffen W.O. Jr. (1976) Colorectal adenocarcinoma in patients less then 40 years old. Dis Colon Rectum 19: 529

48. Welch J.P., Donaldson G.A. (1974) Management of severe obstruction of the large bowel due to malignant disease. Am J Surg 127: 492

49. Welch J.P., Donaldson G.A. (1974) Perforative carcinoma of the colon and rectum. Ann Surg 180: 734

50. Welch J.P., Donaldson G.A. (1974) Recent experience in the management of cancer of the colon and rectum. Am J Surg 127: 258

51. Welch J.P., Donaldson G.A., Welch C.E. (1976) Carcinoma of the colon and rectum. Curr Probl Cancer (July) 1: 1

52. Welch J.P., Welch C.E. (to be published) Carcinoma of the colon. In: Maingot R. (ed) Abdominal operations, 7th edn. Appleton-Century-Crofts, New York

53. Wilson S.M., Beahrs O.H. (1976) The curative treatment of carcinoma of the sigmoid, rectosigmoid, and rectum. Ann Surg 183: 556

7 Polypoid Lesions of the Rectum

Polypoid lesions that occur within the limits of observation of a 25-cm sigmoidoscope include adenomatous (tubular) polyps, villoglandular polyps, villous adenomas, polypoid carcinomas, and a variety of other small polypoid lesions such as hyperplastic polyps, inflammatory polyps, sessile mamillations, and mucosal excrescences. The very small lesions of less than 0.5 cm are essentially of no practical importance, but the larger polypoid lesions pose very important and difficult problems in many instances. In general, all polypoid lesions are removed. One exception is the inflammatory polyp, which may be an early sign of ulcerative colitis and will recur after excision. Gilbertsen and Nelms' data indicate that polypectomy will help to prevent cancer of the rectum.[4] The risk of the recurrence of polyps has been studied by Henry et al.[5]

The surgeon has a choice of many methods for the removal of polyps. Lesions less than 1 cm in diameter can be removed with biopsy forceps or a curette, and the base can be treated with the electrodesiccating unit. These small lesions will not be considered further. Various methods for the removal of larger polyps will be described in this chapter. The choice of method must be based upon the location, histologic type, and size of the polyp, as well as general considerations such as the patient's age and other diseases.

Excision Through the Dilated Anal Canal

Under satisfactory general or regional anesthesia, the patient is placed in the lithotomy position and the anal canal is dilated widely. Retractors are then introduced (Fig. 7.1). If the mucosa is somewhat redundant, polypoid lesions as high as 8–10 cm may be intussuscepted down close to the anus and removed from this position. The polyp is grasped with Allis forceps above and below, and mucous membrane above and below is grasped in a similar fashion. A 0 chromic suture is then placed above the lesion and one is placed below it. They serve as guy ligatures to maintain traction as the tumor is removed. An incision is then made through the mucous membrane in such a fashion as to surround all of the polyp. The incision is begun from

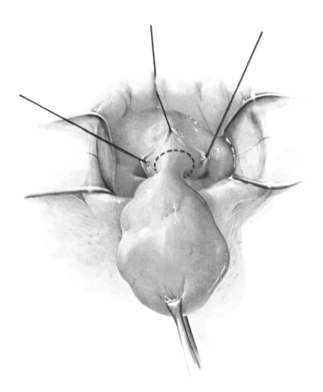

Fig. 7.1. Exposure and excision of polypoid lesion of the rectum through the dilated anus. Guy ligatures are placed at each quadrant and the lesion is excised along the broken line. Interrupted catgut sutures are placed after each cut to avoid hemorrhage.

above and additional interrupted 0 chromic catgut sutures are placed as soon as a cut is made. Submucous infiltration of normal saline will show whether or not the mucosa is attached to underlying muscle. If it is attached, the lesion probably is cancer and the incision must extend through the rectal wall. Usually when the lesion is soft and apparently benign, the dissection only extends down to the muscle. The entire polypoid lesion is removed by means of this cut–suture technique. If hemostasis is not complete, a second continuous suture may be used to reinforce the interrupted sutures. The wound should be entirely dry at the conclusion because continuing bleeding may form a large hematoma that will dissect between the mucosa and muscularis.

The pathologist's examination can be based on a fixed specimen, since diagnosis by frozen section of cancer in polyps is difficult. If the polyp is found to be entirely benign, no further procedures are carried out. If the lesion is shown to be cancer with definite invasion below the submucosa and into the muscle, we believe that the lesion should be treated as an invasive cancer and some type of radical resection should be performed (see Chapter 5). This decision may be modified on other bases, e.g., the age of the patient, histologic type of the cancer, and location of the tumor (i.e., whether or not a permanent colostomy would be necessary).

If the polypoid lesion was low in the rectum and the final specimen shows carcinoma confined to the tip of the polyp with invasion through the muscularis mucosae but minimal involvement of the stroma, an adequate local excision such as that described above is recommended. There is some possibility of metastasis, but this must be weighed against the additional mortality and morbidity and the quality of life that would follow a combined abdominoperineal resection in this location. After local excision the base of the polyp can be examined very easily either by palpation or through the sigmoidoscope and recurrence in that area could be detected; a further operation could be carried out at a later date if necessary.

Excision Through Divided Anal Sphincters

This operation is similar to the one described above except that a better exposure is obtained by division of the sphincters. It has recently been revived and recommended enthusiastically by Mason.[6] The patient is placed in the lithotomy position and the sphincters are divided in the midline pos-

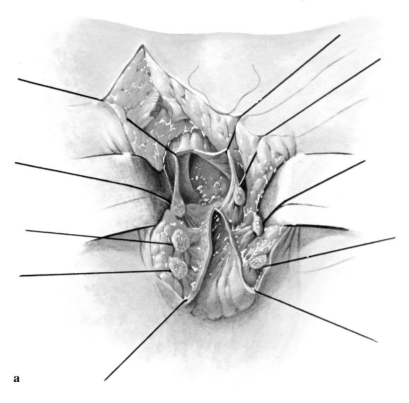

Fig. 7.2a–c. Excision of rectal lesion after division of sphincters (Mason technique). Mason advises a temporary protective colostomy for all but small cancers. The patient lies prone on the table in the jackknife position. The incision is carried upward to the side of the coccyx. a. Exposure after dilatation of anal canal and posterior division of sphincters. Note that all muscle bundles of the external and internal sphincters have been carefully marked. b. The polypoid tumor is now clearly visible. c. Method of excision using four guy ligatures. After full-thickness excision of the entire rectal wall, the defect is closed and the incision is sutured carefully, uniting the muscle bundles accurately.

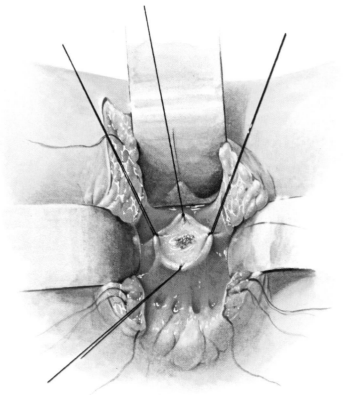

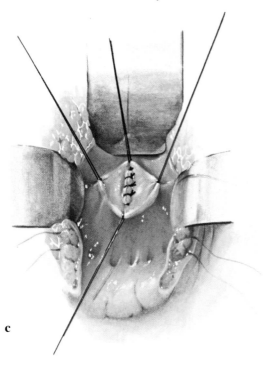

76

teriorly (Fig. 7.2a). Wide retraction is then obtained and the lesion can be excised under essentially direct vision (Figs. 7.2b and c). Caution should be exercised, however, because if the lesion extends to a high level, for example, above the peritoneal floor, it may be impossible to secure adequate mobilization that dehiscence of the line of closure may lead to extensive sepsis. Mason has recommended this procedure for cancers as well as polyps; we are not enthusiastic about its use for cancer.

After the lesion has been removed the sphincters are reconstituted by absorbable sutures and the skin is closed. The introduction of a drain may invite the formation of a fistula. It is essential that antibiotic coverage be provided with this operation because sepsis can be a dangerous complication.

Posterior Proctotomy

An incision is made lateral to the anus and to the coccyx. The coccyx may be removed to provide better observation. The rectum is identified after division of the levators (Fig. 7.3a). The bowel is opened, the polyp is excised, and the continuity of the bowel is restored by two layers of sutures (Fig. 7.3b).

Although this may be a comparatively simple operation in some instances, it introduces definite hazards. It is difficult to mobilize the rectum from this exposure, and the exact location of the tumor may be hard to identify before the bowel is opened. Infection in the retrorectal space or in the peritoneal cavity can be a serious problem.

Although some surgeons have advocated this method, we have not used it and prefer one of the following methods.[1,8]

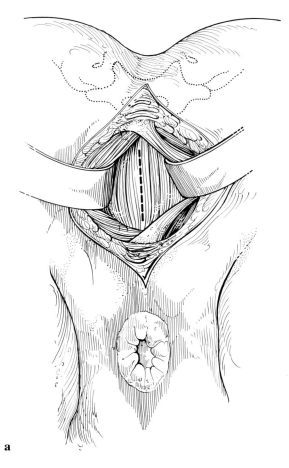

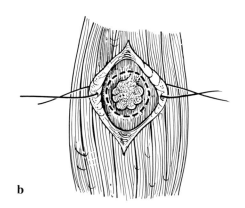

Fig. 7.3a and b. Posterior proctotomy. a. The rectum is through a posterior incision. The levators are retracted and the posterior wall of the rectum is opened along the broken line. b. An anterior wall tumor is exposed. After excision, the mucous membrane will be closed and the posterior incision will be closed in layers with drainage.

77

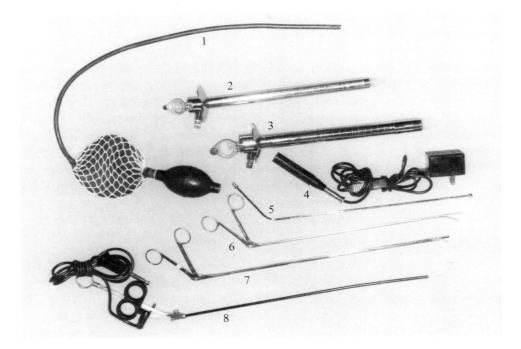

Fig. 7.4. Equipment for removal of polypoid lesions through the sigmoidoscope. The instruments from above downward are (1) inflator, (2) and (3) Welch-Allyn fiberoptic sigmoidoscopes, (4) lighting source, (5), (6), and (7) biopsy forceps, and (8) snare.

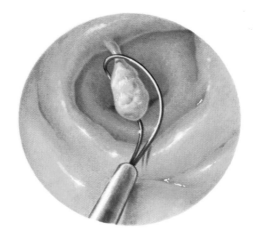

Fig. 7.5. Snaring of rectal polyp through the sigmoidoscope.

Excision Through the Sigmoidoscope with the Snare

This is the favorite method for lesions that are pedunculated or for small sessile polyps (also see Chapter 5). The snare is passed through a large-bore sigmoidoscope (Fig. 7.4); after the polyp has been snared (Fig. 7.5), the pedicle is coagulated with alternating bursts of cutting and coagulating current. Preferably the snare is used to obtain as long a section of the pedicle as possible. Sessile polyps require multiple biopsies and piecemeal removal. Large pedunculated polyps in which the pedicle cannot be visualized may have to be removed partially or wholly in the same fashion. Electrocoagulation of large villous adenomas is not likely to be successful because they tend to recur.

The most common complication after polypectomy is bleeding. It usually can be controlled by further electrocoagulation, adrenalin pledgets, or silver nitrate cauterization.

Perforation is not likely to be a problem when the lesion is below the peritoneal reflection. However, above that level great care must be taken to avoid this catastrophe. Perforations can occur not only into the peritoneal cavity, but also into the bladder in the male or the vagina in the female. Any intraperitoneal perforation requires immediate laparotomy with closure of the perforation. Whether or not complementary colostomy will be required depends upon the extent of the contamination.

Other Procedures

Anterior Resection
Low anterior resection and anastomosis is an excellent operation for the large villous adenomas that occur frequently near the level of the peritoneal floor. By this method an adequate mobilization of the bowel can be obtained and anastomosis at a low level is possible (see Chapter 9).[3]

D'Allaines Procedure
This also is an excellent procedure for villous adenomas of the rectum that are extensive and extend to a low level (see Chapter 9).[2]

Combined Abdominoperineal Resection
Combined abdominoperineal resection by the Miles technique has been employed for some of the very large villous adenomas in which the differential diagnosis of adenoma versus cancer is difficult to determine (see Chapter 8).[7]

Soave Procedure
The Soave procedure (see Chapter 9)[10] has been employed by the senior author in one very extensive lesion extending down to the anal verge in a male 51 years of age. Although this procedure has not been used frequently in adults, in this instance it turned out to be very satisfactory. Three years after the operation the patient was entirely continent of feces. While there were some unexpected expulsions of gas, he was able to prevent this by voluntary control for protracted periods if necessary. No protection of the anal area was necessary and no soiling occurred after 1 year.

Whitehead Operation
A very low villous adenoma of the rectum extending to the anal verge and upward for only a short distance may be treated by the Whitehead operation for hemorrhoids.[12] The mucosa is elevated and dissected upward for approximately 4 cm from the anal verge. Further undermining of the mucosa may take place at a higher level and then the mucosa is sutured to the anal verge with interrupted 00 catgut sutures in two layers. Postoperatively frequent dilatations must be carried out to prevent contracture.

Additional Procedures
Other methods that have been described involve the removal of the villous adenoma by a series of operative procedures removing approximately one-

third of the circumference of the lesion at each operation; Parks and Stuart have used this method.[9] Some surgeons have left the rectal wall denuded of mucosa and expect normal mucosa to grow back over it; Mason has documented this remarkable regeneration. Others have attempted removal by electrodesiccation; this may be a valuable procedure for a small lesion, but for very large ones recurrence is almost certain to be the rule.

In a series of 258 villous adenomas treated in the Massachusetts General Hospital and described by the authors, combined abdominoperineal resections were carried out in 32 instances; invasive cancer was present in 22.[11] The sacrifice of anal sphincters in 10 patients with benign disease can be criticized; on the other hand, many of these lesions were large and in a position that would have been difficult to handle in any other fashion. There were no deaths that could be ascribed to the operation when it was done for benign adenoma.

References

1. Crowley R.T., Davis D.A. (1951) Procedure for total biopsy of doubtful polypoid growths of lowest large bowel segment. Surg Gynecol Obstet 93: 23
2. D'Allaines F. (1946) Traitement Chirurgical du cancer du rectum. Éditions Médicales Flammarion, Paris
3. Dixon C.F. (1939) Surgical removal of lesions occurring in the sigmoid and rectosigmoid. Am J Surg 46: 12
4. Gilbertsen V.A., Nelms J.M. (1978) The prevention of invasive cancer of the rectum. Cancer 41: 1137
5. Henry L.G., Condon R.E., Schulte W.J., et al (1975) Risk of recurrence of colon polyps. Ann Surg 182: 511
6. Mason A.Y. (1977) Transsphincteric surgery for lower rectal cancer. In: Malt R.A. (ed) Surgical techniques illustrated, Vol 2, No 2. Little, Brown, Boston, p 71
7. Miles W.E. (1908) A method of performing abdomino-perineal excision for carcinoma of the rectum and of the terminal portion of the pelvic colon. Lancet 2: 1812
8. O'Brien P.H. (1976) Kraske's posterior approach to the rectum. Surg Gynecol Obstet 142: 412
9. Parks A.G., Stuart A.E. (1973) The management of villous tumors of the large bowel. Br J Surg 60: 688
10. Soave F. (1964) Hirschsprung's disease: New surgical technique. Arch Dis Child 39: 116
11. Welch J.P., Welch C.E. (1976) Villous adenomas of the colorectum. Am J Surg 131: 185
12. Whitehead W. (1882) The surgical treatment of hemorrhoids. Br Med J 1: 148

Cancer of the Rectum and Anus

8

Combined Abdominoperineal Resection

Combined abdominoperineal resection is the standard operation for a cancer of the rectum that is palpable by rectal examination or, if the lesion is deemed to be curable, for a cancer located so near the peritoneal floor that a margin of 5 cm cannot be obtained below it. [7, 13, 15, 18, 21, 24] It also has been used for extremely large villous adenomas, even if they are benign, and as a portion of the operation of total proctocolectomy for ulcerative colitis or familial polyposis. The classification and prognosis of rectal cancer has been discussed in Chapter 6.[1,8,9]

Procedure

The abdomen is opened through a left paramedian incision. The preliminary examination is designed to see whether or not the carcinoma is palpable above the pelvic floor and to assess the possibility of its removal. The remainder of the colon is palpated carefully to discover other lesions. The liver and the gallbladder are examined for metastasis or for any concomitant gallstones. Every attempt is made to remove the local lesion whenever possible, even in the presence of liver metastases because the patient will be saved the problems of severe tenesmus and hemorrhage, which occur if the tumor remains in place. A palliative transverse colostomy may have to be employed if there are widespread peritoneal metastases. A transverse colostomy in the absence of obstruction, however, may make a patient more miserable and is not recommended.

Assuming that the lesion is operable, the sigmoid and intraperitoneal rectum are mobilized first along the left gutter (Fig. 8.1). It is desirable to retain enough peritoneum to effect a later closure of the peritoneal floor. The pelvic peritoneum is divided and reflected laterally. The left ureter is identified and retracted along with the peritoneum to which it is adherent. Dissection is carried down laterally to the base of the pelvis. By blunt dissection the fingers may be placed behind the intraperitoneal rectum and its mesentery, freeing it from the iliac vessels. The peritoneum on the right side of the mesosigmoid is then divided and the incision is carried upward to an area near the origin of the inferior mesenteric artery (Fig. 8.2). The

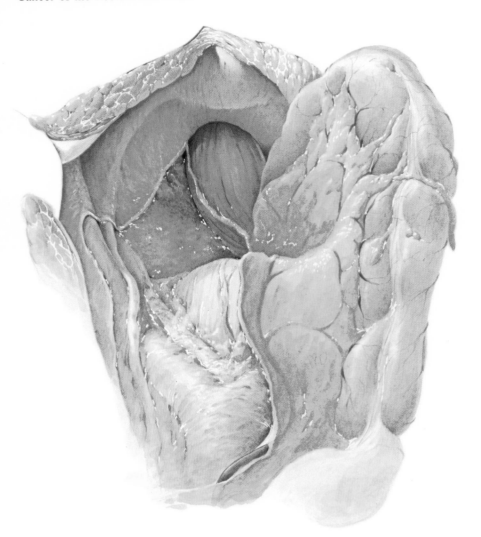

Fig. 8.1. Combined abdomeno-perineal resection. The sigmoid and intraperitoneal rectum are mobilized from the left side. The peritoneum is opened near the left ureter and the ureter is retracted.

inferior mesenteric vessels are clamped just distal to the left colic branch and divided between clamps. At times the left ureter may be intimately adherent to this area; it must be identified and retracted before clamps are applied. The inferior mesenteric vessels are both clamped doubly on the proximal side and tied doubly as well. The mesentery of the sigmoid is divided in such a fashion as to leave a satisfactory length of colon for the sigmoid colostomy.

The peritoneum on the right side is divided down to the pouch of Douglas. The incision is carried anteriorly, dividing the peritoneum overlying the bladder. A plane of cleavage may then be established anteriorly that in males lies immediately posterior to the seminal vesicles and anterior to the rectum, and in females lies posterior to the vagina (Fig. 8.3). The posterior dissection proceeds in a blunt fashion, separating all of the mesorectum from the sacrum (Fig. 8.4). By blunt dissection with the hand this plane can be established down as far as the coccyx. Attention is then turned to the lateral attachments. The middle hemorrhoidal vessels are identified by blunt dissection, clamped, and tied. As this is done, the rectal tumor may be elevated to a surprising degree and occasionally a lesion that was thought to have required a combined abdominoperineal resection may be available for an anterior resection and anastomosis.

After this dissection has been completed to as low a level as feasible, it is necessary to divide the rectum so that the pelvic floor can be recon-

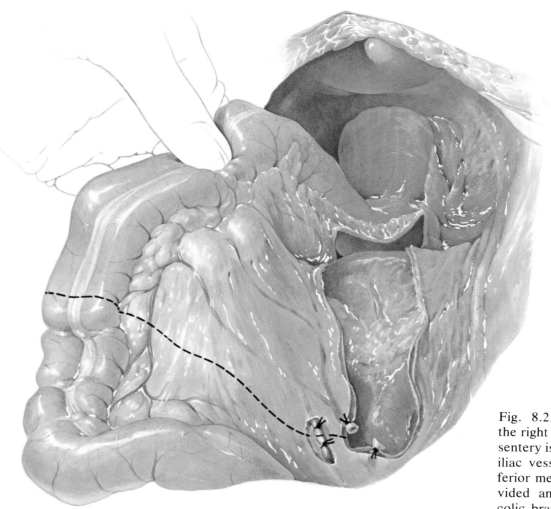

Fig. 8.2. The peritoneum on the right side of the sigmoid mesentery is opened, displaying the iliac vessels and aorta. The inferior mesenteric vessels are divided and tied below the left colic branch. The broken black line shows the line of division of the sigmoid mesentery.

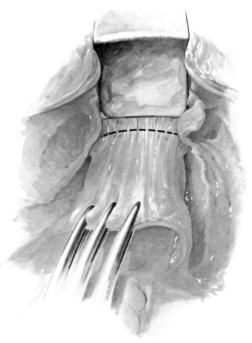

Fig. 8.3. The dissection is carried anteriorly on the prostate or vagina after the peritoneum is divided. The broken black line shows the upper margin of the palpable rectal cancer.

83

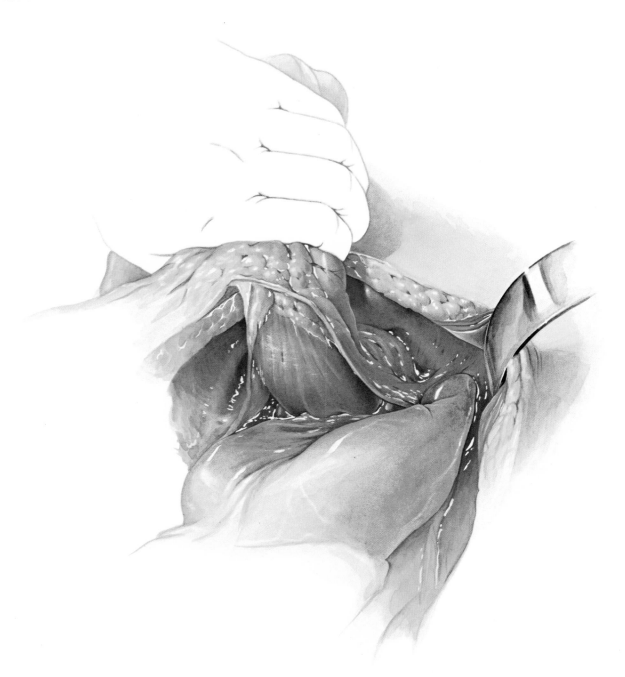

Fig. 8.4. By blunt dissection posteriorly the rectum is mobilized from the sacrum down to the coccyx.

structed. This is usually done above the tumor using a DeMartel clamp (Fig. 8.5). When the mesentery is fatty or edematous it must be divided and the vessels must be ligated as well. Alternative methods of closing the distal segment include the use of a stapler or an open closure with catgut. At times a bulky tumor is elevated to a point where the line of division can be placed below the tumor. In any instance, the colon is divided with the cautery to destroy any viable cancer cells at the line of anastomosis.

A lateral oblique incision is then made in order to withdraw the sigmoid for a left-sided colostomy, which will be made at a site corresponding to McBurney's point. A Kocher clamp is introduced through the stab wound; the bowel is divided between Kochers with the cautery and the proximal end is brought out as a colostomy (Fig. 8.6). Occasionally, because

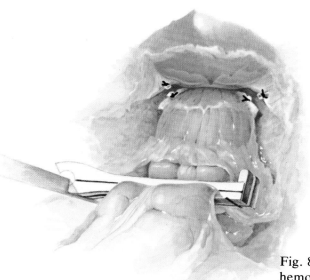

Fig. 8.5. After lateral dissection and ligation of the middle hemorrhoidal vessels a DeMartel clamp is applied and the bowel is divided with the cautery.

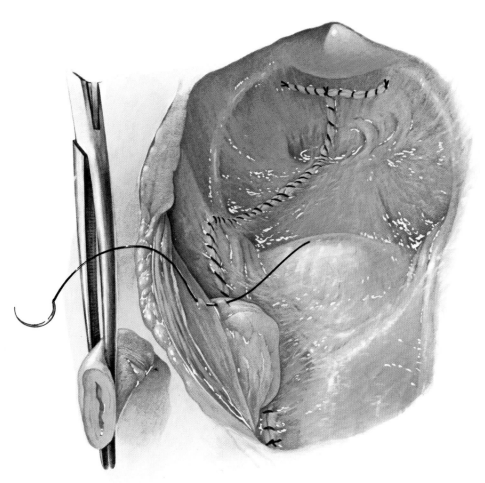

Fig. 8.6. The sigmoid mesentery is divided below the left colic branch. A stab wound colostomy is made. The trap laterl to the sigmoid is closed by suture. The clamp will be left on the bowel for 24 hr, or the mucosal margins alternatively may be sutured to the skin after the laparotomy wound is closed.

of the bulk of the tumor or the difficulties of the distal dissection, it will have been necessary to have divided the sigmoid between clamps well before this stage; if so, the proximal end is merely withdrawn through the stab wound. The colon is withdrawn for a distance of 2–3 cm and held in place by sponges beneath the Kocher clamp. The clamp will be removed in 24–48

85

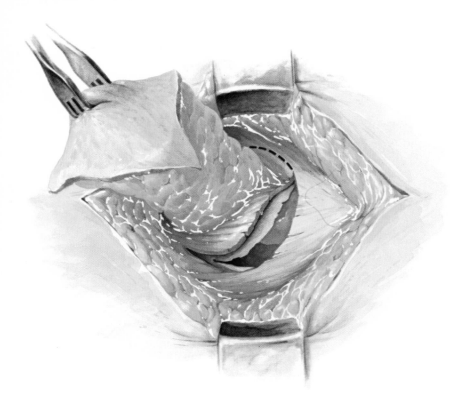

Fig. 8.7. The patient has been placed on the right side and the anus has been closed with a suture. A wide incision about the anus is deepened through the ischiorectal fat. The retrorectal space is entered by dividing Waldeyer's fascia below the coccyx.

hr. Some surgeons open the stoma and suture it to the skin as soon as the abdominal wall is closed.

The pelvic floor is reperitonealized using one layer of continuous 00 chromic catgut sutures and a second layer of interrupted 00 catgut. The pelvic organs in the female furnish an excellent peritoneal floor and will compensate for any absent peritoneum; however, oophorectomy is usually advisable. The trap between the sigmoid and the lateral abdominal wall is closed with several interrupted 00 chromic catgut sutures. The abdominal wall is closed in layers.

The patient is placed on his right side with the buttocks on the very edge of the table and the left knee elevated on a pillow. Both knees are flexed toward the abdomen. The anus is closed with a purse-string suture. An incision is made about the anus (Fig. 8.7). This should be wide if the tumor is located close to the anal orifice but may be less radical if the tumor is at the level of the peritoneal floor. Dissection is carried down through the perirectal fat until the levators are reached. Posteriorly dissection is carried down to the coccyx and the anterior portion of the incision is deepened for 3–4 cm. At this time the precoccygeal fascia of Waldeyer is opened. There is a precoccygeal artery just anterior to the coccyx that requires clamping and ligature. The presacral space is entered and the previous plane of dissection is identified. A finger inserted lateral to the rectum will identify the levators. On the left side they are clamped and divided close to the pelvic wall. A similar procedure is then carried out on the right side. After the levators have been divided downward for 4–5 cm the upper end of the rectal specimen can be withdrawn and dissection carried from above downward on the prostate or the vagina (Fig. 8.8). It is rare for a cancer to penetrate the fascia of Denonvilliers, so that in the male the prostate is involved very rarely. The dissection continues down laterally on both sides; in males, as the rectum is lifted away from the prostate, the urethra, which contains a No. 16 Foley catheter, can readily be identified by palpation and protected.

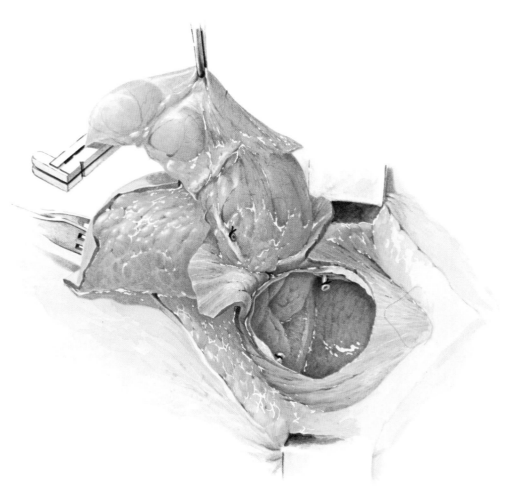

Fig. 8.8. After division of the upper portion of the levators the sigmoid and rectum are withdrawn. Dissection from above downward is preferable in the male since the prostate is easy to identify. In the female the perineal dissection usually is done with the patient in the lithotomy position and the posterior wall of the vagina removed along with the rectum.

The entire specimen is removed. Hemostasis is secured by catgut. In general, there will be a moderate amount of oozing from various vessels in the perineum, and usually four stuffed Penrose drains are left in the perineum and the wound is closed about them. In certain instances the whole area will be comparatively dry. Under these circumstances it is possible to close the skin and leave a sump sucker in place. However, in many instances hematoma or lymph will collect and a secondary opening will be necessary a few days later.

In the female it is possible to make a somewhat more radical resection. When the tumor is located on the anterior wall it is wise to remove the posterior portion of the vagina en bloc with the rectum. The vaginal mucosa can be reconstructed after the excision has been completed.

Some surgeons prefer to carry out the perineal portion of the operation with the patient in the lithotomy position; this may be easier but does not give as good a posterior exposure as the lateral position. However, in females with anterior tumors in whom the posterior portion of the vagina may be sacrificed it gives excellent exposure.

Two-Team Technique
The two-team technique for the combined abdominoperineal operation has

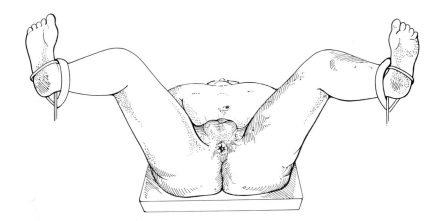

Fig. 8.9. Lloyd-Davies stirrups are used to position the patient for the two-team combined abdominoperineal resection.

become a favorite in many areas. It originated in St. Mark's Hospital. The patient's legs are elevated and separated on the Lloyd-Davies table so that the team working in the perineum can proceed simultaneously with the one working in the abdomen (Fig. 8.9).[12] There are obvious advantages to such a procedure: the operating time is reduced, better control of bleeding is possible, and very bulky tumors can be handled much more simply than by the other method. However, there also are some disadvantages. There may be a good deal of confusion, particularly if the operating room is small. The exposure in the perineum is not as good as by the other method and a less adequate excision may be done. The elevation of the legs may also cramp the surgeon who is working deep in the pelvis from the abdominal side.

Complications Arising During the Operation

Damage to the Left Ureter   At times the ureter may be so involved with tumor that it is necessary to resect a long section of it. Under these circumstances, assuming that the right kidney is known to be functional, the left ureter is doubly tied with catgut and left in place. In most instances no secondary infection will occur and the kidney will undergo atrophy in an asymptomatic fashion. If infection does supervene, a nephrectomy will be necessary at a second stage.

At times a normal left ureter is inadvertently damaged, particularly as the ties are being placed on the inferior mesenteric vessels. If this is the case, every attempt should be made to re-establish continuity of the ureter. A drain is necessary after an anastomosis has been carried out.

Short Sigmoid Mesentery   The sigmoid mesentery may be so short that the stoma cannot be made in the lateral position. In this case the stoma must be brought out through the main incision. Since such wounds are more likely to dehisce or lead to hernias, this is not the preferred method of colostomy.

Bleeding   Severe bleeding from the presacral veins may be encountered. This is a very troublesome complication; fortunately, it occurs very rarely. Attempts to control the bleeding by almost any known method are likely to be incomplete at best. The methods that can be considered include bilateral ligation of the internal iliac arteries, which can be done without hazard if the patient is to have a combined abdominoperineal resection. If there is to be any anastomosis in the perineum, however, ligation should not be done since extensive necrosis may result. Every attempt must be made to try to isolate any open veins and ligate them or control them with clips. Bone wax generally has been ineffective in plugging the interstices. In many instances it will eventually be necessary to apply gelfoam or to put on a large pack, which then will be drawn out through the perineum. This pack is withdrawn 2–3 days later.

Insufficient Pelvic Peritoneum   In some patients there may not be sufficient pelvic peritoneum to effect a closure of the peritoneal floor. Under these circumstances it is best to insert through the perineum a rubber dam that is held up in position with large packs. The packs can be removed after 7 days, at which time the bowel will have become fixed in its normal position. The alternative to this procedure is to leave the pelvic floor wide open but to close the perineal skin; this then allows the small bowel to drop down into the pelvic cavity and fill the whole area from which the rectum has been removed. While this method has been advocated by some surgeons and is necessary after exenterations, early postoperative obstruction is quite possible because of the wide denuded areas. Furthermore, after the wounds have healed there is certain to be a perineal hernia that occasionally can be troublesome.

Contiguous Organs Involved with Carcinoma   Concomitant resection of the uterus, tubes, and ovaries will be required in a number of female patients. It has been suggested that routine oophorectomy should be done with combined abdominoperineal resection because the ovary furnishes a fertile spot for metastatic disease to grow. If the bladder is involved above the trigone, a wide section can be removed in continuity and the bladder can be closed with a suprapubic cystostomy catheter. If the trigone is involved and the lesion is otherwise favorable, a pelvic exenteration must be considered as the only possible method of cure. Involvement of the seminal vesicles and prostate, though very rare, can be treated by simultaneous excision of these organs and reconstruction of the urinary tract.

A loop of adherent small bowel often has to be resected along with a carcinoma of the intraperitoneal rectum. Continuity is re-established by an end-to-end anastomosis.

Postoperative Complications

Urinary Retention   This is a common complaint in the male. An inlying catheter is left for approximately 12 days after surgery. If the patient cannot void thereafter he is usually sent home with a catheter in place to be checked again by the urologist at the end of 3 weeks. If he still cannot void, a transurethral resection is done.

Intestinal Obstruction   This is the most serious complication that can occur after the Miles operation. The small bowel may prolapse through the pelvic floor or lateral to the colostomy or merely be adherent at some other area within the abdominal cavity. A second laparotomy is necessary because of the possibility of strangulating obstruction, particularly with a loop that is caught in one of the two positions noted above.

Bleeding from the Posterior Wound   This is not uncommon in the first 24 hr after surgery. At times re-exploration of the perineal wound will be necessary. Identification of a bleeding vessel high in the pelvis may be difficult but is essential. Control often may be secured more easily by clips than by any other method. If no specific bleeding point can be identified, a large gauze pack is necessary.

Hernias about Colostomies   These are almost routine late complications and rarely produce any difficulty. Since any attempt at repair is usually followed by a second hernia, unless there is incarcerated bowel and symptoms of obstruction, repair of these hernias is rarely carried out.

Perineal Hernia   This complication is not uncommon. When the small intestine is retained only by skin, at times there may be a rupture of the perineal skin with evisceration of the small bowel through the perineum. Obviously repair will be necessary. This is difficult but can be done through the perineum by the insertion of a Marlex mesh.

Impotence   This nearly always follows the Miles operation and occurs in at least 50% of males after the D'Allaines procedure.[23] It is attributable to the wide pelvic dissection, since it is rare after total proctocolectomy for ulcerative colitis.

Perianal Cancers

Cancers near the anus include lesions in the perianal area that are near the anal verge; they may be extrinsic to the sphincters or involve the anal sphincters. They are squamous cell cancers that often originate from the basiloid cells of the epidermis and may in unusual instances be found even higher than the anal canal (Fig. 8.10). Such tumors have been described as cloacogenic cancer.[20] They vary greatly in degree of malignancy, as shown by Grodksy.[10] It should be noted that even adenocarcinomas that appear just above the pectinate line follow the same pattern of metastasis as the squamous cell carcinomas of the anus; thus the possibility of metastasis to the groins must be entertained in both instances.

The treatment of cancer of the anus will vary depending upon its location and physical characteristics.[2,5,6,16,17,19,22,25] Despite the fact that these lesions are often small, the rate of cure is only about 50% in combined series. Combined abdominoperineal resection with a wide excision of the perianal tissues is the accepted method of therapy. A combination of chemotherapy and radiation has been effective in a small series reported by Buroker et al.[4] Though small lesions of the perianal skin are often treated first by radiation therapy, it must be admitted that the recurrence rate is higher than it is elsewhere in the body and that a secondary abdominoperineal resection may be necessary. Deeper lesions or those that involve the sphincters require abdominoperineal resection. This is done according to the usual technique described above.

The main problem with perianal cancer is that it tends to metastasize to the inguinal lymph nodes. These metastases are usually primarily to the superficial inguinal nodes and secondarily to the deep nodes located above Poupart's ligament. This raises the question as to whether or not a prophylactic node dissection would be advisable in patients with such tumors. Inasmuch as the involvement of deep nodes is frequent, this would involve a radical groin dissection. Since this procedure has led to incapacitating edema in many patients who have had to have a bilateral procedure performed, prophylactic groin dissection is not recommended for these patients.

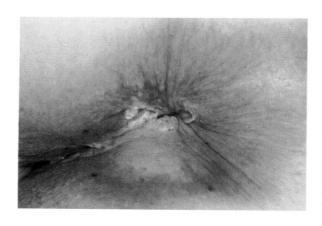

Fig. 8.10. Perianal squamous cell carcinoma recurrent after x-ray treatment. Site of origin was at the anal verge.

Inguinal node dissections may involve removal of the superficial nodes or both superficial and deep nodes.

Superficial Groin Dissection

An oblique incision is made just below Poupart's ligament and skin flaps are reflected widely. The dissection is begun laterally and from below. Subcutaneous fat is divided down to the anterior muscle fascia. The saphenous vein is divided and ligated. The femoral sheath is identified and dissection is carried upward on it. The saphenous vein is divided and ligated at its origin. All of the tissues inferior to the inguinal ligament down to the level of the femoral sheath are then removed en bloc, including fat and lymph nodes. The skin is closed about a suction catheter, which is maintained for several days. Unless there has been careful ligation of lymphatics a lymphocele may form and there may be a profuse discharge of lymph for a matter of several days or even weeks.

Deep Groin Dissection

In this procedure, in addition to the superficial dissection, all of the deep nodes up to the bifurcation of the iliac vessels are removed as well. The combined dissection can be made through an S-shaped incision running across Poupart's ligament or else by the use of two parallel oblique incisions. The essential portion of the upper dissection is the retraction of the peritoneum medially with the exposure of the external iliac artery and vein. Dissection is begun from above and lymph nodes and vessels are removed down to the inguinal ligament. Cloquet's node is located just above the inguinal ligament and is frequently found to contain cancer. It may be possible to excise the obturator node through this incision; an attempt should be made to do this because it may also be involved. Postoperative suction drainage is maintained through a sump catheter for several days.

Pelvic Exenteration

A pelvic exenteration occasionally may be required for a carcinoma of the rectum that has penetrated anteriorly into either the uterus and/or vagina in females or into the base of the bladder in males. A complete exenteration for cancer of the rectum that includes bladder as well as rectum is rare because such tumors usually extend posteriorly as well as anteriorly and involvement of the sacrum occurs so rapidly that there is relatively little advantage gained, particularly in males, by the addition of the removal of the bladder. Females, however, frequently have tumors attached to the uterus or posterior vagina and a posterior exenteration can be carried out; this includes removal of tubes, ovaries, uterus, and the entire posterior wall of the vagina, but retention of the bladder.

Removal of periaortic, peri-iliac, and obturator lymph nodes is a feature of pelvic exenteration as it has been developed for cancer of the cervix. Probably the same philosophy should be followed with cancer of the rectum; the lymph nodes and lymphatic tissues should be cleanly dissected from the bifurcation of the aorta down to the base of the pelvis. It is recognized, however, that whenever the iliac nodes are involved with cancer of the cervix the chances of a cure by exenteration have been very low, and probably the same will be true with cancer of the rectum.

Posterior Pelvic Exenteration in the Female

This operation combines the techniques of the Miles operation, total salpingo-oophorectomy, posterior vaginectomy, and pelvic node dissection. The dissection is begun at the upper level with ligation of the inferior mesenteric vessels just below the origin of the left colic artery. The colon is divided at an appropriate location in order to provide an adequate sigmoid colostomy. The mesentery is divided down to the site of the mesenteric pedicle ligation. The peritoneum is incised laterally near the level of the ureters, stripping lymphatics and lymph nodes from the vessels. The ovarian arteries are tied as they originate from the internal iliacs. The dissection is carried posteriorly down to the coccyx by blunt dissection. The middle hemorrhoidal vessels are divided. The bladder flap is developed and the round ligaments divided; then the entire cardinal ligaments together with the uterus and rectum are freed from all attachments. The vagina is entered anteriorly, and if the posterior wall of the vagina is to be removed appropriate incisions are made posteriorly for this purpose. Careful control of the blood supply is necessary because this area is extremely vascular. If necessary, the internal iliac arteries may be ligated. The obturator nodes should be removed at the anterior portion of this dissection.

The perineal portion of the procedure can be carried on by the other member involved in the two-team technique; if the whole operation is to be performed by one team, a sigmoid colostomy is established through a stab wound and the abdominal wall is closed.

If the one-team technique is used, the patient is then placed in the lithotomy position. The usual Miles operation is carried out, except in this instance the posterior wall of the vagina will be included in the specimen. After the plane of the upper dissection has been reached, the entire specimen may be withdrawn through the open pelvis.

No attempt is made to reconstruct a pelvic floor because all supporting structures have been removed. It is necessary to allow the small bowel to prolapse deep into the pelvis. It will be protected only by the soft tissues and skin, which should be brought together in the midline and closed primarily except for drainage by a sump sucker.

Total Pelvic Exenteration in the Male or Female

In the male a pelvic exenteration involves the removal of the rectum, bladder, and prostate. It is very uncommon to find an operable lesion in the female that will be amenable to total exenteration. It is obvious that this is an exceedingly difficult procedure that will require the establishment of a sigmoid colostomy and an ileal loop as a urinary receptacle. This operation will not be described in detail because it is performed so rarely. The ileal loop is made from the distal ileum by Bricker's technique. The exact details may be obtained from his description.[3]

Local Excision

Local excision of a very small carcinoma may be considered, especially in older, poor-risk patients. For example, a 2-cm lesion that shows only minimal invasion beneath the muscularis mucosae may be excised as described in Chapter 7. Excision is done by drawing the lesion through the dilated anus and making a deep incision through all coats of the bowel with an adequate margin. If the pathologist confirms the fact that it is a low-grade lesion, this procedure will have a high expectation of cure. If the cancer exists in the tip of a pedunculated polyp, local excision also is recommended. Exposure also may be obtained by the Mason or Soave techniques (see Chapters 7 and 9).[11,14] Other methods applicable in special instances include sphincter-saving operations (Chapter 9) and electrocoagulation (Chapter 23).

Palliative Operations

Palliative operations for cancer of the rectum are designed to relieve the symptoms of tenesmus, obstruction, or bleeding. The most satisfactory procedure is a resection of the tumor whenever this is possible. Patients are judged to be incurable either when there is wide local extension or when there are distant metastases, as in the liver or lung. Advanced age is often considered a reason to call a rectal cancer "inoperable"; however, the operation is remarkably well tolerated even in the elderly.

The carcinoma may be judged to be inoperable prior to operation because of extensive fixation of the tumor. Under such circumstances preoperative radiation therapy may reduce the bulk of the tumor and make it possible to carry out a palliative combined abdominoperineal resection. Preoperative chemotherapy to date has not been valuable.

Prior to operation a patient may be shown to have a liver that almost certainly contains metastatic masses secondary to a cancer of the rectum. In such instances, if the patient is otherwise comparatively healthy, we advocate laparotomy; a combined abdominoperineal resection usually will be necessary but a low anterior anastomosis with a narrow margin of normal bowel may be possible. Resection will eliminate the problems of tenesmus and hopefully of pain of local recurrence. Metastatic tumor localized in the liver is more amenable to chemotherapy than tumor elsewhere in the peritoneal cavity.

A simple colostomy occasionally will be all that is possible in some patients because of extensive tumor found in the pelvis. A colostomy done prior to the development of the symptoms of tenesmus or obstruction is not likely to be easily accepted by the patient. If such a colostomy is made, it preferably should be in the transverse colon because the sigmoid may be difficult to mobilize.

In old, poor-risk patients cancer of the rectum proved by biopsy to be metastatic to the liver has been treated by electrocoagulation by some surgeons.

It is well to remember that what is presumed to be metastatic cancer of the liver should be proved to be so by histologic study. For example, liver scans commonly give an erroneous impression. Furthermore, diseases such as multiple liver cysts or benign lesions such as multiple hemangiomas can be mistaken for metastatic carcinoma; in such instances the avoidance of a possible curative resection may lead to unnecessary death from cancer.

Metastatic disease in the liver or lung does not preclude cure, although it makes it unlikely. This matter is considered further in Chapter 23 in the section on Operations Related to Cancer.

References

1. Astler V.B., Coller F.A. (1954) The prognostic significance of direct extension of carcinoma of the colon and rectum. Ann Surg 139: 846
2. Beahrs O.H., Wilson S.M. (1976) Carcinoma of the anus. Ann Surg 184: 422
3. Bricker E.M. (1970) Pelvic exenteration. Adv Surg 4: 13
4. Buroker T.R., Nigro N., Bradley G., et al (1977) Combined therapy for cancer of the anal canal: A follow-up report. Dis Colon Rectum 20: 677
5. Corman M.L., Haggitt R.C. (1977) Carcinoma of the anal canal. Surg Gynecol Obstet 145: 674
6. Cortese A.F. (1975) Surgical approach for treatment of epidermoid anal carcinoma. Cancer 36: 1869
7. DeCosse J.J., Block G.E., Hughes E.S.R., et al (1977) Controversial issues in management of carcinoma of the rectum. Arch Surg 112: 558
8. Dukes C.E. (1932) The classification of cancer of the rectum. J Pathol Bacteriol 35: 323
9. Gilchrist R.K., David V.C. (1938) Lymphatic spread of carcinoma of the rectum Ann Surg 108: 621
10. Grodsky L. (1969) Current concepts on cloacogenic transitional cell anorectal cancers. JAMA 207: 2057
11. Itaya H., Osawa N. (1976) Application for Duhamel's operation for the surgical treatment of rectal cancer. Jpn J Surg 6: 49
12. Lloyd-Davies O.V. (1939) Lithotomy–Trendelenburg position for resection of rectum and lower pelvic colon. Lancet 2: 74
13. Lockhart-Mummery H.E., Ritchie J.K., Hawley P.R. (1976) The results of surgical treatment for carcinoma of the rectum at St. Mark's Hospital from 1948 to 1972. Br J Surg 63: 673
14. Mason A.Y. (1976) Selective surgery for carcinoma of the rectum. Aust NZ J Surg 46: 322
15. Miles W.E. (1908) A method of performing abdomino-perineal excision for carcinoma of the rectum and of the terminal portion of the pelvic colon. Lancet 2: 1812
16. Newman H.K., Quan S.H.Q. (1976) Multi-modality therapy for epidermoid carcinoma of the anus. Cancer 37: 12
17. O'Grady J.F., Bacon H.E., Koohdary A. (1973) Squamous-cell carcinoma of the anus. Dis Colon Rectum 16: 39
18. Patel S.C., Tovee E.B., Langer B. (1977) Twenty-five years of experience with radical surgical treatment of carcinoma of the extraperitoneal rectum. Surgery 82: 460
19. Sawyers J.L. (1977) Current management of carcinoma of the anus and perianus. Am Surg 43: 424
20. Sink J.D., Kramer S.A., Copeland D.D., et al (1978) Cloacogenic carcinoma. Ann Surg 188: 53
21. Stearns M.W. Jr. (1974) Abdominoperineal resection for cancer of the rectum. Dis Colon Rectum 17: 612
22. Stearns M.W. Jr., Quan S.H.Q. (1970) Epidermoid carcinoma of the anorectum. Surg Gynecol Obstet 131: 953
23. Weinstein M., Roberts M. (1977) Sexual potency following surgery for rectal carcinoma. A followup of 44 patients. Ann Surg 185: 295
24. Welch J.P., Donaldson G.A. (1974) Recent experience in the management of cancer of the colon and rectum. Am J Surg 127: 258
25. Welch J.P., Malt R.A. (1977) Appraisal of the treatment of carcinoma of the anus and anal canal. Surg Gynecol Obstet 145: 837

Sphincter-Saving Operations

9

Many kinds of sphincter-saving operations have been reported.[19] They vary depending upon the amount of tissue that is removed distally. It is possible to excise the entire rectum and anal sphincters and anastomose the colon or the ileum to the anal verge. This is the principle of Swenson's operation for Hirschsprung's disease.[29] It is possible to leave the external and internal sphincters, remove the rectal mucosa, and bring the upper sigmoid or ileum down through this muscular tube with anastomosis to the anus; this is the Soave procedure.[27] The D'Allaines procedure combines a low anterior dissection and an anastomosis of the sigmoid to the rectum in the perineum; the anal canal and 3–4 cm of the lower rectum are retained.[6] Black has described an endorectal approach that retains the lowest 2–3 cm of rectal mucosa and the lower portion of the sphincter mechanism[4]; Bacon has retained the sphincters after a combined abdominoperineal dissection.[1]

These operations usually have been done for villous adenomas or for comparatively small, localized cancers of the rectum. A major problem has arisen when they have been used for carcinomas of the rectum located below the pelvic floor in which the lesions are definitely invasive and the line of resection is located only 2–3 cm beyond the cancer. These operations carry a very definite risk of recurrence. Although published figures would show that the risk is no greater than after the ordinary Miles operation, it must be recognized that these operations are done for more favorable tumors and that the incidence of recurrence should be distinctly less than after the Miles procedure.

Pull-Through Operations with Sacrifice of the Sphincter Mechanism

One of the earliest operations was the pull-through procedure; it was originally described by Hochenegg.[13] The colon is freed very widely from within the peritoneal cavity. The inferior mesenteric vessels are divided and a wide area of mesentery is removed along with the intraperitoneal rectum. A sufficient length of colon is maintained to bring down through the anal canal. It is necessary that the anastomosis through the pericolic ves-

95

sels be adequate. At the time of dissection this area of adequate vascularization is marked by the surgeon so that the proper spot for anastomosis may be noted. The anterior dissection is otherwise exactly the same as for a combined abdominoperineal resection; the lateral rectal stalks are cut and the rectum is freed down to the coccyx.

The perineal phase, done with either the same or a second team, involves excision of the entire anorectum along with surrounding supporting tissues, including the levators. The sigmoid colon is then brought down through the resulting cavity and the incision is closed about it. It is possible to leave excess bowel projecting through the new anus and the redundant portion can then be excised a few days later.[30] Other surgeons have resected the bowel at this time and anastomosed it to the new anus.[1,9]

The complications of pull-through operations are those common to operations in the perineum: sepsis and necrosis of the bowel loop due to inadequate circulation, and, at a later date, fecal incontinence. This procedure is not recommended for cancer in adults; there may be many complications and the patient is left with a perineal colostomy that is difficult to control.

Low Anterior Resection

A low anterior resection of the colon is indicated most frequently for carcinoma of the rectum with a lower margin 2–3 cm above the peritoneal floor.[7,12,14] It is also valuable for extensive sessile villous adenomas located at or just below the peritoneal floor. Occasionally a resection for diverticulitis must go this low, but it is very rare that a dissection for that disease has to be carried beneath the peritoneal floor.

Standard Operative Procedure
A Foley catheter is inserted into the bladder and, if irrigation of the rectum is to be carried out prior to the anastomosis, a large rectal tube is inserted into the rectum and attached to an irrigating apparatus. Distilled water will be used for the irrigation.

The abdomen is opened through a left paramedian incision. The characteristics of the pelvic tumor are ascertained and the colon, liver, and gallbladder are carefully palpated.

If possible, a heavy tie is placed around the intraperitoneal rectum above the tumor and another is placed below. The second tie is rarely possible with a low lesion. Assuming that the tumor is favorable for an anterior resection, the left leaf of the mesentery is freed to identify the ureter and to retract it well back from the inferior mesenteric pedicle (Fig. 9.1). The inferior mesenteric pedicle is isolated after an incision through the right side of the mesocolon. The inferior mesenteric vessels are divided between clamps just below the left colic artery unless there are enlarged nodes at this area. If they are present the left colic artery must be taken, but then the anastomosis will require freeing the transverse colon to bring it down for adequate anastomosis.

The dissection is carried distally along the margin of the right mesosigmoid. The right ureter is observed as this is done. The dissection is then carried anteriorly and the peritoneum is divided in the female along the posterior wall of the vagina, and in the male along the base of the bladder. The posterior dissection is carried down on the sacrum and the rectum is freed down essentially as far as the coccyx.

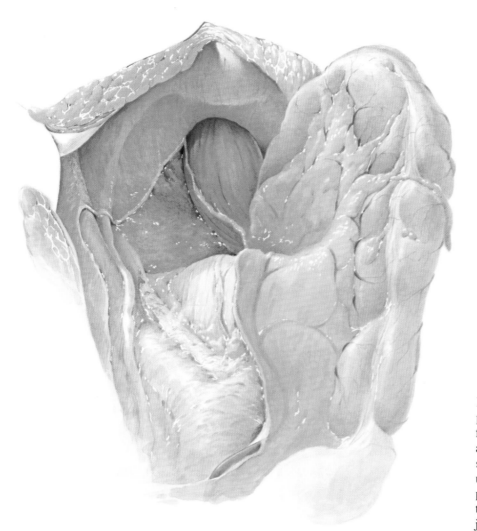

Fig. 9.1. The sigmoid and intraperitoneal rectum are mobilized from the left side. The peritoneal attachments have been cut and the sigmoid retracted to the right. The ureter and the iliac vessels are exposed. Dissection is carried anteriorly in the pouch of Douglas just anterior to the rectal wall.

The lateral ligaments that contain the middle hemorrhoidal vessels are then divided (Fig. 9.2). Care must be taken to avoid the ureters at this time. The middle hemorrhoidal vessels are ligated as they are identified. As soon as this is done the specimen usually can be elevated a considerable distance, and what may have previously appeared to be a tumor too low for a successful anastomosis is now available for an anastomotic procedure.

The sigmoid is divided with the cautery at an appropriate level at least 10 cm above the tumor. Prior to the application of a distal clamp, it is necessary to divide the posterior pedicle of the rectum. There is no true mesentery at this level and the superior hemorrhoidal pedicle is often very adherent to the rectum itself. It usually can be mobilized by blunt dissection with the finger and then the pedicle can be tied at a low level. In very difficult cases it may even be necessary to divide the rectum in an open fashion, seizing the cut margins with long Allis clamps and then dividing and ligating the mesentery secondarily. Hemostasis at this level is extremely important because any oozing vessels can produce a deep pelvic hematoma. The distal end of the bowel is then seized with a Wertheim clamp at least 5 cm below the tumor when the bowel is not on a stretch. At this time the rectum can be thoroughly irrigated with distilled water. A second clamp is applied distally and the bowel is divided between the clamps with the cautery.

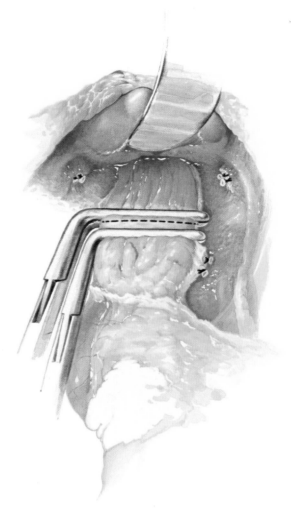

Fig. 9.2. The final dissection. The extraperitoneal rectum has been mobilized essentially down to the coccyx. The middle hemorrhoidal vessels are divided and ligated and the rectum is elevated. A clamp is applied 5 cm below the tumor, the rectum is irrigated, a second, lower clamp is applied, and the bowel is divided along the broken black line.

Preferably the anastomosis is made end-to-end in two layers with an outer layer of interrupted 000 silk and an inner layer of interrupted 000 absorbable sutures (Fig. 9.3). At times, however, it will be found that the lumen of the rectum is very large and that of the sigmoid quite small. In this case it is necessary to close the end of the sigmoid and carry out a side-to-end coloproctostomy (Fig. 9.4).[2] This anastomosis is made in the same fashion, except that since it is a long anastomosis a running suture may be employed on the mucosal side. This should be locked posteriorly and continued around anteriorly as a Connell suture. The outer layer again is of interrupted silk.

After completion of the anastomosis, the medial leaf of the peritoneum is sutured to the mesentery of the sigmoid and to the rectal stump. This peritonealizes the medial half of the abdominal cavity and allows less opportunity for small bowel to become entrapped or adherent. The lateral leaf, however, is left open for drainage so that any blood that collects deep in the pelvis will not be loculated in that area.

Whether or not to drain such an anastomosis and whether or not to carry out a transverse colostomy are decisions that must be made in each individual case. Our opinion is that if the anastomosis goes perfectly without contamination and without any uncontrolled bleeding a transverse colostomy is not necessary. On the other hand, if there is contamination, the

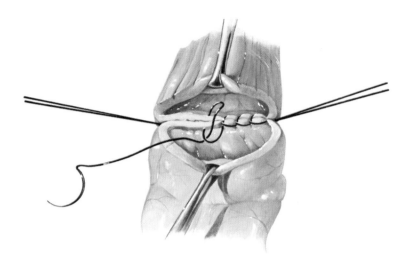

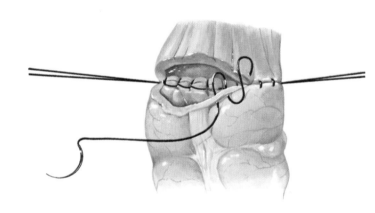

Fig. 9.3. In this instance the sigmoid and rectum were of approximately equal size and thus an end-to-end anastomosis was possible. Since the bowel was wide, running sutures were employed. The posterior row is locked and the anterior is made with a Connell suture. The outer layer is of interrupted silk both anteriorly and posteriorly.

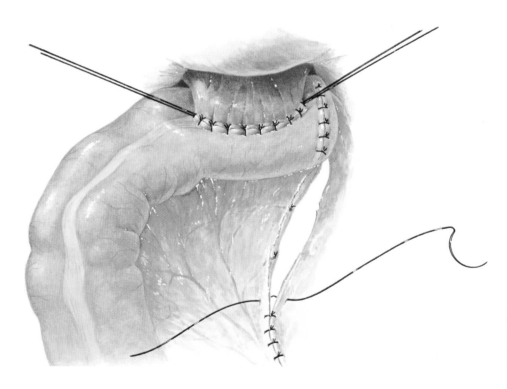

Fig. 9.4. In this instance the reconstruction has been by a side-to-end technique, often known as the Baker anastomosis. The end of the sigmoid has been closed and a two-layer anastomosis made.

anastomosis is not perfect, or there is still some pelvic ooze, it is wise to carry out a loop transverse colostomy that is placed through a transverse incision in the right upper quadrant.

Drainage will be necessary in certain circumstances. If there is wide mobilization of the rectum and there is slight tension on the anastomosis (obviously something that should be avoided whenever possible), there will be a cavity left behind the anastomotic line in the retrorectal space. This is certain to fill with blood or lymph, and in these circumstances we usually place a Shirley sump drainage catheter into this pocket, keep it on suction for 48 hr, and then remove it. J.H. Remington (personal communication) has advised leaving the sump in place and irrigating it regularly with kanamycin solution; he has reported excellent results with this procedure. McLachlin et al. have shown the advantage of the use of omentum to fill this dead space; in experimental dogs it reduced suture-line leakage significantly.[23] Omentum has also been used by Goldsmith.[11]

Variations in Operative Procedure

When it is necessary to carry out a left colectomy because there are suspicious nodes high along the inferior mesenteric pedicle, the distal transverse colon must be brought down for anastomosis. This can prove to be difficult at times, particularly when the mesocolon is extremely short. In very rare instances the mesocolon is so short that it is necessary to do a total colectomy and use the ileum for the anastomosis. However, in nearly every case it will be possible to carry out an end-to-end anastomosis. One of the difficulties that arises with this procedure, however, is that it may be impossible to close the trap that is left behind the colon after the mesentery has been excised widely. If possible, this trap should be closed; however, if this closure compresses the small bowel or if the closure is not adequate, it is far better to leave the trap wide open. The colon will usually lie comfortably behind the small bowel. It may be possible to insert a few sutures drawing the mesentery together close to the anastomosis.

Another problem arises when there is profuse bleeding from the presacral vessels that is impossible to control by any means short of packing. Ligation of the internal iliac arteries should not be carried out because there is a danger of necrosis of the rectum. In one instance in which such profuse bleeding occurred it was necessary to pack the entire area with a handkerchief gauze, bring the end out through the lower end of the incision, and do a transverse colostomy. The pack was removed without incident after 48 hr and, except for a late hernia in the abdominal incision, there was no problem. This method should be used only as a last resort.

Some surgeons have recommended the insertion of a rectal tube that passes through the anastomosis into the lower sigmoid.[26] They have reported good results with this method. It has the clear advantage that if such a tube is used it will be impossible to make the technical error of suturing the anterior wall to the posterior one at the time of the anastomosis. It may also relieve a certain amount of ileus that might occur otherwise. We have not used this method despite the enthusiastic comments of some surgeons.

Some surgeons faced with a low anterior resection for a cancer of the rectum prefer to pass ureteral catheters prior to the dissection. While this may occasionally be necessary, we have used it only in very rare instances in which a very difficult dissection was expected. Even this method may not give perfect results because there may be a double ureter that could fail to be identified and could be injured during the operative procedure. However, illuminated catheters are now available and should be valuable in case a difficult dissection is likely.

A Salem sump tube is placed in the stomach by the anesthesiologist at the time of the operation, and suction is maintained until bowel sounds are reasonably active and gas is passed by the rectum; this usually occurs on the fourth or fifth day. At that time it can be removed and fluids and diet can be advanced cautiously. The inlying Foley catheter is left in place until a bowel movement occurs. With anterior resection there very rarely is any difficulty with postoperative urinary tract obstruction in the male unless there has been disease of the prostate, which may require a transurethral resection. It is unusual for difficulties with erection and ejaculation to occur.

The postoperative bowel habit is likely to be changed significantly by this procedure. Usually evacuations do not occur on a regular schedule for a matter of many months. Removal of the sigmoid and upper rectum appear to remove the time clock of evacuation.

D'Allaines Procedure

The D'Allaines procedure consists of an anterior dissection of the intra- and extraperitoneal rectum combined with a perineal incision and anastomosis.[6] It is indicated particularly for large villous adenomas that are benign and very rarely for small, relatively noninvasive cancers. When this procedure is performed for cancer there is a definite hazard of recurrence because the length of bowel obtained in the resection beyond the cancer is likely to be less than optimal.

The procedure may be performed with the patient in the usual prone position, with a subsequent shift to a right lateral position for the perineal portion.[8] It may also be done with the patient placed obliquely on the table with his hips elevated approximately 45° according to Localio's technique.[15–18,25] Our preference has been for the first method; however, with the Localio exposure, it is not necessary to move the patient.

The usual dissection is similar to that for low anterior resection (Fig. 9.5a). The rectum is freed to as low a level as possible from above. The superior hemorrhoidal and middle hemorrhoidal vessels are divided and ligated. The colon is freed to as high a level as necessary for the projected excision and anastomosis. The colon is not divided but is left intact. A suture is placed to make the projected line of division. The wound is closed temporarily with several heavy wire sutures.

The patient is then placed upon his right side. An incision is made running up from the anus just to the side of the coccyx (Fig. 9.5b). It may be necessary to excise the coccyx for further exposure. The rectum is identified. Tissues surrounding the rectum are included if the lesion is carcinoma, but if it is apparently a benign villous adenoma, wide excision of the levators is not necessary. It is important to maintain the lower portion of the anorectal canal intact. The sphincter mechanisms and the mucosa remain undisturbed.

After the dissection is complete, the excess colon is drawn down from above. The projected site of removal had been previously marked with a suture, and this again is identified. The rectum is then divided just above the sphincters, preferably between clamps with the cautery, and at the upper end in a similar fashion. An open end-to-end anastomosis is then carried out using two layers of sutures—the inner one of interrupted catgut, the outer of interrupted silk (Fig. 9.5c). The perineum is then closed in layers.

101

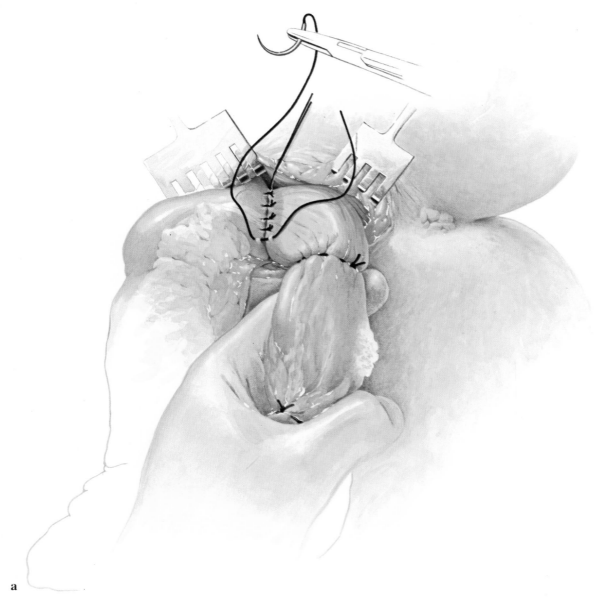

a

Fig. 9.5a–c. D'Allaines perineal anastomosis. a. The abdominal dissection has been carried out exactly as for a low anterior resection. The patient has then been placed upon his left side. Through a vertical incision lateral to the anus running up beyond the coccyx, the coccyx is excised, the levators are cut, and the sigmoid colon is delivered. The anastomosis is begun by suturing the posterior wall with interrupted silk sutures.

The patient is then returned to the abdominal position. The wound is reopened. A loop transverse colostomy is formed. The peritoneum is closed at the pelvic floor so that a loop of small bowel will not prolapse deep into the pelvis. The abdominal wall is closed in layers.

The major complications that follow this procedure are anastomotic leakage, formation of a fistula from the anastomotic line, sepsis, and impotence. Since anastomotic leakage is common, a transverse colostomy is recommended as a concomitant procedure.

The dissection of the rectum is likely to be rather difficult and hemostasis not as perfect as after the usual low anterior resection. Consequently,

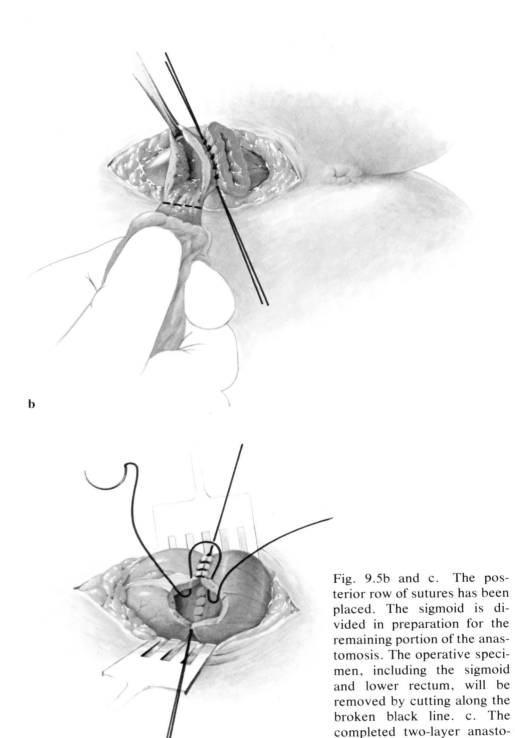

b

c

Fig. 9.5b and c. The posterior row of sutures has been placed. The sigmoid is divided in preparation for the remaining portion of the anastomosis. The operative specimen, including the sigmoid and lower rectum, will be removed by cutting along the broken black line. c. The completed two-layer anastomosis lies a very short distance above the anus.

accumulations of blood are somewhat more common and secondary sepsis is more likely. If there is any persistent ooze in the pelvis, the insertion of a sump catheter from above will aid in the decompression of this collection. It is put in at the time of the operation and can be removed a few days later.

The incidence of impotence in males after this operation is less than after a combined abdominoperineal resection but in reported series approaches 40%.

103

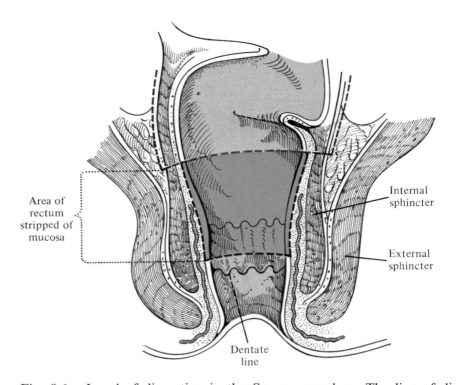

Fig. 9.6. Level of dissection in the Soave procedure. The line of dissection shown by the broken black line lies between the mucosa and the muscular wall of the lower rectum. Dissection is begun at the dentate line and proceeds upward for at least 5 cm. Dissection may be facilitated by the submucosal infiltration of salt solution. The entire rectal wall will be removed at a desirable level. When this procedure is done for Hirschsprung's disease, the colon is resected as far as necessary to a spot where ganglia are present. When it is done for a large villous adenoma, the line of resection can be made above the villous adenoma. The extraperitoneal rectum is divided above the level of the sphincters (broken red line). In young children nearly all of the operation for aganglionosis can be done through an abdominal exposure.

Soave Procedure

This procedure was developed by Soave in 1963 for the treatment of Hirschsprung's disease.[27] However, it has a much wider application and may be considered as a type of pull-through operation that can be used for multiple or familial polyposis, large villous adenomas, and possibly ulcerative colitis. Actually the operation was described first by Yancey et al. in 1952 for multiple polyposis.[31]

The essential feature of the operation is that the entire muscular tube of the anus and lower rectum is preserved (Fig. 9.6); thus after a resection of either the rectum or the colon a higher segment of bowel may be withdrawn through the sphincters and an anastomosis of mucosa to the skin of the anal canal can be performed. This procedure therefore is more likely to lead to continence than one in which the sphincter mechanism is excised.

The mechanism of continence is an extremely complicated one. Undoubtedly there are afferent fibers that run from the level of the anal canal that permit the patient to differentiate between gas and feces. Furthermore, in the normal person this reflex arc maintains an active, competent internal sphincter so that voluntary attention need not be paid to the retention of either gas or feces. On the other hand, when this mucosa is excised

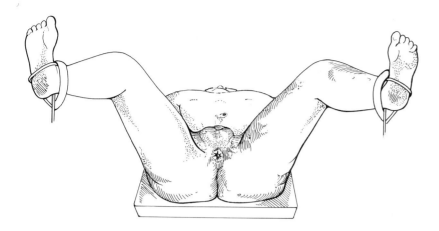

Fig. 9.7a–c. Soave procedure and endorectal anastomosis. a. Position for the Soave operation. It is very helpful to use the two-team technique. The legs are extended on the Lloyd-Davies stirrups. The abdominal incision is left paramedian. The perineal dissection can be done easily through this exposure.

the voluntary retention of fecal contents becomes more difficult. It is interesting to note that recovery of competence is comparatively easy in young patients but becomes progressively more difficult in the elderly.

The procedure may be carried out with either the one- or two-team technique. There are definite advantages in the two-team technique, although the maneuvers will be the same in either circumstance (Fig. 9.7a).

The abdominal portion is exactly the same as for low anterior resection; it consists of the wide mobilization of the colon, carrying the dissection down, if possible, to the levator sling from above. It is important that blood supply be very carefully maintained.

The perineal portion of the operation is begun by a digital dilatation of the anal sphincter. An incision is made at or just above the dentate line and the mucosa is removed from below upward as a cuff (Fig. 9.7b). Dissection may be facilitated by the submucous injection of normal saline solution to which a small amount of epinephrine has been added. The dissection is carried upward for a distance of approximately 6–10 cm. At this time the plane developed by the abdominal dissection will be encountered and the muscle of the intraperitoneal rectum above the internal sphincter is divided at that level. Alternatively, mucosa can be separated from muscle starting at the upper end.

The colon is brought down through the muscular tube that comprises the muscular wall of the extraperitoneal rectum, including the internal and external sphincters and the surrounding levator sling. A two-layer interrupted catgut anastomosis is then employed using interrupted 00 chromic catgut sutures (Fig. 9.7c).

The main complication is bleeding from the muscular walls of the rectum. This may lead to an accumulation of blood between the ileum and the rectal wall. Therefore, it may be necessary to insert a drainage catheter or sump drain past the suture line into this potential space for suction drain-

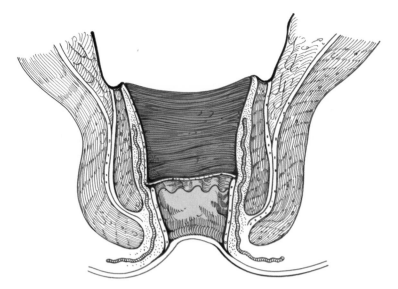

Fig. 9.7b. Exposure of the internal sphincter after resection. A circular incision is begun just above the dentate line. The section of mucosa to be removed is shown in blue, and the line of dissection by the broken blue lines in Fig. 9.6.

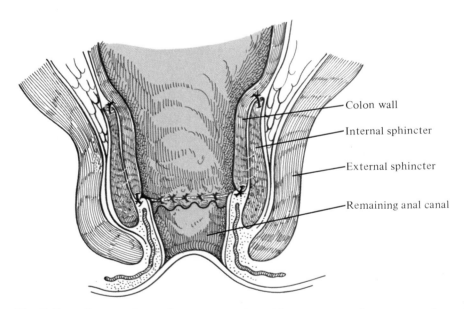

Colon wall

Internal sphincter

External sphincter

Remaining anal canal

Fig. 9.7c. Intraperitoneal rectum or sigmoid anastomosed to mucosa just above the dentate line. The bowel may be sutured at a higher level to the internal sphincter. If there is any bleeding, a drain should be left between the bowel and the surrounding sphincters.

age to prevent formation of an abscess. A deficient blood supply to the colon may lead to infarction of the conduit. If the blood supply is not adequate there also may be dehiscence of the anastomosis at the anus.

The same operation may be used for many other purposes. Soper (personal communication) has used it for familial polyposis in about a dozen cases; this is the largest individual group that has been reported. He removes the entire colon and rectal mucosa and anastomoses the ileum to the anal verge. He has found that in children or teenagers total continence is attained in 1–2 years. Extensive villous adenomas of the rectum that descend very close to the sphincter may be handled in this fashion (Fig. 9.8). Since they occur in adults and if benign require only a resection of the rectal mucosa, the sigmoid may be used to anastomose to the anus. Furthermore, in order to avoid the problems of delayed healing, a temporary transverse colostomy can be employed.

For Hirschsprung's disease in children, the dissection and coring out of mucosa can be done almost entirely by the abdominal route. Dissection is aided by the injection of saline between mucosa and muscle, and a posterior section of the muscular tube. Coran and Weintraub have described a similar method.[5]

The same procedure could be carried out for a low carcinoma of the rectum but we do not advise it because this would be a local procedure and would be likely to fail to remove an adequate amount of the full thickness of rectal wall.

When this operation is used for ulcerative colitis, many other problems appear. Martin et al. have described a small series of patients.[20] Eventually they have achieved good results, but the operation has been difficult and there have been many complications associated with it. In many patients there is a very extensive inflammatory reaction that extends far below the mucosa, and there are multiple problems of sepsis. It is inadvisable to use the operation for either ulcerative colitis or Crohn's disease unless the rectal segment is completely free of gross evidence of the disease. Furthermore, when it is done, adequate drainage of the space between the muscular tube and the bowel, as well as a diverting loop ileostomy, are essential. The ileostomy must be maintained for several weeks until perineal healing is complete. The total time devoted by the patient to this operation and full recovery must be measured in terms of several months.

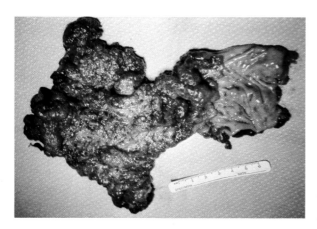

Fig. 9.8. Operative specimen of an enormous villous adenoma extending from the anal verge up for over 12 cm. Three years after a Soave procedure this 50-year-old patient was entirely continent of feces and only incontinent of gas about once a month.

Other Endorectal Resections

Black has used a wide anterior dissection that is then combined with a dilatation of the anus, section through the rectum about 3 cm above the dentate line, and withdrawal of the proximal colon through the anus.[4] The excess tissue can be amputated at this time and an anastomosis made, or the excess can be excised several days later. Parks has used a modified Soave procedure.[24]

In unusual instances a cancer originating in a polyp or of low grade may be treated by local excision through the dilated anus or after division of the sphincters[21,22] (see Chapter 7).

Postoperative Care

Following recovery from any of these operations and any immediate complications, the patient is placed upon a relatively bulky, constipating diet. This will promote continence of feces more rapidly than a low-roughage or soft diet. The patient is taught voluntary contraction of the external sphincter and practices this several times a day.

Eventually, bowel function will vary depending upon the age of the patient, the presence or absence of any sphincter mechanism, and the amount of mucous membrane and anal canal left distal to the anastomotic line.[3,26] Thus the results vary from perfect control in children who have had a Soave procedure to what is essentially a perineal colostomy in adults who have had an extensive operation for cancer. On the other hand, adults who have a rectal segment of 6 cm above the dentate line will be continent.

Patients who have had a complete excision of the sphincter mechanism essentially end with a perineal colostomy. Generally fecal continence can be aided by a constipating diet and a rectal irrigation to start the fecal stream every 2 days. Incontinence is common, however, and in general this type of colostomy is unsatisfactory.

If any of these procedures are carried out for cancer, an adequate margin may be difficult to obtain; hence suture-line recurrence may be an important problem. This occurs only if an anastomosis has been made; if a pull-through operation has been employed without any anastomotic line, this complication is avoided. However, there may be implantation in the perineal wound. The incidence of recurrence in the perineum in Bacon's series was approximately 20%.

Anastomosis with the Stapler

The end-to-end anastomosis (EEA) surgical stapler can be employed for an end-to-end anastomosis anywhere in the gastrointestinal tract. However, in the colon it is chiefly used to secure a low anastomosis. The instrument is extremely effective. It appears to be deceptively simple but in practice a number of technical problems may arise. The essential feature of the operation is that the two ends of intestine to be anastomosed are each tied over a circular piece of metal, one of which carries two circles of staples, and the upper one of which acts as an anvil (Fig. 9.9). When these two are brought together and locked in position by a tightened screw, a knife automatically cuts the inverted ends of the intestine and fires two rows of staples, producing the anastomosis. The entire instrument is then withdrawn from the rectum.

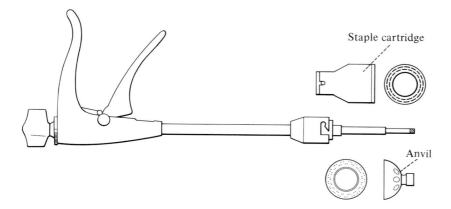

Staple cartridge

Anvil

Fig. 9.9. Anastomosis with the stapler: surgical stapling instrument and disposable loading unit EEA-31. The permanent portion of the instrument consists of a handle equipped with a twist lock and a center rod. There is a wing nut at the outermost portion of the handle. The staple cartridge is reloaded for each operation and is locked on the twist lock. The anvil eventually is attached to the center rod and tightened in place by use of the wing nut.

All of the technical details must be scrupulously followed. The dissection is carried out as for a low anterior resection but can be carried to a much lower level if necessary. After this has been completed it is necessary to place purse-strings about the open end of the distal rectum and the open end of the proximal colon. The purse-string can be of 00 polyolifin. It must incorporate only a relatively small amount of the wall of the bowel. The purse-strings must not be tightened at this stage. The insertion of the purse-string may be facilitated at the upper end by using a special clamp through which the suture may be passed with a Keith needle (Fig. 9.10). It may be difficult or impossible to use this instrument on the lower end.

The operative field is prepared by placing the patient's legs in the Lloyd-Davies stirrups so that the abdominal incision and the perineum will be exposed. After resection of the bowel the surgeon's assistant inserts the instrument through the anus. The wing nut at the distal end of the instrument is then turned to separate the anvil and cartridge. It then will be possible to tighten the purse-strings so that the lower end is tied about the cartridge and the upper end about the anvil (Fig. 9.11). The bowel should

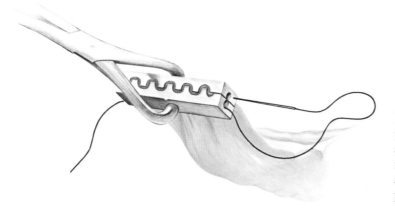

Fig. 9.10. The clamp may be used to insert a purse-string suture if the bowel is mobile. It is applied to the cut end of the colon and a Keith needle is used to draw a suture through both arms of the clamp. An accurate purse-string is produced by this method.

109

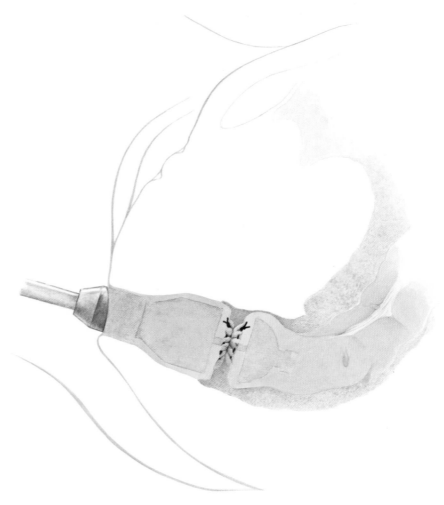

Fig. 9.11. The stapler now is placed within the anal canal. The end of the distal rectum is tied around the center rod above the cartridge and the end of the proximal colon is tied below the anvil. The anvil is tightened on the cartridge in preparation for firing the staples. This instrument can also used for an end-to-end colocolic anastomosis. The instrument is inserted through a colotomy incision proximal to the line of resection; after the anastomosis is complete it is withdrawn and the colotomy incision is closed. Two smaller heads have been used for this purpose: the usual cartridge is 31 mm in diameter; the smaller heads are 25 and 28 mm.

be inspected to be certain that there are no gaps through which mucosa is extruding. The safety latch on the anvil is released; the handle is squeezed to complete the stapling and the cone of tissue is excised by the blade. The instrument is withdrawn from the anus. The anvil can then be disconnected from the center rod. Two complete "doughnuts" of tissue should be present within the instrument.

Several problems may arise with the stapler. The diameter of the bowel to be anastomosed should be equal to or larger than the outside diameter of the cartridge (31.6 mm). If the upper limb to be anastomosed is smaller than this, either some other method should be used or an end-to-side anastomosis may be feasible. No clips or ties should be placed close to the anastomotic line because they will interfere with the action of the instrument. If the bowel wall is greatly thickened, the staples are not likely to catch. All fat must be cleared from the bowel wall before the purse-string is applied.

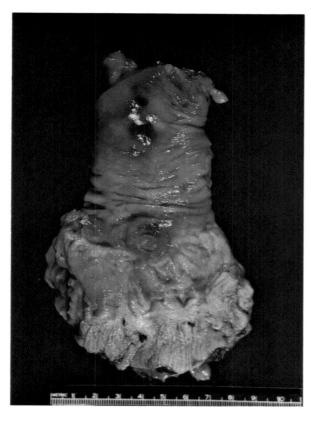

Fig. 9.12. Operative specimen of a cancer of the rectum recurrent after low anterior anastomosis. This was treated by a combined abdominoperineal resection. This recurrence at the suture line indicates the hazard of tumor cell implantation in an anastomotic line. present.

The most difficult problem is the placement of the purse-string suture. While the special instrument designed for this purpose is valuable for the upper end it may be impossible to use in the pelvis and great care must be taken to be certain that all of the mucosa will be drawn within the instrument when the tie is completed. Another problem has been concerned with the removal of the instrument from the bowel; the line of anastomosis must be drawn gently over the anvil and then the instrument can be withdrawn.

After the instrument is withdrawn the anastomosis may be inspected from above and also palpated with the finger in the rectum. The presence of any bleeding should be noted immediately because if a suture line does bleed it would be appropriate to identify the bleeder at this time.

This instrument is attractive and may prove to be the most valuable stapler for use in the large intestine.

References

1. Bacon H.E. (1949) Anus–rectum–sigmoid colon. Diagnosis and treatment, 3rd edn, Vol 1. Lippincott, Philadelphia
2. Baker J.W. (1977) Side-to-end colorectal anastomosis. In: Malt R.A. (ed) Surgical techniques illustrated, Vol 2, No 2. Little, Brown, Boston, p 31
3. Bennett R.C., Buls J., Kennedy J.T., et al (1973) The physiologic status of the anorectum after pull-through operations. Surg Gynecol Obstet 136: 907
4. Black B.M. (1969) Combined abdomino-endorectal resection. In: Turell R. (ed) Diseases of the colon and anorectum, 2nd edn, Vol 1. Saunders, Philadelphia, p 555
5. Coran A.G., Weintraub W.H. (1976) Modification of the endorectal procedure for Hirschsprung's disease. Surg Gynecol Obstet 143: 277
6. D'Allaines F. (1946) Traitement chirurgical du cancer du rectum. Editions Médicales Flammarion, Paris

7. Dixon C.F. (1939) Surgical removal of lesions occurring in the sigmoid and rectosigmoid. Am J. Surg 46: 12

8. Donaldson G.A., Rodkey G.V., Behringer G.E. (1966) Resection of the rectum with anal preservation. Surg Gynecol Obstet 123: 571

9. Gardner B., Kottmeier P., Harshaw D. (1973) A modified one-stage pull through operation for carcinoma or prolapse of the rectum. Surg Gynecol Obstet 136: 95

10. Gilchrist R.K., David V.C. (1938) Lymphatic spread of carcinoma of the rectum. Ann Surg 108: 621

11. Goldsmith H.S. (1977) Protection of low rectal anastomosis with intact omentum. Surg Gynecol Obstet 144: 584

12. Goligher J.C. (1977) Anterior resection of the rectum: One-layer and two-layer anastomoses. In: Malt R.A. (ed) Surgical techniques illustrated, Vol 2, No 2. Little, Brown, Boston, p 13

13. Hochenegg J. (1900) Meine Operationserfolge bie Rektumkarcinom. Wien Klin Wochenschr 13: 399

14. Kratzer G.L., Win M.S. (1970) Low anterior resection in cancer of the rectum. Am J. Surg 119: 649

15. Localio S.A. (1971) Abdominal–transsacral resection and anastomosis for midrectal carcinoma. Surg Gynecol Obstet 132: 123

16. Localio S.A. (1977) Abdominosacral rectal resection (right lateral exposure). In: Malt R.A. (ed) Surgical techniques illustrated, Vol 2, No 2. Little, Brown, Boston, p 37

17. Localio S.A., Eng K. (1975) Malignant tumors of the rectum. Curr Probl Surg (Sept) 12: 1

18. Localio S.A., Eng K., Gouge T.H., et al (1978) Abdominosacral resection for carcinoma of the midrectum: 10 years experience. Ann Surg 188: 475

19. Malt R.A. (ed) (1977) Surgical techniques illustrated, Vol 2, No 1. Little, Brown, Boston

20. Martin L.W., LeCoultre C., Schubert W.K. (1977) Total colectomy and mucosal protectomy with preservation of continence in ulcerative colitis. Ann Surg 186: 477

21. Mason A.Y. (1976) Selective surgery for carcinoma of the rectum. Aust NZ J Surg 46: 322

22. Mason A.Y. (1977) Transsphincteric surgery for lower rectal cancer. In: Malt R.A. (ed) Surgical techniques illustrated, Vol 2, No 2. Little, Brown, Boston, p 71

23. McLachlin A.D., Olsson L.S., Pitt D.F. (1976) Anterior anastomosis of the rectosigmoid colon: An experimental study. Surgery 80: 306

24. Parks A.G. (1977) Endoanal technique of low colonic anastomosis. In: Malt R.A. (ed) Surgical techniques illustrated, Vol 2, No 2. Little, Brown, Boston, p 63

25. Rodkey G.V. (1977) Abdominosacral resection of rectum (d'Allaines' exposure). In: Malt R.A. (ed) Surgical techniques illustrated, Vol 2, No 2. Little, Brown, Boston, p 49

26. Schweiger M., Schellerer W., Kiypers G. (1977) Continence after low anterior resection of the rectum. Langenbecks Arch Chir 343: 281

27. Soave F. (1964) Hirschsprung's disease: New surgical technique. Arch Dis Child 38: 116

28. Stewart W.R.C., Samson R.B. (1968) Rectal tube decompression of left-colon anastomosis. Dis Colon Rectum 11: 452

29. Swenson O. (1950) A new surgical treatment for Hirschsprung's disease. Surgery 28: 371

30. Waugh J.M., Miller E.M., Kurzweg F.T. (1954) Abdominoperineal resection with sphincter preservation for carcinoma of the midrectum. Arch Surg 68: 469

31. Yancey A.G., et al (1952) A modification of the Swenson technique for congenital megacolon. J Natl Med Assoc 44: 356

Diverticular Disease

10

Diverticular disease is an important cause of disability. It was rare a few decades ago, but at present, perhaps due to diet or genetic factors, it has become exceedingly common and has created very difficult problems in the management of colonic disease. The term includes the disease of diverticulosis, which is rarely symptomatic except for the occasional occurrence of massive hemorrhage, and diverticulitis, which is associated with all of the symptoms of inflammation as well as perforation, obstruction, and fistulization. In many instances the borderline between the two is very hazy and for that reason the term diverticular disease is preferred.

The disease is believed to arise because of hypertrophy of the muscle of the sigmoid (Fig. 10.1).[11] Segmental contractions eventuate that are believed to become so powerful that they cause the extrusion of mucosa through weak areas in the bowel wall, particularly along blood vessels.[13] Inflammation then follows with the attendant complications. Whether or not all cases follow this pattern is not clear. In many instances at operation the colonic muscle appears to be essentially normal but numerous diverticula are present. In other instances the muscle of the colon is extremely hypertrophic; such patients are quite symptomatic but there are relatively few diverticula. The latter condition has been described by several authors as the "prediverticular state," although there is no evidence that all cases of diverticulitis have progressed in this sequence.

The indications for operation are numerous.[12,16–18] Emergency procedures are required for perforation, obstruction, or hemorrhage, and elective procedures are performed for fistulization[6] or repeated episodes of discomfort due to the disease. With decreasing mortality there has been a broadening of the indications for operation, but it is important to emphasize that surgery for very loose indications will automatically lead to increased deaths from operations that possibly could have been avoided.

There is little question of the necessity for operation in patients with acute complications.[1–6,8,20–22] The indications for operation in other patients may have to be quite flexible; they are mediated by many factors, such as the patients' age, ability to follow a good regimen, general habitus and other diseases, and accessibility to the hospital. It is difficult, therefore, to lay down hard and fast rules concerning the indications for elective surgery. However, some of the features that we have found of importance will be listed.[22]

113

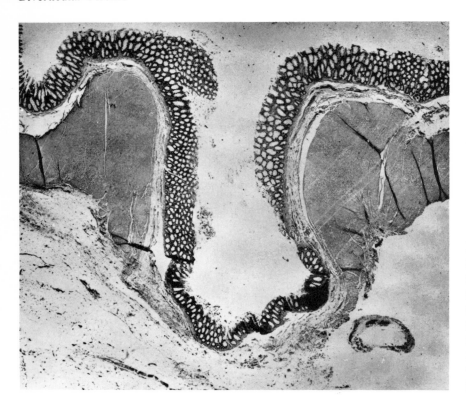

Fig. 10.1. Micrograph of a sigmoid diverticulum. Note the hypertrophy of the colon adjacent to the diverticulum and the absence of muscle in the diverticulum. An artery and vein lie in close apposition to the diverticulum, which is shown extending into the mesentery.

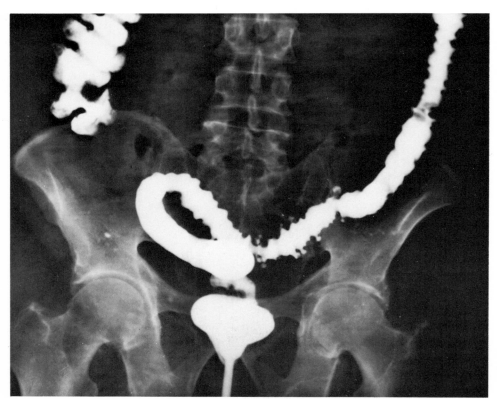

Fig. 10.2. Barium enema showing a typical picture of diverticulitis with obvious diverticula and spasm.

Certainly one attack of uncomplicated diverticulitis is not sufficient to warrant an operative procedure. The subsequent history of such patients is so variable that many of them can go many years or even indefinitely without another attack. However, two attacks with severe left lower quadrant pain, fever, and hospital admission for a few days with antibiotic treatment

114

within a period of 1–2 years would indicate a severe type of disease. Ordinarily such a patient should be operated upon in the belief that a one-stage operation could be done rather than a staged procedure, which might be required at a later date. The onset of diverticulitis in youth or in middle age below age 50 has also indicated severe disease, and such patients generally have required operations. The onset of urinary symptoms in a patient with known diverticulitis, usually noted in males or in females who have had a hysterectomy, may portend a bladder fistula and must be regarded as an indication for resection. Pneumaturia may occur with diabetes but usually means there is a vesicosigmoidal fistula. Some patients develop a subacute inflammatory process and a subsequent mass is palpable. Although some of these masses subside spontaneously, most patients who develop inflammation of this severity require an operation. Repeated attacks of minor bleeding for which no other cause can be found or chronic left lower quadrant discomfort, often alternating with diarrhea or constipation, may become so bothersome that operation is requested by the patient. Finally, in some instances, the barium enema shows severe deformity of the sigmoid (Fig. 10.2); since cancer may produce a very similar picture, operation is indicated on this basis alone. Unfortunately, colonoscopy cannot always differentiate between cancer and diverticulitis as severe deformity may limit the passage of the scope.

Operative Procedures

The operative procedures required for the acute complications of diverticulitis will be discussed in more detail in Chapters 15–17 and 20. However, the essential feature of all operations, whether elective or emergent, is the removal of the segment of bowel that has led to the disease.

The underlying problem of muscular hypertrophy has led Reilly and some other surgeons to consider the possibility of a long sigmoid myotomy as a curative procedure for the disease.[10,15] This operation is somewhat similar to the Rammstedt pyloromyotomy. However, because this operation has been followed by many complications and some mortality, it has lost popular support.

Except in some instances of perforation or obstruction, the proper operation involves a resection and anastomosis. There are several points in the technique that should be considered.

First, the differential diagnosis between diverticulitis and cancer may be difficult. Since an operation for diverticulitis does not necessarily involve the removal of large amounts of mesentery it is in some respects a much less radical procedure than that for cancer. Consequently, the surgeon usually will save a reasonable portion of the mesentery and in particular retain the inferior mesenteric artery. The specimen that has been resected should be examined immediately by the pathologist so that if any unsuspected carcinoma is present a proper cancer operation may be carried out.

The second consideration involves the peculiar difficulties of the anastomosis. If the anastomosis is made through an area of muscular hypertrophy, the lumen is much smaller than it is with cancer, and thus the anastomotic technique must be more delicate. Every attempt must be made to isolate a section of bowel that does not contain diverticula. Assuming that a two-layer anastomosis is made, it should be done in such a fashion that an obstructing diaphragm is not formed. Interrupted sutures in both layers of the anastomosis are essential if the bowel is narrow.

115

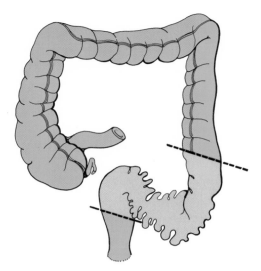

Fig. 10.3. Extent of resection for diverticular disease localized to the sigmoid. The lower line of resection is above the pelvic floor. (Excised area is tan.)

The third consideration is the amount of colon that should be removed. At least 90% of all diverticula that require operation occur in the sigmoid colon. The surgeon must obtain essentially normal bowel both above and below for the anastomosis. With diverticulitis there is often a redundant loop of sigmoid stuck deep in the pelvis. This must be elevated and the anastomosis placed below any obvious pathology. Since diverticula very rarely exist below the peritoneal floor, it should always be possible to have the anastomosis at least a few centimeters above the pelvic floor (Fig. 10.3). If a longer distal stump is to be left, it is essential that the inferior mesenteric artery remain in position to ensure an adequate blood supply.

The appropriate area for anastomosis in the proximal colon must be determined by the presence of an adequate lumen, minimal muscular hypertrophy, and a limited number of diverticula. For this reason it is often necessary to free the splenic flexure and anastomose the distal transverse colon to the rectum.

The fourth consideration, the amount of colon that should be removed, depends upon the above features. As time has passed, more radical operations have been carried out for diverticular disease; in many instances a total left colectomy has turned out to be a safer procedure than a localized sigmoid resection (Fig. 10.4). A total colectomy with ileorectal anastomosis is recommended for massive bleeding if there are diverticula throughout the colon (Fig. 10.5; see also Chap. 20).

Finally, the applicability of the one-stage resection and anastomosis must be considered. Frequently small pericolonic abscesses are encountered that are excised totally. As long as both ends of the colon to be anastomosed are normal, a one-stage operation may be done. On the other hand, in the presence of extensive local or general peritonitis, anastomosis is likely to be followed by leakage, as shown by Schrock et al.[19] A staged operation, described in Chapter 16, is much more satisfactory.

If an anastomosis has been made correctly the patient should be entirely relieved of symptoms. This occurs even though there are proximal diverticula left. In all cases it is to be expected that further diverticula will develop in other sections of the bowel with advancing age. There seems, however, to be no reason to consider a total colectomy for patients with

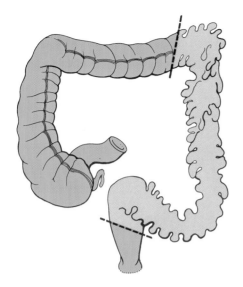 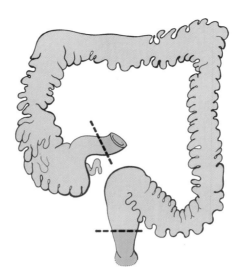

Fig. 10.4.   Left colectomy for diverticular disease. The proximal resection line is in the distal transverse colon and the lower one is just above the pelvic floor. (Excised area is tan.)

Fig. 10.5.   Total colectomy for diverticular disease with massive hemorrhage. The distal line of resection should be within the reach of the sigmoidoscope; but if no diverticula are present in the distal end, it is preferably 20 cm above the anal verge in order to diminish postoperative diarrhea. If the sigmoid is involved with diverticular disease the resection line must be just above the pelvic floor. (Excised area is tan.)

diverticular disease except under very special circumstances—for example, when the operation is carried out for massive bleeding, when the diverticular disease is extremely extensive, or when technical problems make it impossible to secure an anastomosis between proximal colon and distal rectum, making it necessary to use the ileum for this procedure.

After the patient has recovered from the original resection and anastomosis, the necessity for a second operative procedure for further diverticular disease is extremely rare, despite the fact that further diverticula do form in the bowel. This lends a good deal of credence to the theory that the mechanical shape and comparatively narrow lumen of the sigmoid are very important contributing factors to the symptomatology of the disease.

Giant Cysts of the Sigmoid

Giant cysts of the sigmoid average 5–15 cm in diameter and may be large enough that, on a plain abdominal film, they appear to fill the entire upper abdomen. They are presumed to comprise a variety of diverticular disease.[7,9] In our experience two distinct types can be identified. In the first the whole colonic wall is present in the diverticulum. It becomes greatly thickened from inflammation and may contain a large fecalith. Such a giant diverticulum is illustrated in Figure 10.6; this is much more typical of a congenital diverticulum of the ileocecal region since it contains all coats of the bowel.

The second type consists of a very thin-walled, gas-filled cyst (Fig. 10.7). Ferrucci has speculated that it is produced by a ball-valve mecha-

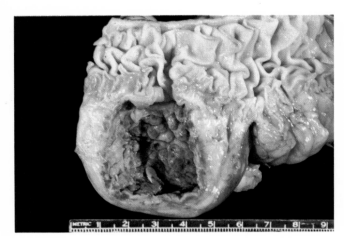

Fig. 10.6. Operative specimen of a resected sigmoid showing a giant diverticulum containing a fecalith. This patient, whose only symptoms were recurrent attacks of chills and fever, was cured by a sigmoid resection.

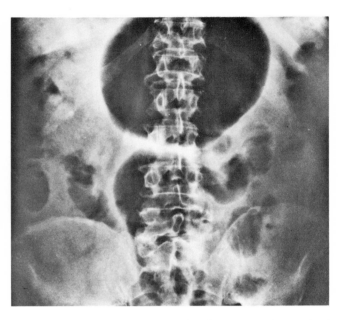

Fig. 10.7. Plain abdominal film demonstrating a giant sigmoid diverticulum.

nism at the mouth of a diverticulum.[9] The intracolonic pressure forces gas into the diverticulum but the ball valve prevents deflation; consequently, the cyst gradually becomes larger and larger. It is necessary to carry out a resection of the area that is involved by diverticular disease for cure.[6a]

Diverticular Disease of the Right Colon

Diverticular disease of the right colon is comparatively rare in the continental United States and comprises only about 3% of all the cases that we have seen. On the other hand, in the state of Hawaii it is extremely common and has often required emergency operation.

The disease is easily confused with appendicitis or, intraoperatively, with carcinoma. The surgeon may be in a quandary as to the proper operative procedure. We believe that an emergency right colectomy can be done with much less hazard than any attempt to define the lesion more accurately by such maneuvers as opening the bowel or biopsy. The extent of the resection is shown in Figure 10.8. The safety of immediate one-stage resection and anastomosis in the unprepared colon has been shown by the figures of Peck et al.: of 108 operative cases, 70 had resections, often as emergencies with unprepared colons, and there were no operative deaths.[14]

It is of interest that none of the patients in our series who have had operations for diverticulitis of the right colon have returned with later complications of the disease originating on the left side.

There are instances in which a truly congenital diverticulum of the right colon is found. This is usually a single diverticulum located just above the ileocecal valve. It may be encountered in young people as well as those in middle age. There have been some reports of local resection and closure of the bowel; however, it seems apparent that if there is a great deal of inflammation around such a diverticulum it would be safer to consider a resection and anastomosis of the right colon.

118

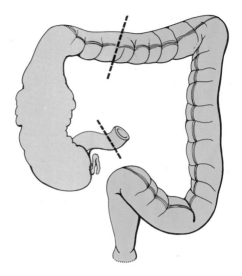

Fig. 10.8. Extent of resection for diverticular disease of the right colon. (Excised area is tan.) The anastomosis will be between terminal ileum and mid-transverse colon.

Postoperative Complications and Mortality

The most prominent postoperative complication peculiar to surgery for diverticular disease is anastomotic dehiscence. Often there is a tendency to push the use of a one-stage resection and anastomosis too vigorously, and unless operative conditions are ideal there may be leakage from the anastomosis a few days after operation. An immediate transverse colostomy and drainage of the local abscess is wise at the first indication of unusual pain or localized tenderness. If the surgeon delays and an abscess or peritonitis results, the outcome is likely to be poor even with wide drainage.

If the anastomosis has been made through inflammatory tissue, at the site of a diverticulum, or in the presence of peritonitis, the major signs of an anastomotic leak may not appear but a fistulous tract may develop. This may be an unsuspected finding, demonstrated only by a barium enema. Occasionally it will be large enough to burrow out through the abdominal incision or to form a fistula at some other site. In such instances it is necessary to carry out a second resection and anastomosis of the colon, probably under the protection of a transverse colostomy.

Late strictures of the anastomosis have been noted. The most important predisposing conditions are the involvement of the very narrow lumen of the bowel by diverticulitis and the presence of concomitant inflammatory disease such as Crohn's disease.

The mortality of operations for diverticular disease has fallen greatly in the last few decades. Prior to 1942 the mortality of resection and anastomosis determined by Smithwick at the Massachusetts General Hospital was nearly 20%.[20] The last compilation of figures by Rodkey and Welch showed that for elective operations the mortality was 0.8%, although for emergency operations it was approximately 10 times greater.[17] At St. Mark's Hospital Morson reported only 1 death in some 200 cases. This low mortality and the disability incurred by staged operations have led some surgeons to be quite radical in their advocacy of early operation for diverticular disease. We believe, however, as discussed above, that such an attitude must be accepted with caution.

119

References

1. Bacon H.E., Shindo K. (1971) Surgical management of peridiverticulitis of the colon. Surg Gynecol Obstet 132: 1049
2. Botsford T.W., Zollinger R.M. Jr. (1969) Diverticulitis of the colon. Surg Gynecol Obstet 128: 1209
3. Canter J.W., Shorb P.E. Jr. (1971) Acute perforation of colonic diverticula associated with prolonged adrenocorticosteroid therapy. Am J Surg 121: 46
4. Case Records of the Massachusetts General Hospital (1977) Weekly Clinicopathological Exercises. Case 18-1977. Fever, jaundice and right-upper-quadrant tenderness in a 69-year-old woman. N Engl J Med 296: 1051
5. Ching-Shen L. (1973) Suppurative pylephlebitis and liver abscess complicating colonic diverticulitis: Report of two cases and review of literature. Mt Sinai J Med 40: 48, 1973
6. Colcock B.P. (1971) Diverticular disease of the colon. Saunders, Philadelphia
6a. Gallagher J.J., Welch J.P. (1979) Giant diverticula of the sigmoid colon: A review of differential diagnosis and operative management. Arch Surg 114(9): 1079
7. Johns E.R., Hartley M.G. (1976) Giant gas filled cysts of the sigmoid colon: A report of two cases. Br J Radiol 49: 930
8. Juler G.L., Dietrick W.R., Eisenman J.I. (1976) Intramesenteric perforation of sigmoid diverticulitis with nonfatal venous intravasation. Am J Surg 132: 653
9. Kempczinski R.F., Ferrucci J.T. Jr. (1974) Giant sigmoid diverticula: A review. Ann Surg 180: 864
10. Kettlewell M.G.W., Moloney G.E. (1977) Combined horizontal and longitudinal colomyotomy for diverticular disease: Preliminary report. Dis Colon Rectum 20: 24
11. Morson B.C. (1963) The muscle abnormality in diverticular disease of the sigmoid colon. Br J Radiol 36: 385
12. Oetting H.K., Kramer N.E., Branch W.E. (1955) Subcutaneous emphysema of gastrointestinal origin. Am J Med 19: 872
13. Painter N.S., Truelove S.C. (1964) Intraluminal pressure pattern in diverticulosis of the colon. Gut 5: 365
14. Peck D.A., Labat R., Waite V.C. (1968) Diverticular disease of the right colon. Dis Colon Rectum 11: 49
15. Reilly M. (1969) Sigmoid myotomy: Interim report. Proc R Soc Med 62: 715
16. Rodkey G.V., Welch C.E. (1969) Diverticulitis and diverticulosis of the colon. In: Turell R. (ed) Diseases of the colon and anorectum, 2nd edn, Vol 2. Saunders, Philadelphia, p 697
17. Rodkey G.V., Welch C.E. (1974) Colonic diverticular disease with surgical treatment. A study of 338 cases. Surg Clin North Am 54: 655
18. Rugtiv G.M. (1975) Diverticulitis: Selective surgical management. Am J Surg 130: 219
19. Schrock T.R., Deveney C.W., Dunphy J.E. (1973) Factors contributing to leakage of colonic anastomoses. Ann Surg 177: 513
20. Smithwick R.H. (1942) Experience with the surgical management of diverticulitis of the sigmoid. Ann Surg 115: 969
21. Watkins G.L., Oliver G.A. (1971) Surgical treatment of acute perforative sigmoid diverticulitis. Surgery 69: 215
22. Welch C.E., Allen A.W., Donaldson G.A. (1953) An appraisal of resection of the colon for diverticulitis of the sigmoid. Ann Surg 138: 332

Ulcerative Colitis and Crohn's Disease

11

Ulcerative colitis and Crohn's disease are closely related.[20,21,50] By clinical symptomatology and later confirmation by pathologic examination, a differentiation between the two is possible in approximately three-quarters of the cases. In the others the differentiation may be very difficult or impossible. The diagnostic criteria have been considered by Schachter et al.[42]

Ulcerative Colitis

From the surgical point of view several features of ulcerative colitis are extremely important.[22] First, the terminal ileum and the remainder of the small bowel are always normal and remain so after excision of the colon. Second, since all cases of ulcerative colitis ultimately will involve the entire colon, any operative procedures that are designed to save a portion of the colon almost certainly are doomed to later failure.

Ulcerative colitis usually begins in the rectal segment and extends rather rapidly throughout the remainder of the colon. Manifestations include diarrhea, bleeding (which may be massive), toxic megacolon, perforation, and the late development of cancer. Intestinal obstruction, fistulas, and large inflammatory masses are typical of Crohn's disease rather than ulcerative colitis. As the disease progresses systemic symptoms become much more common. Loss of weight and failure to thrive are common. Later systemic symptoms include the development of ulcers of the skin, particularly in the lower legs. These ulcers may progress to deep involvement including the underlying fascia or even muscle. Bacteriologic studies are unrewarding since the cultures usually are sterile. Relief can be obtained only when the colon has been removed. Uveitis likewise responds satisfactorily to colectomy. Rheumatoid arthritis is a frequent accompaniment of the disease; although colectomy cannot ensure relief from the symptoms of arthritis, they are often greatly relieved by it.

The onset of acute idiopathic ulcerative colitis often occurs in teenagers or very young adults.[12,13,15,17,47] Nevertheless, it may occur in children or adults in middle or later life. The first attack may be fulminant and require colectomy at the time of the first admission. However, with the advent of steroid therapy most patients can be relieved of the first symptoms and remarkably enough may do well thereafter. Since there is often a favorable response to steroids, many physicians may be tempted to carry on such therapy beyond reasonable limits, particularly when the patient realizes that colectomy will mean a permanent ileostomy. Thus, except in emergency situations, the patient's acceptance of an ileostomy becomes an important consideration prior to operation.

Indications for surgery include diarrhea refractory to medical therapy, repeated attacks of hemorrhage, toxic megacolon, perforation, and cancer. The development of extensive pseudopolyposis does not necessarily warrant colectomy since there may be a remarkable degree of recovery in many such colons; however, in general, extensive pseudopolyposis indicates adamant disease that requires surgery.

Whether or not prophylactic colectomy should be carried out to prevent later cancer of the colon is a moot question.[14] All studies indicate that the colon involved with ulcerative colitis is much more likely to develop cancer than the normal colon. Estimates of the late development of cancer run as high as 40%. Occasionally cancer of the colon may develop in bowel that previously had been involved by ulcerative colitis. In general, however, the features conducive to the development of cancer include wide involvement of the entire colon, onset at an early age, and unremitting symptoms. Cancer can develop before the age of 10 in such colons and remains a threat throughout the life of the patient. Prophylactic colectomy to avoid cancer should be considered in this group of patients. Morson and Pang have indicated that biopsies of rectal mucosa may identify the colons at risk of developing cancer[36]; to date our pathologists have not found this possible. The colonoscope will secure even more satisfactory biopsies.

Crohn's Disease

Crohn's disease is much more complex than ulcerative colitis.[6,8,10,11,46,52] In many instances it may be localized entirely to the colon, in which case the operation of total proctocolectomy with permanent ileostomy may be expected to give excellent results. In other cases there may be isolated areas of involvement of the colon. The disease may be limited, for example, to the right colon, the transverse, the descending colon, or even the rectum. When the rectal segment appears to be entirely normal, a segmental resection and anastomosis often can lead to relief for many years. When the rectal segment and lower sigmoid are involved, a combined abdominoperineal resection with a sigmoid colostomy may likewise be the proper operation.

Unfortunately, many cases of Crohn's disease of the colon also involve the small intestine. A typical pattern consists of Crohn's disease of the terminal ileum and the right colon, in which case segmental resection is desirable. Severe involvement of the terminal ileum may be accompanied by skip areas in the upper small bowel; resection of the ileum may lead to regression of the upper areas. Sometimes the whole intestinal tract is so widely involved with the disease that no surgical procedure is possible; intravenous hyperalimentation and a period of complete rest may be the most satisfactory treatment under these conditions.[41]

The indications for surgery for colonic disease, according to Farmer et al., are as follows: in 26% of patients, poor response to medical therapy, in 23% internal fistula and abscess, in 20% toxic megacolon, and in 19% perianal disease.[15]

Crohn's disease is much more likely to be complicated by fistulas and large inflammatory masses than is ulcerative colitis. On the other hand, massive hemorrhage is uncommon and toxic megacolon occurs much less frequently than with ulcerative colitis.[26] The development of cancer has been reported in both the terminal ileum and the colon in cases of long-standing Crohn's disease. For example, Greenstein et al. reported seven cases that occurred in excluded segments of bowel; one occurred in the cecum and two in the sigmoid.[24] However, the danger of cancer of the colon is not nearly as great as it is in longstanding cases of ulcerative colitis.

Because there is a high incidence of recurrence and of these other complications, approximately 75% of cases of Crohn's disease eventually require surgery, compared to 25% of those patients with ulcerative colitis. The results of operation likewise vary considerably. With ulcerative colitis, once the entire colon has been successfully removed, the chances of cure are 100%. With Crohn's disease, particularly when anastomoses have been made, the tendency for recurrence is high. The recurrence nearly always takes place proximal to the line of anastomosis. Figures on the incidence of recurrence vary considerably depending upon the economic status of the patients. In the ward population nearly all have demonstrated recurrence. In private patients who are well nourished the incidence of recurrence after segmental resection appears to be at least 25% within a 7-year period. When Crohn's disease has been localized to the colon and treated by total proctocolectomy, the recurrence rate has been reported by Glotzer et al. to be low.[20] However, few observers are so optimistic.[31] Greenstein and co-workers followed 30 patients with Crohn's colitis and 130 with ileocolitis. 100 patients required operation, and by the 15th year after operation there was a cumulative reoperation rate of 89%.[23]

Total proctocolectomy for ulcerative colitis was introduced by Miller and co-workers in 1949.[35] This procedure, which is described below, is applicable to both ulcerative colitis and Crohn's disease.

Staged procedures are still used in certain instances. The hope that an ileostomy will lead to subsidence of colonic inflammatory disease has not been fulfilled.[39] At times the rectum has been left in place after a subtotal colectomy in the hope that continuity can be re-established[1,3,30]; studies of Massachusetts General Hospital patients by Moss and Keddie have shown that this is impractical.[37] In another series Binder et al. found that 73.5% of these patients required later resection of the rectum.[7] It should be noted that it is impossible to examine such rectal stumps carefully and the danger of cancer is always present.

Operative Procedures

Ileostomy

The early surgical attacks on ulcerative colitis were limited to ileostomy alone. In many instances the symptoms were not relieved and the late development of cancer became a very important consideration. In modern days, therefore, if any surgical procedure is to be carried out, a colectomy is a necessary portion of the therapy. With the advent of excellent preoperative preparation, adequate supply of blood, and other adjuvant measures, staged procedures that involve only an ileostomy, and later a subtotal colectomy, have in general been replaced, except in dire emergencies, by a total proctocolectomy with permanent ileostomy.

The permanent ileostomy that is described in this chapter is tolerated extremely well. The development of enterostomal specialists and of numerous appliances has made it possible for almost all ileostomies to be ac-

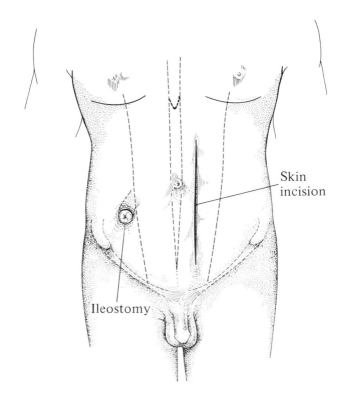

Fig. 11.1. Total proctocolectomy for ulcerative colitis or Crohn's disease: site of incision and ileostomy. The ileostomy is made at McBurney's point in thin patients, but in obese individuals the site should be marked prior to operation when the patient is standing to be certain that the stoma is high enough so that it will not be beneath a skin fold.

cepted by patients. Nevertheless, the permanent application of an appliance still remains a deterrent to certain persons. For this reason further attempts to provide anal ileostomies have been made, and the "continent ileostomy" has been developed.

Total Proctocolectomy with Permanent Ileostomy

This is the operation of choice for ulcerative colitis. The abdomen is opened through a generous left paramedian incision. Right-sided incisions should be avoided since they will interfere with the location of the ileostomy. In the normal person the ileostomy will be placed approximately at McBurney's point (Fig. 11.1). If the patient is unduly obese it is advisable to mark the projected site of the ileostomy on the abdomen when the patient is erect so that when he is on the table accurate placement may be obtained.

After the abdomen is opened careful exploration is carried out (Fig. 11.2). This must be performed with extreme care because of the risk of perforation of a badly inflamed colon. Although the most dangerous spot is immediately below the splenic flexure, perforation may occur at any other area. Concomitant disease of the hepatobiliary tract is not uncommon and may progress after a colectomy has been done. Gallstones, sclerosing cholangitis, or hepatitis may be found. Except in unusual circumstances, even

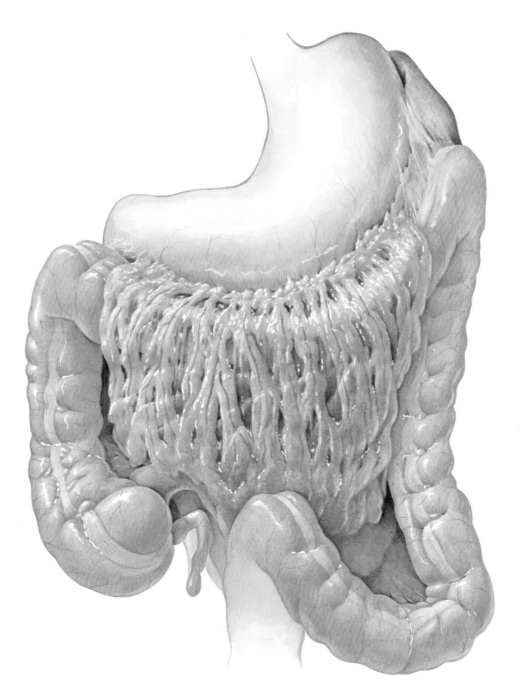

Fig. 11.2. Appearance of the abdomen prior to resection. The dissection is usually begun in the transverse colon. If there is marked distention the colon is decompressed by a long sump sucker introduced through the very distal ileum.

if gallstones are found, no attempt is made to remove them at this time because the colectomy will be a very serious procedure.

Dissection is usually started in the area of the transverse colon where mobilization is easiest (Fig. 11.3). Numerous lymph nodes may be found along the course of the colon, but unless there is some serious question that malignancy may be present, it is not necessary to carry out the wide excision of the mesentery that would be required otherwise. This is partic-

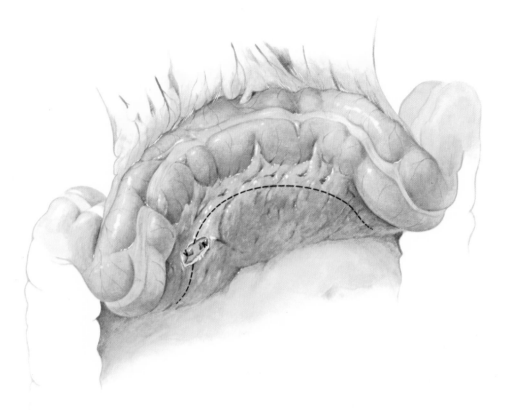

Fig. 11.3.   The omentum must be removed along with the colon if there is a sug-
gestion of cancer. The dissection is started caudad to the gastroepiploic arteries.
The colon is then turned upward and the mesentery is divided along the broken
line. If cancer is present, as much mesentery as possible is removed. If there is no
evidence of cancer, a longer section is left.

ularly true in the region of the right and transverse colons. By saving as
much of the right colonic mesentery as possible it will be possible to fix the
ileostomy in a much better fashion than if a wide excision of the mesentery
had been carried out. Furthermore, if adequate mesentery is left along the
transverse colon it will be possible to close the opening into the lesser peritoneal sac by merely suturing the omentum to the transverse colon mesentery after the colon has been excised. Usually the dissection is carried reasonably close to the bowel in the transverse colon. After the transverse
colon has been freed the right colon is elevated in a similar fashion (Fig.
11.4). The major portion of the mesentery is retained. The sigmoid colon is
mobilized and dissection proceeds upward along the descending colon and
from the midtransverse colon toward the splenic flexure in order that the
most dangerous point of the dissection may be approached with great care
(Fig. 11.5). After the colon is freed down to the intraperitoneal rectum, a
decision can be made as to whether or not the perineal portion of the operation should be carried out simultaneously. If the condition of the patient
has deteriorated it may be advisable to divide the bowel in the lower sigmoid and bring the lower end out through the lower end of the abdominal
incision rather than proceed with a total colectomy. However, any retained
colon may cause persistence of symptoms, diarrhea, and even massive
bleeding so that the retention of an area of inflamed bowel carries hazards
in itself. Except under unusual circumstances it is wise to proceed with the
remainder of the proctocolectomy.

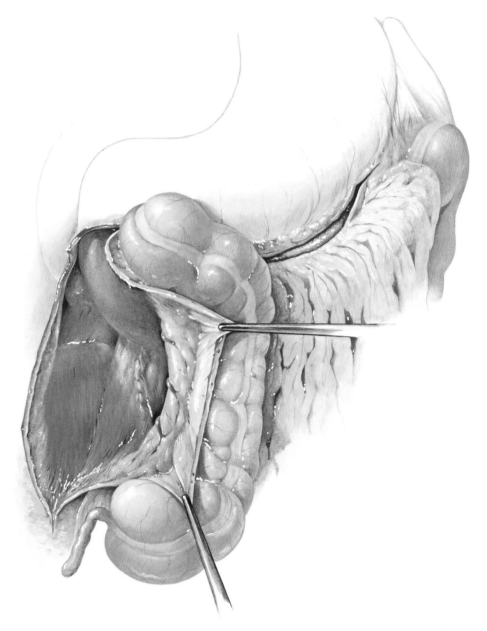

Fig. 11.4. After freeing the transverse colon the surgeon mobilizes the right colon by cutting the lateral white line and turning the colon forward on the duodenum.

The most bloody portion of the operation occurs in the pelvis and several units of blood may be lost. The dissection will differ from that in the combined abdominoperineal excision for cancer since it is advisable to retain as much of the mesentery of the distal sigmoid and intraperitoneal rectum as possible in order to have tissues left to fill the presacral space and to prevent injury to the sympathetic and parasympathetic nerves. This requires repeated division of the smaller vessels: The inferior mesenteric artery will not necessarily have to be removed (Fig. 11.6). Dissection is carried to as deep a level as possible either on the prostate or vagina anteriorly (Fig. 11.7). The middle hemorrhoidal vessels are cut and ligated and dissection is carried distally down to the levators.

The terminal ileum is then divided between clamps 10–15 cm proximal to the ileocecal valve. The lower end of the rectum is divided after

127

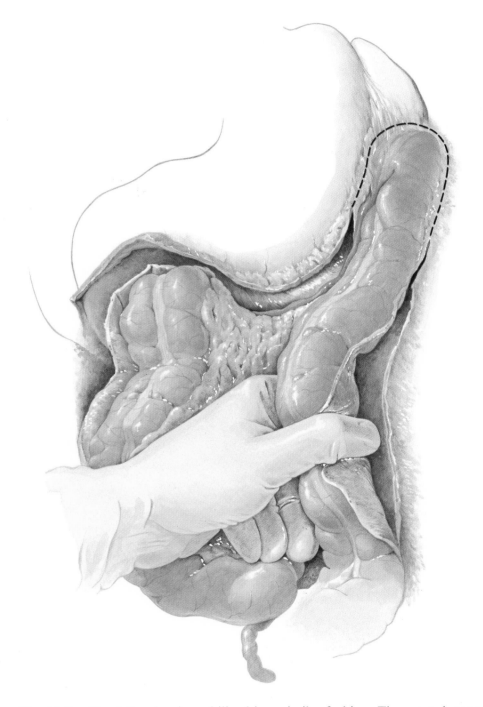

Fig. 11.5. The left colon is mobilized in a similar fashion. The most dangerous portion of the dissection—the splenic flexure (shown by the broken line)—is then approached.

application of a DeMartel clamp and the specimen is removed (Fig. 11.8). An examination should immediately be carried out by the pathologist to be certain that no cancer has been overlooked. The pelvic floor is closed with two layers of sutures (Fig. 11.9).

Attention is then turned to the formation of the ileostomy. A circular incision is made at McBurney's point, and a core of skin and subcutaneous fat down to the rectus fascia is removed. The fascia is incised in a cruciate

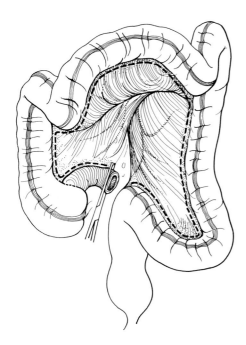

Fig. 11.6. The inferior mesenteric artery and the sigmoid mesentery should be removed if cancer is suspected; otherwise the individual vessels may be divided close to the colon, leaving the inferior mesenteric artery intact. In the absence of cancer the dissection follows the broken line.

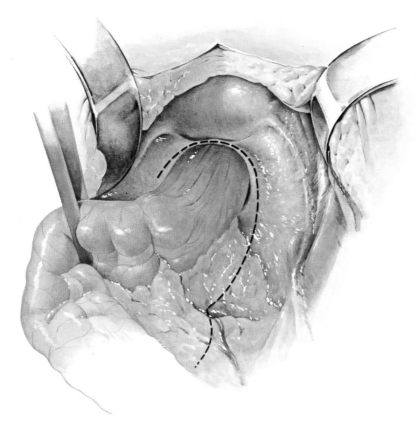

Fig. 11.7. The pelvic peritoneum is incised. The dissection (along the broken line) is kept relatively close to the colon posteriorly, assuming that cancer is not present.

129

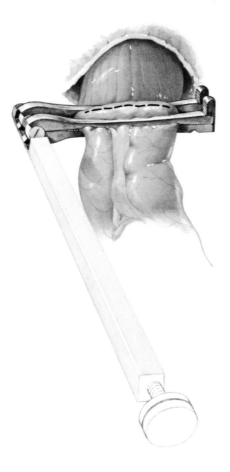

Fig. 11.8. The rectum is mobilized by sharp and blunt dissection down to the coccyx. A DeMartel clamp is applied and the center section of the clamp is removed. The handle is then removed and the bowel is divided between the remaining two clamps along the broken line.

fashion, the muscle is split bluntly, and the peritoneum is opened in this area. Two fingers should be passed through the opening, which should provide an adequate exit for the stoma. The terminal ileum is withdrawn through this area (Fig. 11.10). It should be withdrawn at least 5 cm from the margin of the skin. This will not be difficult unless the mesentery is fat. If it is, some vessels in the mesentery must be divided. Great care must be taken, however, to avoid devascularization of the stoma. The trap lateral to the ileostomy is then closed by a series of silk or cotton sutures that unite the mesentery of the right colon to the lateral peritoneum. Occasionally this closure can be performed caudal to the ileostomy but it will almost always be required cephalad. This measure will completely obliterate any trap and prevent the herniation of bowel around the stoma.

The abdominal wall is closed and the ileostomy is matured by the Brooke technique. The ileum is sutured carefully to the subcutaneous fascia with several interrupted catgut sutures (Fig. 11.11a). Care must be taken to be sure that these sutures do not penetrate the lumen of the bowel. The stoma is then everted and the mucosa is sutured to the skin with a series of interrupted 000 catgut sutures following the technique described by Brooke (Fig. 11.11b).[9] At this time the stoma should be approximately 2.5 cm in length.

The patient is next placed on the right side. The anus is closed with a purse-string suture (Fig. 11.12a). The perineal phase is begun by making a circular incision close to the margin of the rectum and removing as small an amount of perirectal tissue as possible (Fig. 11.12b). Dissection is carried

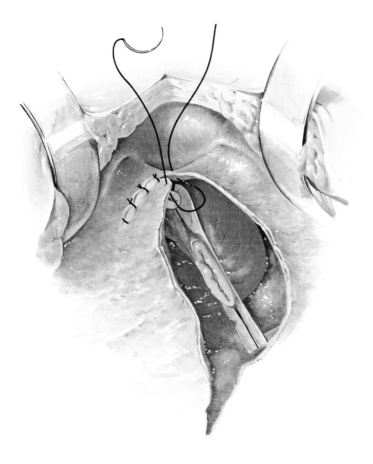

Fig. 11.9. The pelvic peritoneum is closed above the rectum.

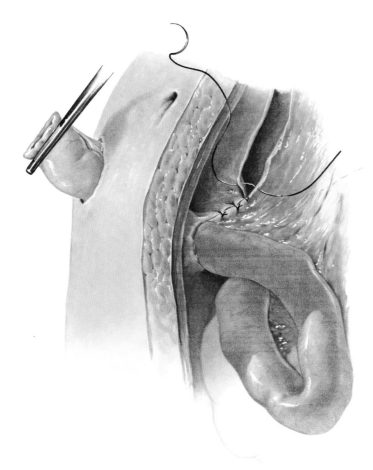

Fig. 11.10. The ileum is then withdrawn through a circular incision that is made near McBurney's point. The trap above the ileac mesentery is closed with interrupted sutures.

131

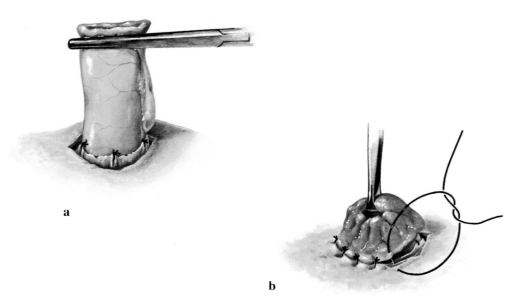

Fig. 11.11a and b.   Abdominal phase of ileostomy by the Brooke technique. a. The ileum has been sutured to the peritoneum prior to closure of the incision. The ileum is withdrawn for a distance of approximately 5 cm. b. The mucosa of the ileum is everted, and the ileostomy is completed by suture of the mucosa to the skin margins.

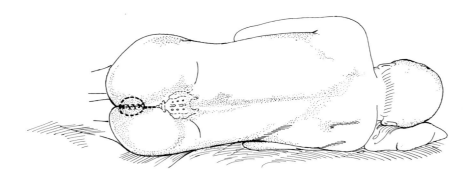

Fig. 11.12a–c.   Perineal phase of ileostomy. a. The patient is placed on the right side, and the anus is closed with a purse-string suture.

upward until the previous plane of abdominal dissection is encountered. The whole specimen is then removed (Fig. 11.12c).

Unless there has been gross contamination, the perineum can be closed with a suction catheter. However, if there has been extensive perirectal inflammation or contamination at the time of operation, it is well to leave the perineum open to prevent any retroperitoneal sepsis.

Several variations in the technique described above have been employed by various surgeons. Some of the important ones are as follows:

1. In cases in which the colon is distended it is advisable to decompress it before starting the operation. This can be done in an aseptic fash-

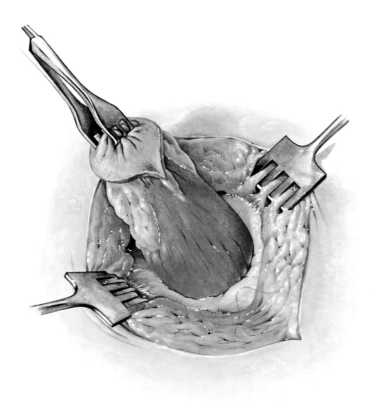

Fig. 11.12b. An incision is made about the anus extending up to the coccyx and a small amount of perirectal tissue is removed. The dissection is kept close to the rectal wall.

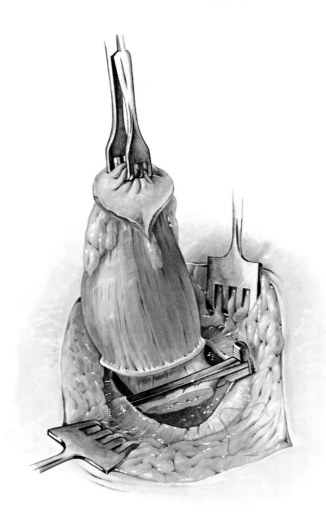

Fig. 11.12c. The rectum and clamp are removed. The incision is closed about one or two stuffed Penrose drains.

133

ion by introducing a sump sucker through the terminal ileum into the right colon through the ileocecal valve. The area in which the sump sucker has been inserted will be excised at the time of the removal of the terminal ileum. This will allow complete decompression of the right colon. If necessary, a similar incision can be made in the transverse and descending colons.

2. Some surgeons have brought the terminal ileum posterior to the peritoneum and then out through the ordinary exit at McBurney's point. This is presumed to prevent prolapse of the ileostomy and pericolostomy hernias. However, since ileostomy prolapse is extremely rare when the mesentery has been fixed by the method described, in our opinion this modification does not seem necessary. Since a retroperitoneal ileostomy is more difficult to take down, it is probably contraindicated after colectomy for Crohn's disease, in which recurrence in the ileum is possible.

3. Closure of the pelvic peritoneum may be omitted. The small bowel is allowed to prolapse into the true pelvis and rest upon the pelvic floor that has been reconstructed from the perineal side by closure of the levators. Such incisions are closed with temporary drainage by a sump placed through the abdominal wall down deep in the pelvis. Warshaw et al. have reported a series of cases in which this method has succeeded very well without any increase in intestinal obstruction.[51] There is, however, the possibility that the risk of adhesive obstruction will be greater if raw spaces are left in the pelvis than if the peritoneal closure had been effected. This method might have the advantage of allowing more rapid healing of the perineum, and, since the peritoneal cavity is much more tolerant of infection than the retroperitoneal space, it might prevent the formation of some of the longstanding retroperitoneal abscesses that sometimes occur when the peritoneum has been closed from above. This method certainly deserves a throrough trial since the early experience has indicated that it is valuable.

4. Some surgeons have advocated the retention of the normal anus and rectal sphincter, having cored out all mucosa down to it. In some instances we have seen retroperitoneal abscesses follow this procedure.

Complications of Total Proctocolectomy

Complications after this operation are so frequent that they will be discussed in detail.

Intestinal Obstruction This is by far the most common serious complication following total proctocolectomy. The incidence of adhesive obstruction is very high due to the wide areas of denuded peritoneum and the numerous ligatures that must be placed along the mesentery. Pelvic adhesions have been particularly troublesome. If the closure of the trap lateral to the ileostomy has not been adequate, prolapse of the loop of bowel around it may lead to a strangulating obstruction and require an emergency operation.

Most of the cases of intestinal obstruction occur within the first 2 weeks after surgery. The possibility of such a problem, however, remains an increased hazard for a protracted period of time; it usually occurs within the first year after operation, but may occur at any time.

Problems Referable to the Ileostomy[4,9,25]

1. Necrosis: If the stoma has been completely devitalized, it may become necrotic and require complete revision. Fortunately, since the blood supply of the ileum is usually remarkably good, even if the stoma appears somewhat blue at the time of operation or during the next few days, sufficient circulation will be regained. Frank gangrene, however, requires immediate revision.

2. Ileostomy prolapse: This has been almost entirely eliminated by the use of the accurate closure of the trap lateral to the ileostomy. If it should occur despite that maneuver and become troublesome, a relaparotomy with the plication of the two or three distal loops of ileum to form a buttress against the abdominal wall has been recommended as a method to prevent it. Retroperitoneal placement of the terminal ileum will eliminate this hazard.

3. Fistula from the ileostomy: This may occur with Crohn's disease but is extremely uncommon after surgery for ulcerative colitis. It nearly always signifies further disease in the terminal ileum. When this is encountered a formal laparotomy with further excision of the terminal ileum is indicated.

4. Peristomal hernia: This is a common complication. A loop of bowel protrudes into the abdominal wall beside the stoma and produces the usual physical findings of a hernia. This may be a serious problem because the hernia may incarcerate or strangulate and require operative intervention. Generally, however, peri-ileostomy hernias are asymptomatic. They are, by the same token, extremely difficult to repair. Transplantation of the ileostomy to another site in the abdominal wall, such as the left lower quadrant, has been required in some instances.

5. Ileostomy stenosis: This was a very common complication before stomas were matured according to the Brooke technique. A rim of granulation tissue appeared near the tip of the stoma. This led to a very marked stenosis and a typical squirting ileostomy in which diarrhea developed with the forceful expulsion of large volumes of intestinal fluid. The problem was easily solved by dilatation of the stoma or by cutting the "bishop's collar" that surrounded the stoma. This complication is not seen at the present time when stomas are matured in the usual fashion. However, if an ileostomy in the early postoperative phase is found to function poorly with the continued discharge of large amounts of fluid rather than the conversion within a few days to semisolid contents, the possibility of obstruction at some point either near the tip of the stoma or at the peritoneal opening must be considered. This can be confirmed by the introduction of a catheter. This maneuver may be definitive since once the immediate postoperative edema subsides, the lumen may be entirely adequate.

6. Persistent diarrhea: Persistent diarrhea is usually a result of partial obstruction. Usually the administration of diphenoxylate hydrochloride with atropine sulfate (Lomotil) and a low-roughage diet will result in improvement. Matolo and Wolfman reversed a segment of terminal ileum in a recalcitrant case, with relief.[34]

7. Bleeding: Adson and Fulton have reported bleeding from an ileal stoma due to portal hypertension.[2]

Late Complications The important late complication after proctocolectomy for ulcerative colitis is slow healing of the perineal incision. Several factors contribute to this delay. If there has been a wide excision of pericolonic and perirectal tissues, a large dead space may be left in the perineum. This is involved in inflammatory change, so that a deep sinus tract may be left running anterior to the coccyx and sacrum. As this cavity becomes thick walled, collapse becomes almost impossible. In appropriate cases the previously mentioned technique of Warshaw and Bartlett could be employed to eliminate this large cavity. However, in instances, particularly of Crohn's disease, in which there has been fistulization and therefore it is impossible to employ such a technique, the possibility of long, continued drainage from the perineum must be entertained.

When such sinuses occur many measures are available. A secondary infection by anaerobes or by fungi may be quelled by specific therapy. If a long tract is present, thorough curetting may lead to healing. When a large cavity is present in the presacral space, Silen and Glotzer advocate removal of the coccyx and distal two segments of the sacrum.[43] Cohen and Ryan have had success by revising the cavity and filling it with a combined skin–gracilis muscle implant.[10]

With the use of these various methods all of these fistulas should heal eventually, even if they were extremely extensive prior to colectomy. A great deal of time may be necessary. We have seen them heal as late as 5 years after colectomy.

Anal Ileostomy

Inasmuch as ulcerative colitis never extends into the ileum, it has been proposed that after total removal of the colon the ileum could be brought down to the perineum and an anal ileostomy could be established. Early attempts to do this by Ravitch and Sabiston[40] and others were not particularly successful. There was a high incidence of complications, and persistent diarrhea made life so miserable for many patients that the usual type of ileostomy had to be re-established. With the development of the Soave procedure, in which the muscular tube of the anal canal is maintained intact, the operation has been re-evaluated.[32] Martin et al. have described its use in a small series of cases.[33] The operation is complicated in the presence of ulcerative colitis. It requires a protective loop ileostomy, careful drainage of the area between the muscular tube and the withdrawn sigmoid, and a protracted postoperative course. They believe that if a patient is willing to spend an additional 6–12 months, possibly with repeated operative procedures, the success rate will be high enough to warrant this operation. It is more likely to be successful in youth that it is in older age because diarrhea can continue to be a problem in the elderly.

Kock Continent Ileostomy

The Kock continent ileostomy has attained a moderate measure of popularity since its introduction in 1971.[28,29] In this procedure the terminal 60 cm of ileum are used to produce a pouch that will hold 8–12 oz of fecal content. Continence is produced by the formation of a valve just proximal to the ileostomy stoma; the pouch is then emptied by means of a catheter approximately every 8 hr.

This procedure is still experimental and patients must recognize the possibility that complications may occur.[19] In general terms it is not advisable to consider it when the colectomy is done under urgent circumstances. The most frequent postoperative complications have been incontinence and prolapse of the valve. Revision has been required in a substantial number of cases. At times it has been necessary to sacrifice the terminal 90 cm of ileum and construct a standard ileostomy. Although perforation of the pouch by introduction of the catheter has not been reported, this possibility must be entertained, particularly when the great number of catheter introductions that will occur within a patient's lifetime are considered. The largest series in the United States was reported by Beahrs et al.; they are cautiously optimistic about the results.[5] The Kock technique is shown in Figure 11.13. His monograph should be consulted for details.[29]

Surgery for Toxic Megacolon

Toxic dilatation of the colon (Fig. 11.14) in the United States is nearly always due to an exacerbation of chronic ulcerative colitis (Fig. 11.15a). It is much less common with Crohn's disease (Fig. 11.15b). In countries in which amebiasis is a serious infection it may occur particularly in association with pregnancy. Under these circumstances it is a very lethal disease.

This disease was not recognized prior to 1950. The causes other than underlying ulcerative colitis are not entirely clear. It has followed the use of opiates and anticholinergic drugs. It may occur after a colonoscopy if air has been used to distend the colon rather than an absorbable gas such as carbon dioxide. It may occur very early in the course of ulcerative colitis.

Strauss et al. collected 604 cases from the literature.[45] The overall medical mortality in this series was 27%, the surgical mortality 19.5%. The greatest hazard occurs when perforation is present; thus the surgical mortality was 41% with perforation and 9% without.

The most important controversy at the present time is concerned with the type of operation that should be employed.[27,38] It is certain that early operation on a toxic megacolon will lead to lower mortality. Occasionally it may also respond dramatically to the use of cortisone. Cortisone, however, is a very treacherous agent because perforations of the colon may occur silently when it is being used.

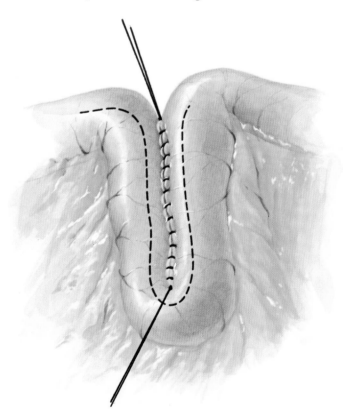

Fig. 11.13a–c. Kock continent ileostomy. a. Line of sutures to prepare the pouch. The terminal 15 cm of the ileum will be used to make the conduit and nipple. Two limbs of ileum, each 15 cm in length, just proximal to the conduit are sutured together and the bowel is opened along the broken line.

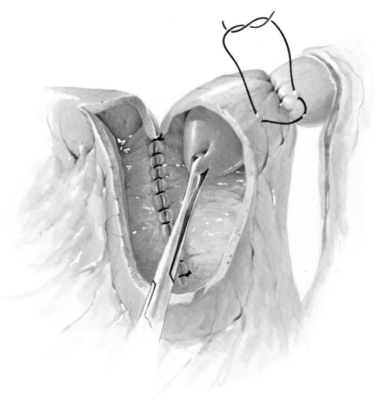

Fig. 11.13b. Formation of the nipple valve. The open pouch is shown. The nipple is formed by intussusception of the terminal ileum in a retrograde fashion into the pouch. Fixation of the nipple is aided by scarification of the serosa and by suture. The pouch is completed by a two-layer suture of the anterior wall.

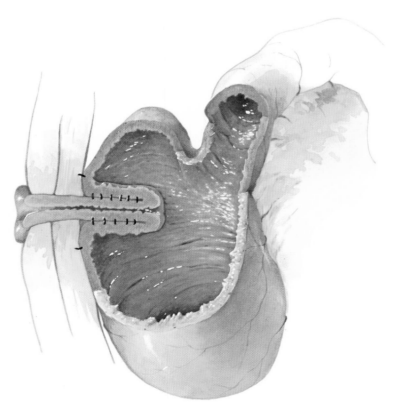

Fig. 11.13c. Cross section of the continent ileostomy. The pouch has been anchored to the abdominal wall, and excess ileum has been amputated. [Adapted from Koch N.G., Darle V., Hultén L., et al (1977) Ileostomy. Curr Probl Surg (Aug).]

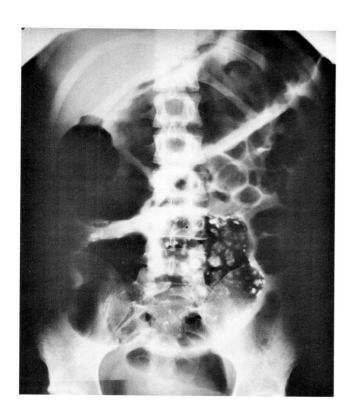

Fig. 11.14.   X-ray film of toxic dilatation of the colon.

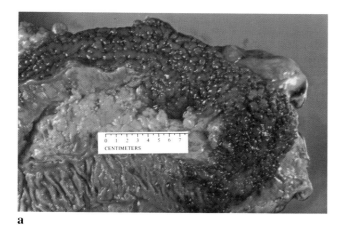

a

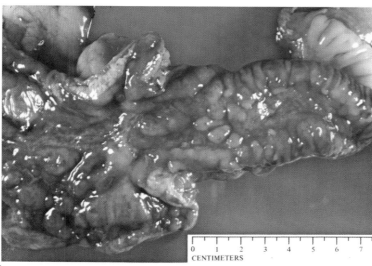

b

Fig. 11.15. a. Operative specimen of toxic dilatation of the colon associated with ulcerative colitis. b. Crohn's disease of the terminal ileum and cecum.

Most surgeons prefer to use a subtotal colectomy with permanent ileostomy, with the lower end of the sigmoid drawn out as mucous fistula, or total proctocolectomy.[18,44] Turnbull et al., however, advocate the use of the "blow-hole" colostomy.[48]

This operation consists of the withdrawal of a loop of terminal ileum as a loop ileostomy and then the formation of a blow-hole either in the transverse colon alone or in the sigmoid as well.[49] An incision is made directly over the dilated colon, the colon is identified, the margins of the colon are sutured to the abdominal wall, and the colon is opened. Immediate decompression is obtained by this method and the patient's symptoms generally subside rapidly.

In certain instances the colitis continues to be very active after this procedure. There is a continued discharge of very watery feces and continuation of toxic symptoms. In such cases a colectomy is required. In nearly all patients, however, the symptoms subside after the blow-hole colostomy; then after a period of several months, when the patient is in optimum condition, the colectomy may be carried out.

It is interesting to note that 16 of Turnbull's 42 patients had a diagnosis of Crohn's disease. The overall mortality was 5%, which is the lowest recorded in the literature. To this figure, however, would need to be added any later mortality following a total proctocolectomy as a second stage.

One of the most successful series is that of Block and co-workers.[8,38] They operated on 23 patients seen over a 5-year period: 16 underwent total abdominal colectomy with ileostomy and 7 underwent total proctocolectomy. Two had perforated colons and both died. There was 1 death among the 21 patients without perforation. The mortality was 4.7% for nonperforated cases, and 8.7% overall.

References

1. Adson M.A., Cooperman A.M., Farrow G.M. (1972) Ileorectostomy for ulcerative disease of the colon. Arch Surg 104: 424
2. Adson M.A., Fulton R.E. (1977) The ileal stoma and portal hypertension. An uncommon site of variceal bleeding. Arch Surg 112: 501
3. Baker W.N.W. (1971) Ileo-rectal anastomosis for Crohn's disease of the colon. Gut 12: 427
4. Barker V.F., Benfield J.R., deKernion J.B., et al (1975) The creation and care of enterocutaneous stomas. Curr Probl Surg (Dec) 12: 1
5. Beahrs O.H., Kelly K.A., Adson, M.A., et al (1974) Ileostomy with ileal reservoir rather than ileostomy alone. Ann Surg 179: 634
6. Binder S.C., Katz B. (1977) Regional enteritis. A review of the literature. Ohio State Med J 73: 661
7. Binder S.C., Miller H.H., Deterling R.A. Jr. (1976) Fate of the retained rectum after subtotal colectomy for inflammatory disease of the colon. Am J Surg 131: 201
8. Block G.E., Moossa A.R., Simonowitz D., et al (1977) Emergency colectomy for inflammatory bowel disease. Surgery 82: 531
9. Brooke B.N. (1952) Management of an ileostomy including its complications. Lancet 2: 102
10. Cohen B., Ryan J.A. Jr. (1979) Gracilis muscle flap for closure of the persistent perineal sinus. Surg Gynecol Obstet 148: 33
11. Crohn B.B., Ginzburg L., Oppenheimer G.D. (1932) Regional enteritis. JAMA 99: 1323
12. Devroede C.J., Taylor W.F., Sauer W.G., et al (1971) Cancer risk and life expectancy of children with ulcerative colitis. N Engl J Med 285: 17

13. Ein S.H., Lynch M.J., Stephens C.A. (1971) Ulcerative colitis in children under one year: A twenty-year review. J Pediatr Surg 6: 264

14. Farmer R.G., Hawk W.A., Turnbull R.B. Jr. (1971) Carcinoma associated with mucosal ulcerative colitis, and with transmural colitis and enteritis (Crohn's disease). Cancer 28: 289

15. Farmer R.G., Hawk W.A., Turnbull R.B. (1976) Indications for surgery in Crohn's disease: Analysis of 500 cases. Gastroenterology 71: 245

16. Foglia R., Ament M.E., Fleisher D., et al (1977) Surgical management of ulcerative colitis in childhood. Am J Surg 134: 58

17. Frey C.F., Weaver D.K. (1972) Colectomy in children with ulcerative and granulomatous colitis: Operative indications and results. Arch Surg 104: 416

18. Fry P.D., Atkinson K.G. (1976) Current surgical approach to toxic megacolon. Surg Gynecol Obstet 143: 26

19. Gelernt I.M., Bauer J.J., Kreel I. (1977) The reservoir ileostomy: Early experience with 54 patients. Ann Surg 185: 179

20. Glotzer D.J., Gardner R.C., Goldman H., et al (1970) Comparative features and course of ulcerative and granulomatous colitis. N Engl J Med 282: 582

21. Goligher J.C. (1977) Surgical aspects of ulcerative colitis and Crohn's disease of the large bowel. Adv Surg 11: 71

22. Goligher J.C., de Dombal F.T., Watts J. Mck., et al (1968) Ulcerative colitis. Williams & Wilkins, Baltimore

23. Greenstein A.J., Sachar D.B., Pasternack B.S., et al (1975) Reoperation and recurrence in Crohn's colitis and ileocolitis. Crude and cumulative rates. N Engl J Med 293: 685

24. Greenstein A.J., Sachar D., Pucillo A., et al (1978) Cancer in Crohn's disease after diversionary surgery. A report of seven carcinomas occurring in excluded bowel. Am J Surg 135: 86

25. Hollender L.F., Meyer C. (1977) L'anus artificiel colostomies et ileostomies. Laboratoire Porgès, Paris

26. Homan W.P., Tang C., Thorbjarnarson B. (1976) Acute massive hemorrhage from intestinal Crohn's disease. Report of seven cases and review of the literature. Arch Surg 111: 901

27. Judd E.S. (1969) Current surgical aspects of toxic megacolon. Surgery 65: 401

28. Kock N.G. (1969) Intra-abdominal "reservoir" in patients with permanent ileostomy. Arch Surg 99: 223

29. Kock N.G., Darle N., Hultén L., et al (1977) Ileostomy. Curr Probl Surg (Aug) 14: 1

30. Korelitz B.I., Dyck W.P., Klion F.M. (1969) Fate of the rectum and distal colon after subtotal colectomy for ulcerative colitis. Gut 10: 198

31. Korelitz B.I., Present D.H., Alpert L.I., et al (1972) Recurrent regional ileitis after ileostomy and colectomy for granulomatous colitis. N Engl J Med 287: 110

32. Lyttle J.A., Parks A.G. (1977) Intersphincteric excision of the rectum. Br J Surg 64: 413

33. Martin L.W., LeCoultre C., Schubert W.K. (1977) Total colectomy and mucosal proctectomy with preservation of continence in ulcerative colitis. Ann Surg 186: 477

34. Matolo N.M., Wolfman E.F. Jr. (1976) Reversed ileal segment for treatment of ileostomy dysfunction. Clinical application. Arch Surg 111: 891

35. Miller C.G., Gardiner C. Mcg., Ripstein C.B. (1949) Primary resection of the colon in ulcerative colitis. J Can Med Assoc 60: 584

36. Morson B.C., Pang L.S.C. (1967) Rectal biopsy as aid to cancer control in ulcerative colitis. Gut 8: 423

37. Moss G.S., Keddie N. (1965) Fate of rectal stump in ulcerative colitis. Arch Surg 91: 967

38. Mungas J.E., Moossa A.R., Block G.E. (1976) Treatment of toxic megacolon. Surg Clin North Am 56: 95

39. Oberhelman H.A. Jr., Kohatsu S., Taylor K.B., et al (1970) Diverting ileos-

tomy for Crohn's disease of the colon. Fourth World Congress of Gastroenterology, Copenhagen, July 12–18

40. Ravitch M.M., Sabiston D.C. Jr. (1947) Anal ileostomy with preservation of the sphincter: Proposed operation in patients requiring total colectomy for benign lesions. Surg Gynecol Obstet 84: 1095

41. Reilly J., Ryan J.A., Strole W., et al (1976) Hyperalimentation in inflammatory bowel disease. Am J Surg 131: 192

42. Schachter H., Goldstein M.J., Rappaport H., et al (1970) Ulcerative and ''granulomatous'' colitis—validity of differential diagnostic criteria: A study of 100 patients treated by total colectomy. Ann Intern Med 72: 841

43. Silen W., Glotzer D.J. (1974) The prevention and treatment of the persistent perineal sinus. Surgery 75: 535

44. Sirinek K.R., Tetirick C.E., Thomford N.R., et al (1977) Total proctocolectomy and ileostomy. Procedure of choice for acute toxic megacolon. Arch Surg 112: 518

45. Strauss R.J., Flint G.W., Platt N., et al (1976) The surgical management of toxic dilatation of the colon. A report of 28 cases and review of the literature. Ann Surg 184: 682

46. Tomkins R.K., Weinstein M.H., Foroozan P., et al (1973) Reappraisal of rectum-retaining operations for ulcerative and granulomatous colitis. Am J Surg 125: 159

47. Truelove S.C. (1971) Ulcerative colitis beginning in childhood. N Engl J Med 285: 50

48. Turnbull R.B. Jr., Hawk W.A., Weakley F.L. (1971) Surgical treatment of toxic megacolon: Ileostomy and colostomy to prepare patients for colectomy. Am J Surg 122: 325

49. Turnbull R.B., Weakley F.L. (1967) Atlas of intestinal stomas. Mosby, St. Louis

50. Van Prohaska J. (1969) The inflammatory diseases of the large and small bowel. Curr Probl Surg (March) 6: 1

51. Warshaw A.L., Ottinger L.W., Bartlett M.K. (1977) Primary perineal closure after proctocolectomy for inflammatory bowel disease. Am J Surg 133: 414

52. Zetzel L. (1970) Granulomatous (ileo) colitis. N Engl J Med 282: 600

Volvulus

12

There are several distinct varieties of volvulus of the colon. For example, in infancy and early childhood an unattached mesentery of the right colon and small bowel may lead to volvulus of the entire right colon and most or all of the ileum and jejunum. This situation is rarely encountered in an adult. In the adult the right colon has usually been fixed to the parietal wall so that only the cecum is subject to volvulus in that section. The sigmoid is a more likely site because it tends to be redundant in many patients. It is necessary for the attachments of a redundant loop to be relatively close together for volvulus to occur. For example, in the transverse colon, which may be long and redundant, fixation of the flexures renders a volvulus of this section of the colon uncommon. Furthermore, since the colon is not commonly held down by adhesions, a major cause of volvulus in the small intestine is not found in the colon; however, Wilson and Cheek found that 50% of their cases of cecal volvulus were secondary to nonfixation and adhesions.[8]

Cecum

A volvulus of the cecum may vary in its severity from a partial twist to a total volvulus causing gangrene of the segment. Gangrene may follow total circulatory occlusion within a few hours. Emergency operation in such patients is necessary.

The symptoms of abdominal pain, nausea and vomiting are accompanied by a mass, generally in the mid- or upper abdomen. The abdominal film shows a large gas shadow that usually lies in the left-upper quadrant (Fig. 12.1a). Confirmation is secured by the barium enema (Fig. 12.1b).

At the time of laparotomy, several options are available. If there is gangrene or ischemia of the cecum, an immediate right colectomy with ileocolostomy is the proper procedure. If the gangrene has progressed to perforation, it is better to exteriorize the two ends of the bowel rather than to attempt an anastomosis.

If the cecum is twisted in the typical clockwise position but the blood supply is adequate, it will be possible to relieve the torsion. The cecum can then be fixed in the right lower quadrant either by suture, which may be rather difficult, or by a cecostomy, which can be done either by the tube

143

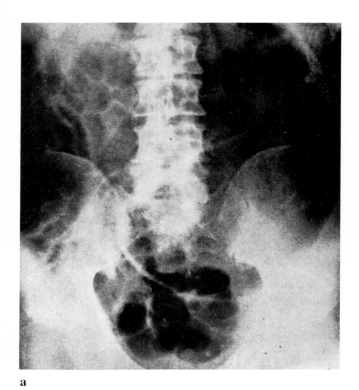
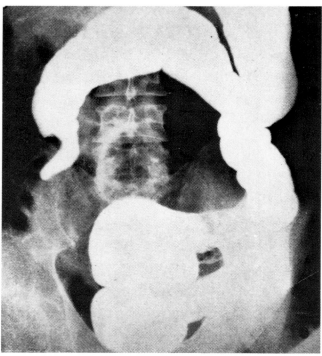

a   b

Fig. 12.1a and b.   Volvulus of the cecum. a. Plain abdominal film demonstrating the greatly enlarged cecum in the left upper quadrant. b. Barium enema showing sharp cutoff at the site of the volvulus.

technique or by suture of the cecum to the abdominal wall, with a subsequent opening of the cecostomy (see Chapter 15). Fixation may not be permanent, and thus may be inferior to a resection of the involved area. If fixation is chosen as a method of treatment, an appendectomy is done as a concomitant procedure.

Sigmoid

Sigmoid volvulus is a very common disease in some sections of the world, particularly in Eastern Europe and in Bolivia, where colons tend to be longer and consequently more subject to torsion than they are elsewhere. Extremely long colons (dolichocolons) are noted in many children in Bolivia. In the United States volvulus is encountered most frequently in psychiatric hospitals or in nursing homes; the reason this occurs is not clear but may be related to poor bowel habits.[7] These patients therefore are likely to be poor operative risks, and in some instances symptoms may not be reported until gangrene of the loop has appeared.

Unfortunately, there is no way to be sure that gangrene has not already occurred in a loop with volvulus. The presence of a greatly distended abdomen that is tender, however, should raise that suspicion. The diagnosis of volvulus can be made by an abdominal film, which shows the large loop of sigmoid (Fig. 12.2a), and is confirmed by barium enema, which shows a typical bird-beak deformity at the site of the twist. The presence or absence of gangrene can only be determined by clinical observation.

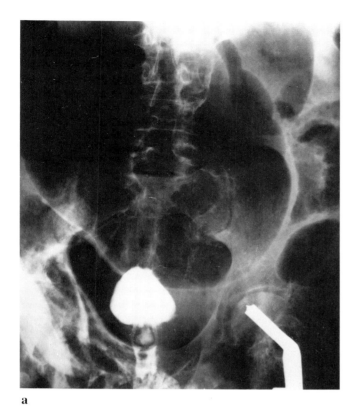

a

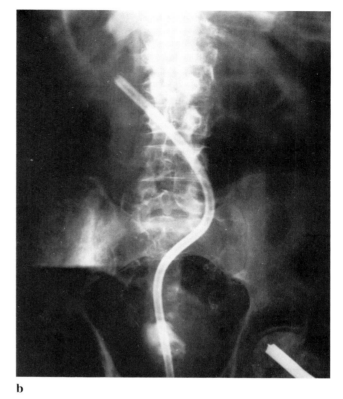

b

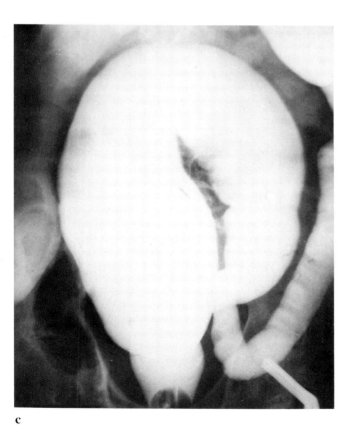

c

Fig. 12.2a – c. Sigmoid volvulus. a. Plain abdominal film showing a greatly dilated loop of sigmoid. b. Complete deflation after passage of the tube through the sigmoidoscope. c. Barium enema taken after reduction, showing huge sigmoid.

Decompression can often be obtained by the insertion of a rectal tube through a sigmoidoscope (Fig. 12.2b,c) or by the passage of the colonoscope beyond the point of torsion.[2,4] Enemas (either barium or saline) may also lead to deflation. If detorsion can be obtained in this fashion and the mucosa appears normal by colonoscopy, a period of observation is warranted.

If pain or tenderness persists or the white blood cell count rises, laparotomy is necessary. In the Charity Hospital (New Orleans) series, 76% of patients with sigmoid volvulus had successful reduction by a combination of sigmoidoscopy, tubes, and enemas.[1]

Several procedures are available to the surgeon if laparotomy is necessary.[5,6] The simplest is merely the detorsion of the loop. Decompression can be secured by an inlying rectal tube placed high in the sigmoid. Frequently the colon is unusually long and may be wider than usual even proximal to the sigmoid. Simple detorsion, while a lifesaving measure, is almost certain to be followed by a later volvulus. Furthermore, attempts at fixation of the sigmoid loop are not likely to be successful. We believe that the wisest plan is to resect the involved area at the time of laparotomy. A decision can then be made as to whether or not an immediate anastomosis can be carried out. If the process has been quite acute and the proximal bowel is essentially normal and not packed with feces, an end-to-end anastomosis may be made. If conditions are not optimum, the surgeon can bring the two ends of the colon out as stomas with the intention of anastomosing them at a later date.

Because there is a high incidence of recurrent volvulus, a second operation to carry out a resection and anastomosis of the involved segment should follow simple detorsion as soon as the bowel has been adequately prepared.

Transverse Colon

Volvulus of the transverse colon is a rare lesion.[3] Patients with this disease usually have a dolichocolon or have had a previous operation for sigmoid volvulus. Symptoms may be chronic or acute. After an unrelated operation, such as hysterectomy, ileus may lead to distention and volvulus.

The therapy will depend upon the patient's condition. Those with chronic symptoms should be amenable to a one-stage resection and anastomosis. Acutely ill patients should have a resection with proximal colostomy and distal mucous fistula; continuity can be restored at a later date.

References

1. Arnold G.J., Nance F.C. (1973) Volvulus of the sigmoid colon. Ann Surg 177: 527
2. Bruusgaard D. (1947) Volvulus of the sigmoid colon and its treatment. Surgery 22: 466
3. Eisenstat T.E., Raneri A.J., Mason G.R. (1977) Volvulus of the transverse colon. Am J Surg 134: 396
4. Ghazi A., Shinya H., Wolff W.I. (1976) Treatment of volvulus of the colon by colonoscopy. Ann Surg 183: 263
5. Greco R.S., Dragon R.E., Kernstein M.D. (1974) Alternatives in management of volvulus of the sigmoid colon: Report of four cases. Dis Colon Rectum 17: 241
6. Hinshaw D.B., Carter R. (1957) Surgical management of acute volvulus of the sigmoid colon. A study of 55 cases. Ann Surg 146: 52
7. Ingalls J.M., Lynch M.F., Schilling J.A. (1964) Volvulus of the sigmoid in a mental institution. Am J Surg 108: 339
8. Wilson H., Cheek R.C. (1972) Volvulus of the colon. In: Hardy J.D. (ed) Rhoads textbook of surgery. Principles and practice, 5th edn. Lippincott, Philadelphia, p 1217

Intussusception of the Colon

13

Intussusception of the colon occurs infrequently in adults.[1-5] The etiology is entirely different from that of the ileocolic intussusception that occurs in infants and children since in adults the disease is nearly always caused by a tumor. The tumor is usually benign or of low-grade malignancy, since invasion of the muscular wall by an invasive cancer may lead to fixation of the mass to the parietal peritoneum. Lipomas of the right colon are the most common cause of intussusception, but villous adenomas or polypoid carcinomas may also be involved. In exceptional circumstances a low-grade carcinoma may be extruded from the anus; in one of our cases such a tumor had originated in the transverse colon.

The diagnosis is generally made because the patient complains of the symptoms of intestinal obstruction. On barium enema typical evidence of obstruction is obtained with the appearance of a ''coiled spring'' of barium distal to the point of obstruction (Fig. 13.1). Occasionally there may be complete obstruction to the retrograde flow of barium, but the patient has no evidence of antegrade obstruction. Colonic intussusception is much more likely to be rather slow in its onset and does not require an emergency operation in adults, as it does in children.

The operation consists of resection of the involved area of bowel. Continuity, except in cases of severe obstruction, can be restored immediately by anastomosis. However, if the proximal bowel is poorly prepared or is full of barium from an unfortunate upper gastrointestinal series, the surgeon may elect the formation of two stomas with restoration of continuity at a later date. One of the considerations that is involved at the time of operation is whether or not the intussusception should be reduced prior to resection. Although this measure may involve some danger if, for example, there has been subacute perforation, it is generally better to do this since it may indicate more clearly which section of the bowel requires removal. An intussuscepting lesion of the sigmoid may progress into the extraperitoneal rectum, and if the intussusception were not reduced the surgeon might believe that a Miles operation was indicated; after reduction, however, a simple resection and anastomosis of the sigmoid could be possible. After reduction lipomas can usually be distinguished by their soft consistency; segmental resection of the bowel and anastomosis can be carried out without sacrifice of a large amount of mesentery. However, if a polypoid lesion

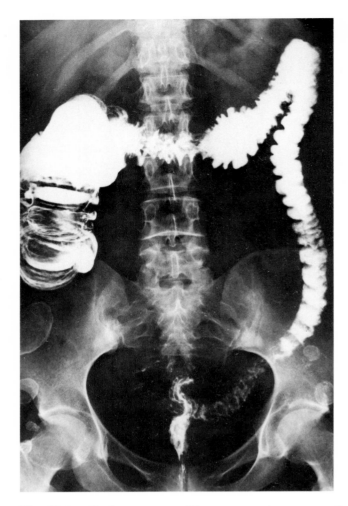

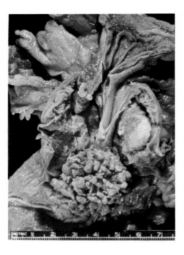

Fig. 13.2. Operative specimen of a large polypoid villous adenoma that had intussuscepted through a narrow area of the bowel; it was found microscopically to be an independent cancer of the colon. (Courtesy of Dr. D. F. Brewster.)

Fig. 13.1. Barium enema of intussuscepting tumor of the cecum. Note the typical bedspring appearance at the site of the intussusception.

or a carcinoma is encountered (Fig. 13.2) the mesentery should be removed.

Gupta reported a small series of intussusceptions in adults in India.[4] Only half were caused by tumors. Amebiasis and mobile cecums were the causes in adults. Worms, chronic dysentery, nonspecific intestinal ulcerations, and high-residual vegetarian diets have been unusual causes of ileocolic intussusception in tropical countries.

References

1. Brayton D., Norris W.J. (1954) Intussusception in adults. Am J Surg 88: 32
2. Dean D.L., Ellis F.H. Jr., Sauer W.G. (1956) Intussusception in adults. Arch Surg 73: 6
3. Donhauser J.L., Kelly E.C. (1950) Intussusception in adults. Am J Surg 79: 673
4. Gupta S. (1977) Treatment of adult intussusception. Chir Gastroenterol 11: 315
5. Stubenbord W.T., Thorbjarnason B. (1970) Intussusception in adults. Ann Surg 172: 306

Wounds of the Colon and Rectum

14

In this chapter perforations of the large bowel secondary to trauma will be considered. Chapter 16, on perforations of the colon, should also be consulted. It is customary to divide traumatic wounds into two groups—those caused by perforating trauma and those caused by blunt trauma.

Perforating traumas include injuries with sharp objects (such as knives) or missiles, and rarely iatrogenic injuries related to foreign bodies or endoscopic manipulation.[1,4,5,9]

The possibility of a perforating injury of the colon exists in nearly all wounds not only of the abdomen, but also of the chest, buttocks, and upper thighs. If possible, the course of the missile or the instrument should be considered, and if there is any possibility that the peritoneal cavity might have been penetrated, we believe that an exploratory laparotomy is safer than delay. We realize that such a course might be impossible to follow if an emergency ward is overwhelmed with patients with traumatic wounds. It is also recognized that there are some hazards involved in early laparotomy. Most of these dangers are associated with the possibility of other undiagnosed injuries or of aspiration from a full stomach during anesthesia. Obviously the stomach should be thoroughly emptied before any anesthesia is administered.

A few diagnostic measures may be helpful. Sigmoidoscopy may reveal blood in the rectum; this would indicate a rectal injury. A peritoneal tap with or without irrigation has been used by many surgeons and can be recommended, particularly when there is a cerebral injury as well. If any blood is present there is a strong indication for laparotomy; on the other hand, a negative tap does not rule out abdominal surgery. A simple test has been used. The peritoneal cavity is irrigated with 1000 ml saline. The return is placed in a test tube; if there is enough blood in it so that a printed page cannot be read through the tube, laparotomy should be done. We have not been impressed with attempts to inject the wound with radiopaque materials to determine whether or not there has been an intraperitoneal perforation.

Injuries due to blunt trauma are much less common than penetrating wounds. The diagnosis may be more difficult, but the operative procedures are the same.

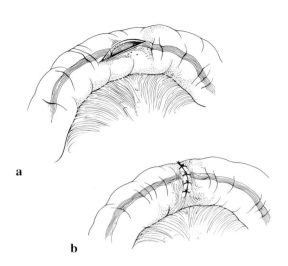

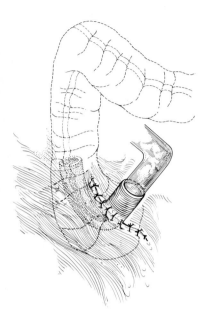

Fig. 14.1a and b. Laceration of the colon. a. Clean laceration of colon. b. Closure by suture.

Fig. 14.2. Closure of cecum about a cecostomy tube.

Injuries to the colon that occur in civilian life can be treated much more definitively than they could be in war time, when there was a possibility of early transportation over rough roads and limited or no postoperative care.[1,2,4] For example, most knife wounds of the colon (Fig. 14.1 a and b) can now be treated by simple suture or by closure about a catheter or tube (Fig. 14.2). During World War II it was advocated that every colon injury be treated by colostomy, either at the site of perforation or proximal to it.[7] Injuries of the right colon may be treated by resection and, in optimal cases, immediate anastomosis (Fig. 14.3 a–c); in others the two ends of the bowel may be brought out for a delayed anastomosis a few weeks later. Extensive injuries of the right colon or concomitant damage to other viscera or parietes make immediate anastomosis dangerous. Bullet wounds that involve the mesentery may produce large hematomas and perhaps later necrosis of the colon wall (Fig. 14.4a); it is best to treat them as if they were more dangerous than they appear and to consider exteriorization in all instances in which it is possible (Fig. 14.4b). Some surgeons have closed the colonic wound and then exteriorized the section of colon containing the suture line (Fig. 14.4c). If the sutures hold, the colon is replaced within the peritoneal cavity in 10 days; if they fail, the exteriorized bowel forms a colostomy. Kirkpatrick reported 61 patients treated in this way; in 70% the suture remained intact.[6]

Wounds of the rectum should be diagnosed by sigmoidoscopy prior to surgery. However, if such a lesion has not been found and at the time of laparotomy the surgeon finds a good deal of blood in the pelvis, particularly in the retroperitoneal area, the possibility of such a wound must be entertained and a transverse colostomy may be a wiser procedure than an attempt to open the retroperitoneal area, where there may be extensive bleeding from large veins that will be impossible to control (Fig. 14.5).

Wounds of the perineum or buttocks that have damaged the extraperitoneal rectum are treated by transverse colostomy: a perineal incision, identification of the wound, closure of the defect, reconstruction of the muscles, and drainage are performed. Wounds of the sphincters also

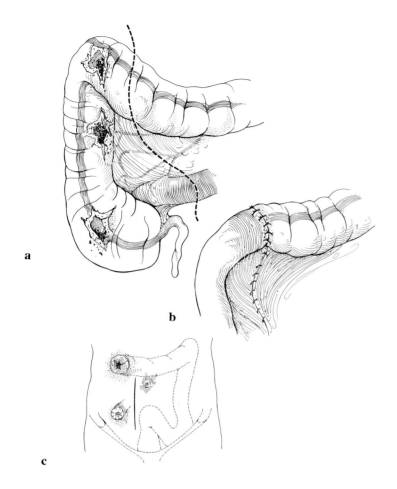

Fig. 14.3a–c. Extensive injury of the colon. a. Extensive wound of the right colon (resection shown by broken line). b. Resection and primary anastomosis. c. Resection with double stomas.

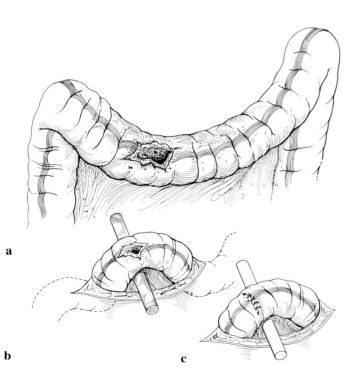

Fig. 14.4a–c. Serious injury of the colon. a. Ragged wound transverse colon. b. Exteriorization of colon. c. Exteriorization with closure of laceration.

151

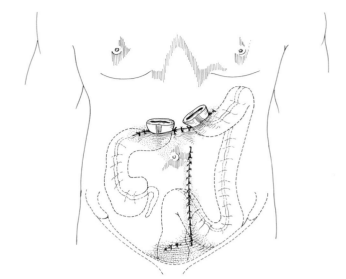

Fig. 14.5. Closure of rectal wound and proximal colostomy.

should be repaired immediately. Very serious wounds of the rectum associated with hemorrhage have a high rate of sepsis and, according to the experience of Getzen et al., should be treated by abdominoperineal resection.[3]

Blunt trauma is not as likely to injure the colon as it is to fracture the solid viscera such as the liver and the spleen. However, the colon may burst as a result of blunt trauma.[5] The principles of therapy are the same as those discussed above.

Fistulas and incontinence are common sequelae to a wound of the rectum. The late repair of sphincter injuries has been described by Parks and McPartlin.[8]

References

1. Beall A.C. Jr., Bricker D.L., Alessi F.J., et al (1971) Surgical considerations in the management of civilian colon injuries. Ann Surg 173: 971
2 Chilimindris C., Boyd D.R., Carlson L.E., et al (1971) A critical review of management of right colon injuries. J. Trauma 11: 651
3. Getzen L.C., Pollak E.W., Wolfman E.F. Jr. (1977) Abdominoperineal resection in the treatment of devascularizing rectal injuries. Surgery 82: 310
4. Haygood F.D., Polk H.C. Jr. (1976) Gunshot wounds of the colon. A review of 100 consecutive patients, with emphasis on complications and their causes. Am J Surg 131: 213
5. Howell H.S., Bartizal J.F., Freeark R.J. (1976) Blunt trauma involving the colon and rectum. J Trauma 16: 624
6. Kirkpatrick J.R. (1977) The exteriorized anastomosis: Its role in surgery of the colon. Surgery 82: 362
7. Ogilvie W.H. (1944) Abdominal wounds in the Western Desert. Surg Gynecol Obstet 78: 225
8. Parks A.G., McPartlin J.F. (1971) Late repair of injuries of the anal sphincter. Proc R Soc Med 64: 1187
9. Sohn N., Weinstein M.A., Gonchar J. (1977) Social injuries of the rectum. Am J Surg 134: 611

Surgery for Obstruction

15

Obstruction of the colon is secondary to cancer in about 80% of cases, to diverticulitis in 15%, and to other causes in the remaining patients. There are some clinical variations in each type. For example, cancer of the right colon may mimic small bowel obstruction. Furthermore, in the presence of a competent ileocecal valve a cancer of the right colon may produce a closed loop obstruction that leads to early gangrene or perforation. Diverticulitis may lead to pure colonic obstruction, pure small bowel obstruction because of adhesive bands to the inflamed colon, or combined large and small bowel obstruction. Volvulus produces a closed loop obstruction in which the hazard of strangulation is high.

A diagnosis is made on the basis of abdominal cramps, distention, and obstipation. Nausea and vomiting usually are late manifestations of colonic obstruction. On physical examination peristalsis is typically high pitched but disappears with the onset of gangrene. Tenderness is absent until strangulation or perforation occurs. Rectal and vaginal examinations are essential. Sigmoidoscopy may demonstrate a cancer of the intraperitoneal rectum. Electrolyte abnormalities are unusual.

The plain abdominal film may indicate the site of the lesion by a sharp cutoff of gas at some part of the colon (Fig. 15.1). However, since liquid feces often fill the bowel proximal to the obstruction, the lesion may be at a different site than expected. The barium enema is very helpful but care should be taken to avoid forcing barium proximal to the point of incomplete obstruction.

One of the most dangerous results of distal colonic obstruction is marked distention of the thin-walled cecum; perforation occurs more easily in the cecum than in any other section of the bowel due to its large diameter. Whenever the x-ray film shows a diameter of 9 cm or more a danger point has been reached.

Acute colonic obstruction generally requires emergency surgery. It is unsafe to wait in the presence of possible perforation. Nasogastric intubation is essential to empty the stomach prior to general anesthesia.

The operative procedures available include (1) a one-stage operation with resection and anastomosis for cancer of the right and transverse colons, and (2) staged operations in which first the bowel is either defunctionalized (transverse colostomy) or decompressed (cecostomy) and at a

153

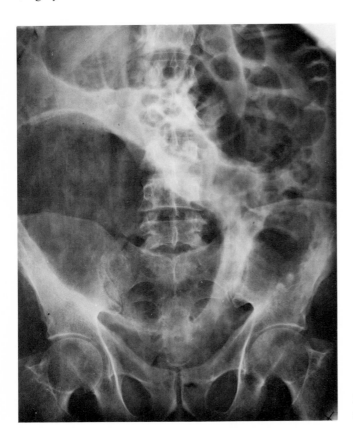

Fig. 15.1. Plain abdominal x-ray film showing obstruction of the sigmoids.

second stage the causative cancer in the distal colon is resected. Whenever a simple colostomy or cecostomy is elected, the possibility of cecal perforation must be considered; exploratory laparotomy is essential in questionable cases. If an exploration is done, the obstructing lesion should not be manipulated unless the surgeon is prepared to proceed with a resection should it be necessary. Biopsy of an offending lesion never should be performed since it may spread cancer or lead to perforation.

Obstruction of the colon may be acute, subacute, or chronic. Acute obstruction requires emergency remedial surgery, since if the ileocecal valve is competent, high pressure may build in the colon and lead to perforation, particularly in the cecum.[4–6,8,10] Mechanical distention may be mimicked by paralytic ileus in which only the colon is involved. The operative measures that will be required are described below.

Cecostomy

Cecostomy has been performed for acute obstruction of the left colon or as a concomitant procedure along with a resection and anastomosis of the left colon.[1] This operation was very popular in the past but in recent years has been used much less frequently.

The advantages of a cecostomy are that it serves to decompress a distended colon and thus provides relief of acute obstruction or, alternatively, prevents pressure upon a fresh anastomotic line. On the other hand, there are a number of disadvantages to the procedure. The operation always invites some contamination and a low-grade fever for several days after the procedure is the rule rather than the exception. Furthermore, unless adequate provision for decompression is made, the cecostomy functions very

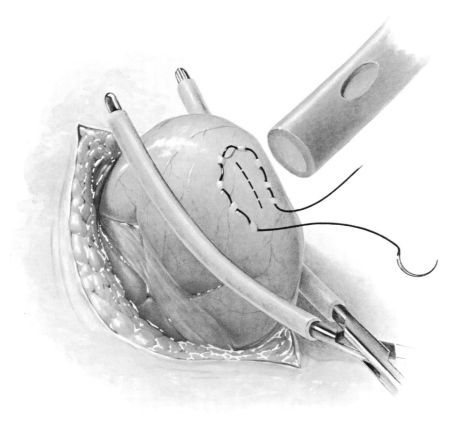

Fig. 15.2a–c. Tube cecostomy. a. A large rubber tube is inserted into the cecum. The cecum is opened along the broken line after insertion of a purse-string suture and application of an occluding clamp.

poorly. It is not, of course, a defunctionalizing operation and cannot be expected to sidetrack the fecal current that will continue to pass behind the stoma.

After the cecostomy has fulfilled its function any inlying tube may be removed. In most instances the stoma will close spontaneously unless the mucosa has been sutured to the skin. However, in our experience about one case in six did require formal closure. Furthermore, hernias occur in cecostomy wounds rather frequently and often require repair.

When transverse colostomy and cecostomy are compared as decompressive procedures for lesions of the left colon, it appears that transverse colostomy is far superior and may be depended upon for both decompression and defunctionalization.

Two types of cecostomies will be described. In the first, a tube is sutured in the cecum; in the second, the cecum is sutured to the abdominal wall and opened.

Tube Cecostomy

Unless the abdomen has been opened for another operative procedure, it is possible to carry out the cecostomy as an individual, separate operation. It may be performed with the patient under local anesthesia if he is quite ill. The line of incision is infiltrated with lidocaine and the peritoneal cavity is entered. The markedly distended cecum should present immediately beneath the McBurney incision. The cecum is withdrawn for a slightly further distance. An inlying tube is prepared. This is made of soft rubber approximately 2 cm in diameter and is designed to lie in the ascending colon (Fig. 15.2a). It is attached to a right angle glass tube that will come out through the abdominal incision. If possible, a curved rubber-covered clamp is applied to the cecum in order to minimize the amount of contamination. A purse-string suture is then placed at the appropriate position and the cecostomy tube is inserted well into the ascending colon. The suture is tied and the tube is sutured in place (Fig. 15.2b). A second inverting suture then completes the closure about the rubber tube. The cecum is then returned to the peritoneal cavity and the wound is closed about it (Fig. 15.2c). Immediate decompression can be obtained.

This operation has been modified by the use of Pezzer or Foley catheters. Unfortunately, in some instances the catheter is so small that it does not function well and may become completely occluded by folds of cecum. We prefer to use the larger tube, which is certain to function.

One caution should be mentioned. This tube cannot be left in the cecum indefinitely without danger of erosion of the cecal wall; it should be removed within 2 weeks. At this time a fistulous tract should have been established, although if necessary a shorter catheter could be reintroduced.

The postoperative complications include failure to relieve the distension, the inability to clean out the previously obstructed colon completely, late failure of the stoma to close, and hernia in the incision.

Suture of Cecum to Skin

A second type of cecostomy is made by withdrawing the cecum, suturing the serosa to the skin of the wound, and then opening the lumen of the bowel. This procedure is similar to that Turnbull popularized in his blowhole technique for toxic megacolon. This type of cecostomy may be employed in difficult cases in which the cecum is greatly distended and any

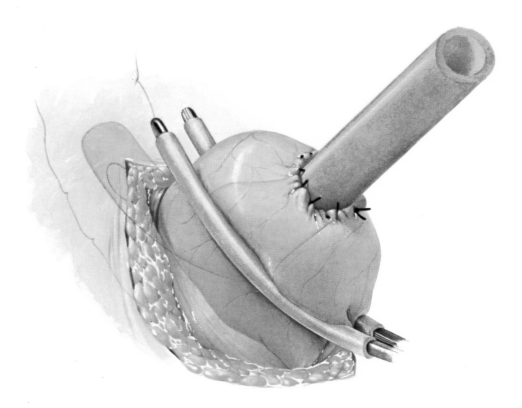

Fig. 15.2b. The tube is held in position in the ascending colon by two purse-string sutures. The outer one includes the tube.

attempt to insert a tube might be met with a great deal of contamination. Although it appears that it would be safer to wait several hours before opening the cecal wall, in practice this can be done immediately and usually is necessary if there is severe distention.

One of the disadvantages of both of these methods of "blind" cecostomy is that the whole cecal wall is not observed. There may be, in the presence of marked obstruction, serosal tears or even perforation of the cecum due to the marked distention. A full-scale laparotomy may be necessary to eliminate this possibility.

Transverse Colostomy

Transverse colostomy now is employed as a preliminary operation for obstructing lesions of the left colon. The colostomy usually is placed in the right upper quadrant. It has numerous advantages over a cecostomy. As mentioned above, it avoids the contamination that is so common with cecostomies. It provides complete defunctionalization of the bowel, thereby preventing further contamination of the left colon by the fecal stream. It can remain for an indefinite period of time without any danger of erosion by tubes. On the other hand, it will require a secondary closure and, unless the colostomy is placed very close to the offending lesion or can be excised at the time of the major reconstructive surgery, it involves a three-stage rather than a two-stage operation.

Transverse colostomy in the presence of large bowel obstruction may be difficult. The transverse colon mesentery may be extremely short or the colon may be in an unusual position. A preliminary plain abdominal x-ray made with a coin placed on the umbilicus may assist the surgeon in accurately locating the transverse colon prior to the abdominal incision. An unduly short mesentery of the transverse colon may make withdrawal of a loop extremely difficult; it always is possible, although a wider incision may be necessary for mobilization. At times a gallbladder full of stones and acutely inflamed will be found as the right upper quadrant transverse colostomy is made. A judgment must be made as to whether or not concurrent

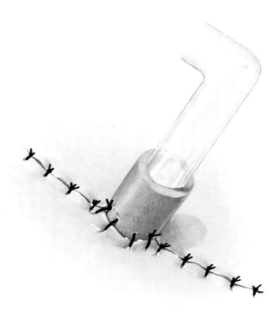

Fig. 15.2c. The abdominal wall is closed about the tube.

157

cholecystectomy or cholecystostomy with removal of stones should be done.

There are two types of transverse colostomies: loop colostomies and divided colostomies.

Loop Colostomy

This operation can be done with the patient under local anesthesia, but then it is impossible to explore the abdomen. In many cases it is advisable to explore through a left lower paramedian incision in order to identify the primary lesion that is causing the obstruction and also to note the presence or absence of any tears of the cecal wall. Under no circumstances should any attempt be made to mobilize or to biopsy any lesion in the left lower quadrant unless the surgeon is prepared to proceed immediately with a one-stage resection. If it appears that this will be necessary for some reason, then the transverse colostomy is abandoned, a left colectomy is carried out, and the decision as to whether or not to make an immediate anastomosis is made at that time.

The transverse colostomy begins with a transverse incision over the right side of the transverse colon (Fig. 15.3a). Omentum is freed from the colon for a distance of several inches. A soft rubber drain is passed about the transverse colon at the projected site of the stoma, and then the colon is drawn back through the abdominal wall. The opening in the wall should be generous enough to admit the colon but no larger than necessary. After the colon has been withdrawn a rod is passed beneath it (Fig. 15.3b). A few skin sutures may be necessary.

The surgeon must then decide whether or not it is necessary to decompress the distended colon immediately. One warning is necessary. If the colon is markedly distended it is not wise to use an electrocautery for this purpose because it can produce an explosion. The stoma should be

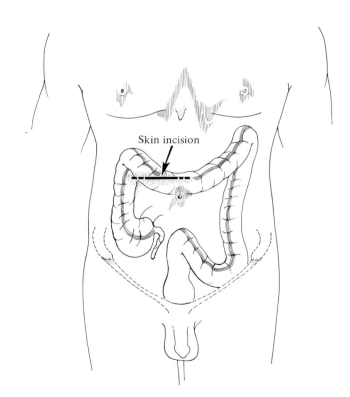

Fig. 15.3a and b. Loop colostomy. a. The incision is made over the right side of the transverse colon.

opened with a scalpel after proper protection of the abdominal wall. A large catheter can then be passed proximally and distally to relieve any gaseous obstruction and any liquid fecal material that is present.

The main advantage of a loop colostomy is that it is made very easily. It is easier to perform in the presence of a markedly distended colon than a divided colostomy. Furthermore, it can be turned into a divided colostomy later merely by cutting the posterior wall of the colon such that the two limbs separate at least a short distance. On the other hand, loop colostomies are a little more likely to retract into the abdominal wall. It is harder to prevent spill-over from the proximal loop into the distal one than with a divided colostomy; consequently, if the bowel is in reasonably good condition and the stoma is expected to be left for several months, it is better to perform a divided colostomy as the primary procedure.

Divided Colostomy

A slightly more generous incision than that used for loop colostomy is necessary in the right upper quadrant. After omentum has been removed from the colon for a short distance (Fig. 15.4a), the transverse colon is withdrawn in a similar fashion. The bowel is grasped with Kocher clamps and divided with the cautery. It is necessary to divide the mesentery downward for a short distance as well (Fig. 15.4b). The two limbs of the bowel are then brought out through opposite ends of the incision (Fig. 15.4c). The peritoneum, fascia, and skin are closed between the two loops. The clamps are removed in approximately 24 hr.

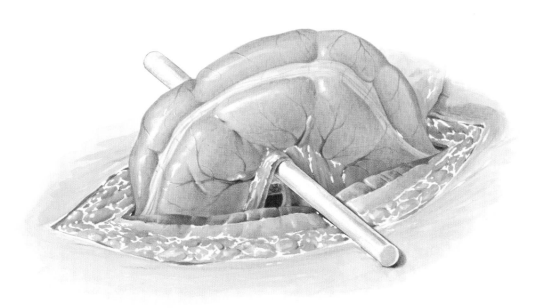

Fig. 15.3b.   A loop of colon is withdrawn, omentum is freed from it, and a glass rod is passed beneath the exteriorized colon.

The complications of transverse colostomy include retraction of the stoma and prolapse of a redundant transverse colon. Prolapse can be very annoying and at times may occur very soon after the primary operation. It

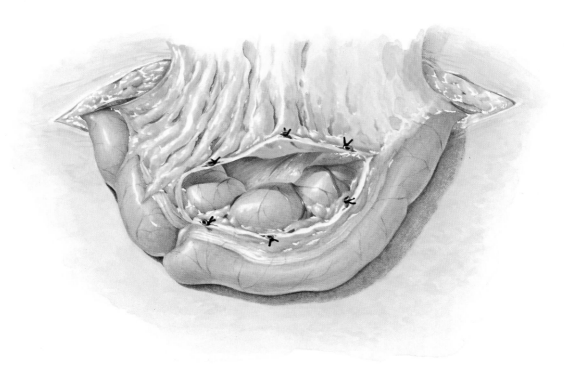

Fig. 15.4a–c. Divided colostomy. a. Omentum is removed from the colon for a short distance.

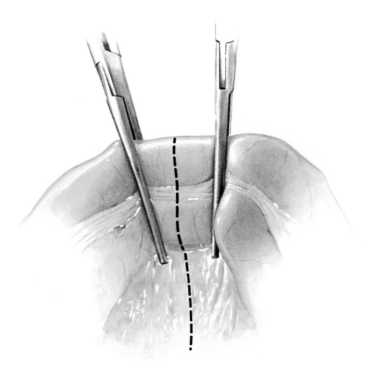

Fig. 15.4b. The mesentery is divided downward for a short distance along the broken line.

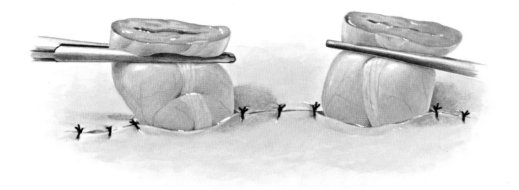

Fig. 15.4c.   The two limbs of bowel are brought out through the lateral margins of the wound.

may be excessive enough to require a very early secondary procedure with resection of the colon.

Closure of Persistent Stomas

Cecostomy

If a persistent stoma with mucosa growing to the surface is left after cecostomy a formal closure is necessary. The mucosa is freed from the abdominal wall and all adhesions to the peritoneum in the immediate neighborhood of the fistula are freed. The cecum is withdrawn for an appropriate distance. The stoma is then closed with two layers of sutures—an inner layer of 000 chromic catgut and an outer layer of interrupted silk. The stoma is then returned to the peritoneal cavity and the wound is closed in layers, preferably with catgut because of the possibility of sepsis.

Transverse Colostomy

Loop transverse colostomies may be closed in two ways. The first is applicable if the lumen of the bowel is large. The stoma is freed entirely from the abdominal wall and surrounding peritoneum. These adhesions must be freed widely because it is essential that the transverse colon be returned to the peritoneal cavity and that there be no kinking. This is at times a somewhat arduous task due to the adhesions of omentum around the stoma. Once the stoma has been completely freed, the colon is withdrawn from the peritoneal cavity and attention is turned to the stoma itself. The margins of the stoma are freshened and any adherent skin and scar are removed. If the lumen appears to be large, a simple closure can be carried out of the opening on the anterior wall of the loop colostomy by an inverting layer of interrupted or continuous Connell 000 chromic catgut and an outer layer of interrupted 000 silk (Fig. 15.5). The stoma is then returned to the peritoneal cavity and the wound is closed.

The above procedure is obviously applicable to loop colostomies. If the colostomy has been divided or the lumen of the colon is found to be too small after loop colostomy, it is necessary to carry out a resection and anastomosis of the transverse colon. The stomas are freed and withdrawn from the peritoneal cavity as described above. Normal transverse colon is

161

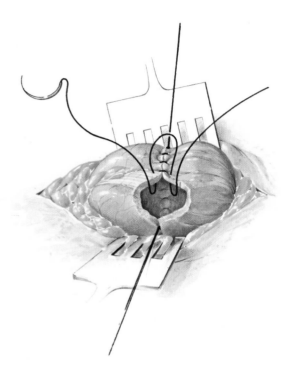

Fig. 15.5. Transverse colostomy closure. The bowel has been freed entirely and will be replaced within the peritoneal cavity. The lumen is so wide that a closure of the anterior wall can be made with two layers of sutures. The inner layer is interrupted catgut, and the outer layer is interrupted 000 silk. The rectus fascia is closed with polyolifin (Prolene) and deep retention sutures are inserted. If a delayed closure is to be employed the wound is packed open at this time. The pack is removed 3–4 days later and the sutures are tied. If primary closure is to be done the sutures are tied immediately and the skin is closed with silk. If the lumen of the colon is small, a resection and end-to-end anastomosis are necessary.

selected and Allen-Kocher clamps are applied both proximally and distally and the portion of the colon that is located immediately adjacent to the colostomy is excised. The corresponding vessels and mesentery also must be divided and ligated. An open end-to-end anastomosis is carried out according to the technique shown in Chapter 3. The colon then is returned to the peritoneal cavity and the incision is closed.

Methods of closure of colostomy incisions have elicited a great deal of comment in recent years. Two problems are involved. One is that there is an increased likelihood of infection because one is working with the open bowel. Second, these wounds are particularly likely to develop ventral hernias. Although there is no way to prevent all of these complications, we have found that the use of broad-spectrum antibiotics such as 1 g cephaloridine preoperatively and 1 g cephalexin or cefazolin sodium intravenously during the procedure reduces the incidence of sepsis and allows primary wound closure. In the preantibiotic days delayed wound closure was commonly used to prevent wound sepsis. Closure of the abdominal wound is preferably done in the following manner: No attempt is made to separate the various muscle layers. At times the peritoneum will even remain very adherent to the posterior muscle. The peritoneum is closed with a running catgut suture and then the rectus or oblique muscles are sutured in one layer with No. 30 steel wire or 00 polyolifin (Prolene). Two Mersilene tension sutures are inserted through the anterior fascia to eliminate dead space and the wound is closed primarily.

This procedure does not entirely eliminate the possibility of sepsis or late hernia but it has proved to be quite satisfactory. On the other hand, many surgeons prefer delayed primary closure after colostomy closure.

Complications of Closure of Transverse Colostomy

Studies of the complications following the closure of colostomies showed that the complications were exactly the same and just as numerous as those after resection and anastomosis of the colon.[9,11] This is not surprising since many of the same factors are present. Complications, including sepsis, late hernia formation, bleeding within the peritoneal cavity, leakage from the anastomosis with the formation of a fistula, intraperitoneal abscess, and rarely intestional obstruction, occurred in almost one-third of the patients. Formerly, when the closed colon remained in the abdominal wall, the formation of a fistula was very common. The return of the colon to the peritoneal cavity has essentially eliminated this complication. Intestinal obstruction may follow if the lumen of the transverse colon is inadequate to transmit gas or feces. This is usually manifested in the first few postoperative days by a good deal of distension of the right colon. For this reason decompression by the Levin tube is used for several days after operation.

Those surgeons who prefer delayed primary closure of such incisions close the abdominal wall by closing the peritoneum with running catgut. The muscle and fascia are then closed in a single layer of interrupted wire or polyolifin. The subcutaneous fat and skin are left open but several deep sutures are placed running through the skin and the anterior fascia. A loose gauze pack is then placed in the wound. This is removed 3–4 days later and the skin is brought together by tightening the tension sutures and inserting a few silk sutures. This secondary closure can be done relatively painlessly if the gauze is soaked with 1% lidocaine (Xylocaine) and the patient is given some intravenous meperidine prior to tying of the sutures.

One-Stage Operations for Colonic Obstruction

While it is our belief that one-stage resections and anastomoses are not indicated for lesions in the left colon, the situation is quite different if there is an obstructing carcinoma of the cecum, right colon, or transverse colon (Fig. 15.6). Under these circumstances it is possible to carry out a one-stage resection and anastomosis, and indeed this operation may be easier than in the normal patient because the terminal ileum may be sufficiently dilated to facilitate the anastomosis.

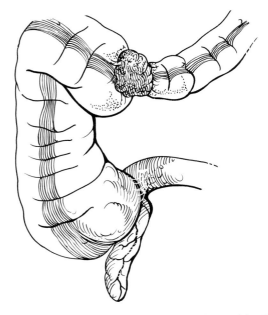

Fig. 15.6. Obstructed transverse colon with distention of right colon.

163

Obstructed Cecum, Right Colon, or Transverse Colon

The colon should be decompressed at the time of operation because the operation will be safer and the extent of the removal of the mesentery will not have to be compromised.

The abdomen is opened through a right or left paramedian incision. It is assumed that the patient already has a nasogastric tube in place. Distended small bowel and colon is encountered running to the site of obstruction. A long sump sucker is introduced through the terminal ileum into the cecum, and the gas and liquid contents of the cecum are removed in this fashion (Fig. 15.7). This opening is then closed with a purse-string suture. The operation can then proceed as a standard right colectomy.

It has been suggested (and frequently done in the past) that obstructions of the right colon could be treated by a diverting ileotransverse colostomy followed by a later resection of the right colon. This operation, however, has definite disadvantages. Since it is a two-stage operation, it is necessary to subject the patient to two procedures, a delay in the removal of the cancer, and a longer period of hospitalization. In addition there are technical problems that interfere with its efficacy. The most important is that behind this side-to-side anastomosis of the ileum to the colon there is a large trap through which small bowel may prolapse and produce obstruction. In addition, if the ileocecal valve is competent, there is essentially a closed loop located between the ileocecal valve and the obstructing cancer. Hence the ileotransverse colostomy may not completely protect against the possibility of perforation of the cecum. Furthermore, if it is used as a

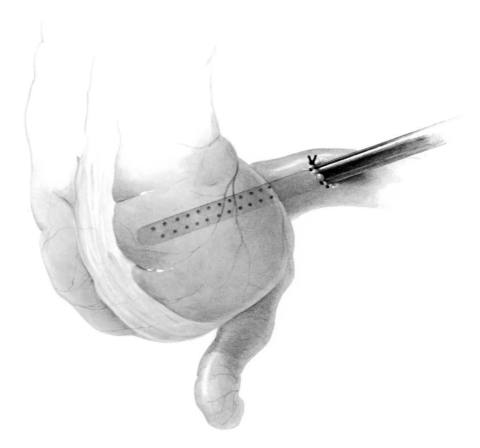

Fig. 15.7. Aspiration of contents of right colon by a sucker inserted through the terminal ileum.

more permanent measure it may not relieve the cramps of continuing right colon obstruction in the patient in whom a palliative sidetrack is carried out. For these reasons we prefer to carry out a resection of the right colon, even as a palliative procedure, whenever possible.

Obstructed Left Colon

The preceding discussion has indicated that we are strongly in favor of a decompressive transverse colostomy in the right upper quadrant for these lesions. Some surgeons have adopted a much more radical attitude. For example, it has been suggested that even in the presence of acute obstruction it will be possible to mobilize the obstructed left colon, bring the proximal limb out over the table, empty out all the feces into a bucket, and then proceed with a resection and anastomosis of the bowel as a primary measure. Needless to say, unless this is done very expertly there will be a great deal of contamination. Furthermore, the surgeon is likely to devote so much attention to the relief of the obstruction that he will carry out a less radical operation for cancer than he would under other circumstances. Consequently, we do not approve of this procedure.

However, it is possible to carry out a primary resection of an obstructed left colon and perform a colostomy rather than attempt an anastomosis. This method is indicated when the obstruction is associated with free perforation of the colon, as occurs occasionally with diverticulitis and less frequently with cancer.

Another variation of the procedures noted above is the performance of a colostomy immediately above the site of obstruction. If the obstruction is in the sigmoid, the descending colon has to be mobilized. This is generally not an easy procedure and may very well lead to contamination. Furthermore, the problems with wound care become much more difficult. The stoma tends to retract into the left paramedian incision. If there is a good deal of infection present around the obstructing lesion, the wound may become septic and delay any secondary procedure. We therefore believe that it is wiser to stay out of the left lower quadrant entirely (unless it is absolutely necessary to enter it to drain an abscess) until the transverse colostomy is functioning well and the intestinal obstruction has been relieved.

Other Manifestations of Obstruction

Apparent Small Bowel Obstruction due to Colonic Cancer

Cancer closely adjacent to the ileocecal valve or cancer of the lower ascending colon may give a clinical picture that is typical of acute small bowel obstruction. X-ray films will show multiple loops of dilated small bowel and no gas will be observable in the colon. At times the obstructing colonic carcinoma may be considerably more distal than the right colon. If the ileocecal valve allows free reflux of gas, the right colon may fill with soft fecal material and the x-ray film will show dilated, gas-filled small bowel loops that closely mimic ileac obstruction. Therefore, a thorough abdominal exploration is necessary at the time of any operation for presumed small intestinal obstruction.

Colonic Ileus and Pseudo-obstruction of the Colon

An unusual type of colonic obstruction may develop from paralytic ileus. In some instances the colon distends remarkably while the small bowel remains essentially normal. These changes have been noted after some abdominal operations, after nailing of a fractured hip, or after retroperitoneal injuries. The patient develops a quiet, distended abdomen. X-ray films show extensive dilatation of the colon. The cecum may become greatly distended and may measure as much as 13 cm in diameter.[6]

The proper treatment is decompression. This can be accomplished by the performance of a cecostomy with the patient under local anesthesia. Once the distention is relieved, spontaneous recovery is the rule. Deflation with the colonoscope has been reported by Kukora and Dent.[3] Hedberg has used colonoscopy successfully for this purpose as well.

A somewhat similar situation has been termed "pseudo-obstruction of the colon" or Ogilvie's syndrome.[6,7] There is marked distention of the right and transverse colons as far as the splenic flexure with collapse of the descending colon. A barium enema, however, shows no intrinsic obstruction. Unless there is some complicating feature or some other associated disease, spontaneous improvement is usual, but not certain.[8] In most instances, however, the differential diagnosis of a cancer of the splenic flexure must be entertained. A colonoscopy may prove to be both diagnostic and therapeutic. If deflation does not occur, a cecostomy is mandatory.

Colonic Ulceration Proximal to Obstructing Cancer

Ulceration and inflammation of the colon may occur proximal to obstructing carcinoma without a prior history of idiopathic ulcerative colitis.[2] The ulcers may be discrete, or in some cases a nonspecific enterocolitis may be present. Unless they are recognized at the time of operation an anastomosis may be made through an inflamed site, and anastomotic dehiscence may follow. Hence it is important for the surgeon or pathologist to open the specimen in the operating room.

Similar ulceration or enterocolitis may occur proximal to a stenosed ileostomy or rectal obstruction secondary to Hirschsprung's disease.

References

1. Allen A.W., Welch C.E. (1941) Cecostomy. Surg Gynecol Obstet 73: 549
2. Glotzer D.J., Roth S.I., Welch C.E. (1964) Colonic ulceration proximal to obstructing carcinoma. Surgery 56: 950
3. Kukora J.S., Dent T.L. (1977) Colonoscopic decompression of massive nonobstructive cecal dilation. Arch Surg 112: 512
4. Lowman R.M., Davis L. (1956) An evaluation of cecal size in impending perforation of the cecum. Surg Gynecol Obstet 103: 711
5. Paine J.R. (1966) Cancer of the colon. Treatment of large bowel obstruction. Postgrad Med 39: 596
6. Søreide O., Bjerkeset T., Fossdal J.E.(1977) Pseudo-obstruction of the colon (Ogilvie's syndrome), a genuine clinical condition? Dis Colon Rectum 20: 487
7. Spira I.A., Wolff W.I. (1976) Gangrene and spontaneous perforation of the cecum as a complication of pseudo-obstruction of the colon. Report of three cases and speculation as to etiology. Dis Colon Rectum 19: 557
8. Welch C.E. (1958) Intestinal obstruction. Year Book, Chicago
9. Welch C.E., Hedberg S.E. (1975) Complications in surgery of the colon and rectum. In: Artz C.P., Hardy J.D. (eds) Management of surgical complications, 3rd edn. Saunders, Philadelphia, p 600
10. Welch J.P., Donaldson G.A. (1974) Management of severe obstruction of the large bowel due to malignant disease. Am J Surg 127: 492
11. Yajko R.D., Norton L.W., Bloemendal L., et al (1976) Morbidity of colostomy closure. Am J Surg 132: 304

Surgery for Perforations

16

Perforations of the colon vary widely in their clinical manifestations. For example, in some instances the perforation may be slow and accompanied by agglutination of the colon to surrounding structures, producing a fistula rather than peritonitis. In other situations a perforation may occur that is walled off immediately by surrounding structures, producing an abscess. In rare instances, perforation into or involvement of a mesenteric vein can lead to pylephlebitis.[2,3,7] Subcutaneous emphysema has been reported.[9,10] In the most severe cases, however, there is free communication of the lumen of the colon with the peritoneal cavity, resulting in fecal peritonitis. In these cases mortality is extremely high unless prompt therapy is undertaken. In this chapter these major perforations will be considered.

The etiology is extremely variable. Perforations can be the result of acute diverticulitis, cancer, gangrene secondary to volvulus or vascular occlusion, acute ulcerative colitis, or wounds of the colon from either penetrating or blunt trauma. Iatrogenic injuries include perforations by the sigmoidoscope, colonoscope, or a foreign body introduced through the rectum, explosions from diathermy, bursting injuries of the colon due to compressed air, and perforation from barium scybalae or amebiasis. Many of these entities are rare and many of them can be prevented. Many are secondary to surgical misadventures, such as undetected injury of the colon at the time of laporatomy or an anastomotic leak several days after anastomosis.

The principles of therapy are the same in all cases, namely rapid preparation of the patient with fluid, blood, electrolytes, and broad-spectrum antibiotics, and immediate surgery. Depending upon the circumstances, the perforations are either repaired, exteriorized, or drained, or the colon is resected with or without an anastomotic procedure. The exact type of operation, as described in preceding chapters, is determined by the type of lesion and the degree of contamination. Since peritonitis militates against healing of an anastomotic line, anastomoses of the colon are performed with a great deal of hazard under unfavorable circumstances such as generalized peritonitis. Irrigation of the peritoneal cavity at the time of operation may be of value if there is gross fecal contamination; in general, however, irrigation of established peritonitis does little good. Appropriate drainage may be required in such areas as the pelvis or the right or left gutters. Antibiotic therapy is continued postoperatively.

TABLE 16.1. Antibiotics for Perforated Colon with General Peritonitis

Surgeon[a]	Antibiotic	Peritoneal irrigation
Beahrs, O. H.	Gentamicin, clindamycin, penicillin	None
Burke, J. F.	Gentamicin, penicillin	None
Cohn, I, Jr.	Gentamicin, clindamycin	Saline, kanamycin
Condon, R. E.	Gentamicin, clindamycin	Kanamycin, bacitracin
Dunphy, J. E.	Gentamicin, clindamycin	Half-strength povidone–iodine
Gallagher, D. M.	Gentamicin, clindamycin	None
Goligher, J. C.	Gentamicin, clindamycin	Saline
Hanley, P. H.	Gentamicin, clindamycin	Kanamycin, bacitracin
Polk, H. C., Jr.	Penicillin, kanamycin; Cephalothin gentamicin (severe cases)	Saline; half-strength povidone–iodine
Remington, J. H.	Cephalothin	Saline
Turnbull, R. B.	Cephalosporins	Cephalosporins
Welch, C. E., Ottinger, L. W., Welch, J. P.	Gentamicin, clindamycin	Saline

[a] All data are from personal communications (1978).

Antibiotic therapy varies in the hands of different surgeons; representative opinions of the proper choice are presented in Table 16.1.

Unusual Perforations of the Colon

Perforations of the colon may form fistulas that track through the peritoneum and appear on the thigh, in the perineum, or in the flanks, or that penetrate the diaphragm and are manifested in the chest.[19]

Perforations of the colon may also occur from feces. A mass of barium may be caught above an area of diverticulitis and produce a rock that cannot be extracted except by open operation. Stercoral perforations also may occur in the cecum.

In patients who are on cortisone therapy there is an increased possibility of perforations of diverticula.[1,17] The patients with ulcerative colitis who are being treated for toxic megacolon with large doses of cortisone may perforate silently without an increase in white blood cell count or fever.

Diverticular disease poses a hazard in patients who have an organ transplant and will require immunosuppressives. Preliminary colon resection has been urged by Sawyerr et al.[14]

An unusual perforation was seen by Shafiroff et al. As a complication of uterine prolapse, there was a spontaneous perforation of the rectum; small bowel prolapsed into it and out through the anal canal. The patient recovered after repair.[15]

Diastatic Perforations of the Cecum

The tension in a hollow cylinder varies directly in relationship to the diameter. Hence the pressure in the distended cecum is higher than that in the left colon. One of the most feared complications of acute colonic obstruction is a diastatic perforation of the cecum, which can split and perforate.

Whenever the cecum is more than 9 cm in diameter this possibility must be entertained, and above 12 cm the danger is excessive.[8] In nearly all of these instances there will be a competent ileocecal valve; thus the ascending colon will not be able to decompress itself back into the ileum.

This type of perforation is so important that whenever it is suspected at the time of laparotomy for intestinal obstruction it is necessary to observe the cecum to be sure that there are no tears of the serosa and no undetected perforations. If they are found, operative decompression on the table and an immediate resection are the wisest procedures. If the cecum is intact but extremely full and a transverse colostomy is contemplated, the transverse colostomy may be done, and the stoma can be opened on the table as soon as the wound has been closed. A catheter is inserted through the open colostomy into the ascending colon to provide decompression.

Acute Perforation Secondary to Diverticulitis

As an example of the numerous considerations that accompany the treatment of perforations associated with a specific disease, diverticulitis will be considered since this is one of the most common causes that is encountered.

These perforations nearly always occur in the sigmoid colon. They are diagnosed by localized pain and tenderness with fever. In many cases an inflammatory mass becomes palpable; this is an indication that the perforation has been walled off and an abscess is forming. In severe cases, however, the signs are those of diffuse peritonitis and surgery is indicated without delay. Several operative procedures are available for the treatment of perforations caused by diverticulitis. It is our belief that the surgeon must judge in individual cases which procedure will be the best to use.

Exploratory Laparotomy, Drainage of Abscess, Closure of Perforation, and Transverse Colostomy

This operation was the favorite procedure for perforated diverticulitis for many years.[4,12] It still is an excellent operation under some circumstances, particularly when there is a localized abscess. In cases of spreading peritonitis, even though the perforation in the bowel is small and the colon relatively flexible, we now prefer primary resection (see below). If a resection is not done, omentum is sutured over the perforation to provide further protection. An abscess can be drained directly by a stab wound and the insertion of drains or a suction catheter (Fig. 16.1). The transverse colostomy preferably is placed to the right of the midline. The second stage of the procedure—resection of the involved colon—will be carried out at an optimum time, usually 2–3 months later. The third stage involves the closure of the transverse colostomy.

This operation has been criticized on several counts.[12,13] First, the perforation may be so large or the walls of the bowel so stiff that it is impossible to close such an opening and any attempt to do so will be ineffectual. It has also been suggested that there is a long column of fecal material between the transverse colostomy and the perforated sigmoid that will provide an opportunity for continued contamination. Furthermore, the three-stage operation entails a long period of hospitalization and potentially increased morbidity due to the three operations that are required.

169

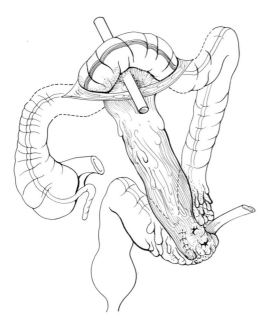

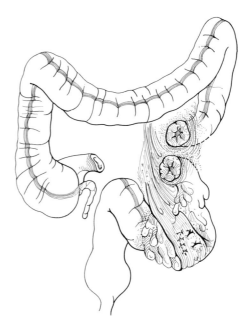

Fig. 16.1. Transverse colostomy, closure of perforation, and drainage of abscess. The colostomy is placed in the right upper quadrant. Identification of the site of perforation often is impossible. If a definite abscess is present, drainage and colostomy are indicated.

Fig. 16.2. Descending colon colostomy, suture of perforation, and drainage of abscess. This operation requires deep dissection and is much more difficult than that shown in Fig. 16.1.

Exploratory Laparotomy, Drainage of Abscess, Closure of Perforation, and Descending Colostomy

This operation is similar to that just described, but the colostomy is placed a short distance above the perforation (Fig. 16.2). This procedure has been advocated because it removes the chance of contamination from the long column of feces proximal to the perforation of the bowel. It also allows a two-stage rather than a three-stage operation since the colostomy can be excised along with the area of diverticulitis during the second stage.

Despite these advantages this procedure has its difficulties. It may be extremely difficult to make a stoma a short distance above the perforation. It would necessarily have to be in the descending colon, which is fixed; in many instances a good deal of dissection is required to bring the left colon to the surface. If the stoma is made in the same incision as the exploratory laparotomy, there is a danger of sepsis, breakdown of the wound, and retraction of the stoma, which can make this operation much more difficult in practice than it appears to be on paper. We do not advise this operation.

Laparotomy, Resection of the Area of Perforation, and Proximal and Distal Colostomies

This operation has been attaining a great deal of favor in the United States and undoubtedly represents one of the great advances in surgery in recent years.[5,9,11] The procedure is decidedly more difficult than that described above because it requires a great deal more dissection, better anesthesia, and more ancillary support (Fig. 16.3). Numerous tissue planes must be opened. Since the bowel may be inflamed, making hemostasis more difficult, this must be regarded as a more major operation than the above operations.

170

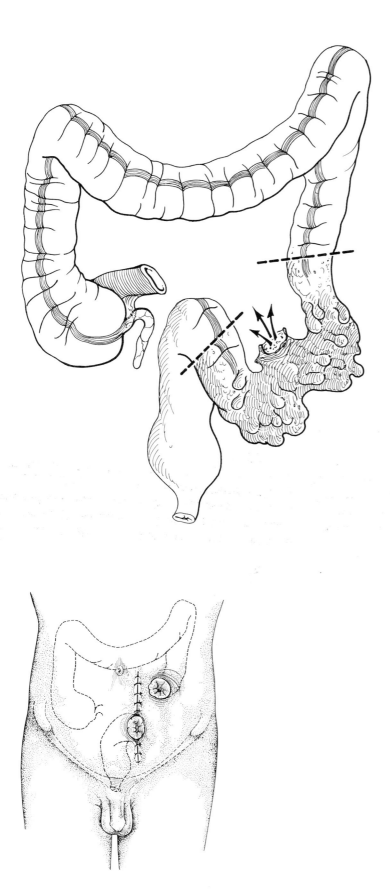

Fig. 16.3.   Resection of colon with double colon stomas. The distal colon must be long enough to be brought to the abdominal wall. The upper stoma should be brought out through a separate incision.

171

However, great advantages are derived from it. It can be employed for perforations that would be impossible to close adequately, and above all it removes the primary site of contamination from the peritoneal cavity. The second stage of the operation, which involves the reconstruction of intestinal continuity, can be carried out when the patient is in good condition.

Most of the reports on this operation have come from large centers, where it may be expected that the operating conditions in each instance were optimal. For example, Himal et al., of Royal Victoria Hospital, compared the three-stage operation (67 patients, 18 deaths) with primary excision and delayed anastomosis (10 patients, 1 death).[6] The advantage of primary excision has been confirmed by other series. Much better results with this procedure than with the three-stage operation have also been reported by Roxburgh,[13] Sweatman and Aldrete,[16] and Watkins and Oliver.[18] If conditions are not satisfactory, in an emergency a surgeon could merely exteriorize the perforated loop and achieve nearly the same objective with less dissection.

Immediate Resection of the Sigmoid, Proximal Colostomy, and Turn-In of the Rectal Stump

In a number of instances in which the area of diverticulitis has been resected, the rectal stump is too short to bring out to the surface of the skin. In this case the stump is turned in with three layers of sutures and the proximal colostomy is formed by withdrawal of the descending colon (Fig. 16.4). This application of the Hartmann operation is excellent for this complication. The surgeon should be certain to make the division of the distal colon in normal bowel but keep it as far above the base of the pelvic floor as possible. This makes the secondary reconstruction much easier than if the bowel has been cut off close to the peritoneal floor.

At the time of restoration of intestinal continuity, identification of a short rectal stump can be helped by filling the rectum with a uterine gauze pack prior to entering the abdomen. The gauze pack can be withdrawn after the stump is opened prior to the anastomosis.

Resection of the Perforated Sigmoid and Immediate End-to-End Anastomosis With or Without a Protective Transverse Colostomy

The presence of peritonitis makes this operation a good deal more hazardous than those described above. Immediate resection and anastomosis without concomitant transverse colostomy is not advised for this reason. There may be occasional instances in which the surgeon may feel that contamination has been relatively minor and the anastomosis can be done without the protection of the colostomy; this is true when small abscesses can be excised along with the colon.

Summary

In summary, we advise immediate segmental colon resection without anastomosis for patients with diffuse, general, or spreading peritonitis from perforated diverticulitis. The three-stage operation is reserved for patients with localized abscesses or with small perforations that can be closed easily, or it is used in instances in which surgery is done under unfavorable circumstances.

172

Acute Perforation Secondary to Cancer of the Colon

Fortunately, acute perforation secondary to cancer of the colon is rare. The areas of colon that are most frequently involved are the sigmoid and the cecum.[20] In these instances, if there is to be any hope of cure whatso-

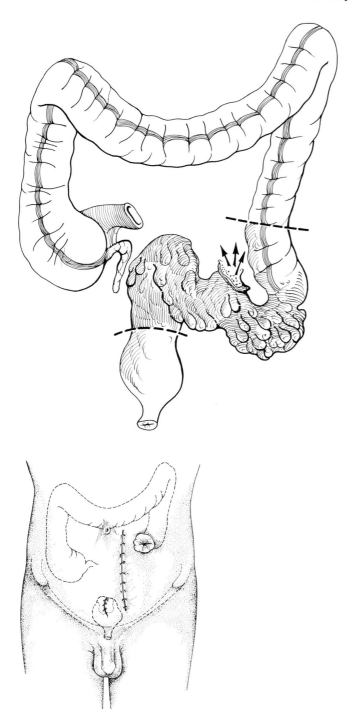

Fig. 16.4.   Hartmann operation. The rectal stump is too short to be exteriorized. The stump should be made as long as possible in order to make the second stage easier. The stump is turned in with three layers of catgut sutures.

ever, it is imperative that the section of bowel containing the cancer be excised at the time of emergency laparotomy. Usually it is wise to avoid an immediate anastomosis and to provide proximal and sital stomas that can, if the patient survives, be closed at a later date. The operative mortality is very high in these instances. One factor that contributes to these rather sorry results is the fact that, particularly in the sigmoid, perforation is often associated with obstruction, making the fecal contamination excessive, and death from peritonitis is likely to follow.

References

1. Canter J.W., Shorb P.E. Jr. (1971) Acute perforation of colonic diverticula associated with prolonged adrenocorticosteroid therapy. Am J Surg 121: 46
2. Case Records of the Massachusetts General Hospital (1977) Weekly Clinicopathological Exercises. Case 18-1977. Fever, jaundice and right-upper-quadrant tenderness in a 69-year-old woman. N Eng J Med 296: 1051
3. Ching-Shen L. (1973) Suppurative pylephlebitis and liver abscess complicating colonic diverticulitis: Report of two cases and review of literature. Mt Sinai J Med 40: 48
4. Classen J.N., Bonardi R., O'Mara C.S., et al (1976) Surgical treatment of acute diverticulitis by staged procedures. Ann Surg 184: 582
5. Eng K., Ranson J.H.C., Localio S.A. (1977) Resection of the perforated segment. A significant advance in treatment of diverticulitis with free perforation or abscess. Am J Surg 133: 67
6. Himal H.S., Ashby D.B., Duignan J.P., et al (1977) Management of perforating diverticulitis of the colon. Surg Gynecol Obstet 144: 225
7. Juler G.L., Dietrick W.R., Eisenman J.I. (1976) Intramesenteric perforation of sigmoid diverticulitis with nonfatal venous intravasation. Am J Surg 132: 653
8. Lowman R.M., Davis L. (1956) An evaluation of cecal size in impending perforation of the cecum. Surg Gynecol Obstet 103: 711
9. Nahrwold D.L., Demuth W.E. (1977) Diverticulitis with perforation into the peritoneal cavity. Ann Surg 185: 80
10. Oetting H.K., Kramer N.E., Branch W.E. (1955) Subcutaneous emphysema of gastrointestinal origin. Am J Med 19: 872
11. Rodkey G.V., Welch C.E. (1969) Surgical management of colonic diverticulitis with free perforation of abscess formation. Am J Surg 117: 265
12. Rodkey G.V., Welch C.E. (1974) Colonic diverticular disease with surgical treatment. A study of 338 cases. Surg Clin North Am 54: 655
13. Roxburgh R.A. (1972) Immediate resection of acute diverticulitis. Proc R Soc Med 63 [Suppl]: 52
14. Sawyerr O.I., Garvin P.J., Codd J.E., et al (1978) Colorectal complications of renal allograft transplantation. Arch Surg 113: 84
15. Shafiroff B.B., Carnevale N., Delany H.M. (1976) Spontaneous rupture of the rectosigmoid colon with anal evisceration: A new complication of uterine prolapse. Surgery 79: 360
16. Sweatman C.A. Jr., Aldrete J.S. (1977) The surgical management of diverticular disease of the colon complicated by perforation. Surg Gynecol Obstet 144: 47
17. Warshaw A.L., Welch J.P., Ottinger L.W. (1976) Acute perforation of the colon associated with chronic corticosteroid therapy. Am J Surg 131: 442
18. Watkins G.L., Oliver G.A. (1971) Surgical treatment of acute perforative sigmoid diverticulitis. Surgery 69: 215
19. Welch, J.P. (1976) Unusual abscesses in perforating colorectal cancer. Am J Surg 131: 270
20. Welch J.P., Donaldson G.A. (1974) Perforative carcinoma of colon and rectum. Ann Surg 180: 734

Surgery for Fistulas

17

Fistulas from the colon may be either external or internal and are associated with a number of diseases.

Internal Fistulas

Internal fistulas from the colon have involved nearly all of the abdominal viscera, including the small intestine, duodenum, stomach, renal pelvis, ureter, uterus, and bladder. In addition, fistulous tracts may burrow into unexpected areas such as the chest, buttocks, retroperitoneal area, or thigh. The gallbladder also may be the site of fistulization, but this is usually caused by a stone eroding through the gallbladder into the colon. In one of our cases, a pancreatitis eroded into the colon and caused massive colonic hemorrhage.

Duodenocolic fistulas may arise from ulcerative disease or cancer of the duodenum penetrating into the colon or, in a reverse direction, from colonic carcinoma or diverticular disease penetrating into the duodenum (Fig. 17.1). Since the fistula is usually comparatively small, it will not lead to the marked nutritional defects that occur with a large gastrocolic fistula.

The presence of a gastrocolic fistula is usually marked by the sudden onset of severe diarrhea. The bowel movement may contain undigested food. A barium enema usually but not always shows reflux into the stomach. Although these fistulas usually follow either a gastroenterostomy or gastric resection with a Billroth II anastomosis for duodenal ulcer, in some instances a benign gastric ulcer leads to perforation of the colon and a gastrocolic fistula.[12] It is more common for a carcinoma of the transverse colon to penetrate into the stomach than a cancer of the stomach to penetrate the colon.

The operative procedures employed for these internal fistulas involve appropriate resections and anastomoses to restore intestinal continuity.[11-13] Inasmuch as some diseases have led to very marked nutritional deficiencies, a period of hyperalimentation is now employed prior to surgery to place the patient in good enough condition so that the old staged operations that were required for such fistulas no longer are necessary.

175

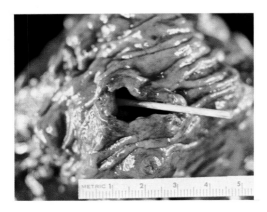

Fig. 17.1.   Operative specimen of duodenocolic fistula secondary to cancer of the colon.

External Fistulas

External fistulas occur when the disease that is primary in the colon produces perforation that eventually tracks through the skin.[1,3,5,8,11] This complication usually follows diverticulitis but also can occur with cancer, Crohn's disease, tuberculosis, actinomycosis, or foreign body perforations. Healing of the tract may be expected to follow removal of the colon segment from which the fistula arises. With inflammatory diseases such as tuberculosis or actinomycosis, specific antibiotic therapy may be extremely important and may avoid the propensity to refistulization.

An important cause of fistulas is anastomotic leakage, with tracking through a drain site to an external area. Placement of a drain next to an anastomotic line increases the risk of fistula formation. Secondary drainage of an abscess that has followed an anastomotic leak will also be followed by fistula formation. Spontaneous healing is the rule provided there is no distal obstruction.

The factors that militate against spontaneous closure of an external colonic fistula include (1) a large fistula, i.e., over 1 cm in diameter, (2) the presence of distal obstruction, (3) the presence of inflammatory disease in the colon, such as Crohn's disease, diverticulitis, or rare infections such as tuberculosis or actinomycosis, (4) epithelialization of a longstanding tract, which allows no opportunity for spontaneous constriction and cure, (5) persistent cancer, and (6) previous radiation therapy. In our experience approximately half of all colonic fistulas close spontaneously. However, in the presence of prolapsed mucous membrane or the other factors mentioned above, spontaneous closure cannot be expected and an operative procedure should be carried out.

The operation involves identification of the area from which the fistula arises. It is usually necessary to resect a section of colon to be certain that normal bowel is selected for any anastomosis.

After low anterior resections some surgeons place drains downward through the perineum. If a fistula forms it tends to persist despite colostomy because of fixation of the bowel to surrounding structures. A difficult resection and anastomosis may then be required.

Sometimes surgery for a fistula requires proximal fecal diversion as a preliminary step. This is indicated particularly if there is a large amount of drainage from the fistula or if a secondary infection is associated with it. Unless there is underlying disease in the colon, this procedure in itself may lead to spontaneous closure of small fistulas. This situation is encountered most often in draining sinuses following resections of the sigmoid colon. A transverse colostomy is made by the usual technique. Closure of the colostomy is deferred until healing is certain and confirmed by barium enema or by sigmoidoscopy. Hyperalimentation is helpful in patients with poor nutrition.[1,3,5]

Sometimes a colostomy may have to serve as the definitive treatment of a fistula. In the presence of a large rectovaginal fistula after radiation treatment for cancer of the cervix it may be impossible to find any normal distal rectum suitable for anastomosis. In cases in which there is a few centimeters of normal distal mucosa, preliminary colectomy may be followed by a D'Allaines or Soave procedure.

Rectovaginal fistulas following childbirth are now extremely rare. Transverse colostomy followed by direct repair through the posterior wall of the vagina is the usual therapy. Mucosal flaps are dissected back, the fistula is excised, and the bowel wall is turned in with one or two layers of catgut sutures. The vaginal mucosa is closed in a separate layer; silver wire was used originally by Sims and still is an excellent material. Rectovaginal fistulas arising above the sphincters due to inflammatory disease are not likely to be cured by this technique.

In a study of colon fistulas carried out in Massachusetts General Hospital by Edmunds et al., it was found that 29 of 55 colonic fistulas were treated expectantly, with cure in 15 of the 20.[4] Operative procedures were used in all the other cases. The lesions were caused by anastomotic failures, surgical injury, appendicitis, diverticulitis, Crohn's disease, ulcerative colitis, chronic abscesses, tuberculosis, perforation by a catheter, and blunt and penetrating trauma. A more recent series by Aguirre et al. led to essentially similar conclusions.[1]

Fistulas Arising from Diverticulitis

Since diverticulitis is the most common colonic disease that leads to both internal and external fistulas, it will be considered separately. The location of these fistulas in a representative series is shown in Table 17.1. It will be observed that the most important is the sigmoidovesical fistula[2,4,7] (Fig. 17.2).

Sigmoidovesical fistulas are more apt to occur in males or in females who have had a hysterectomy because the uterus does protect the bladder effectively when it is interposed between the sigmoid and the bladder. The onset of urinary symptoms in a patient with known diverticulitis may indicate the presence of an incipient fistula. The passage of air by urethra is pathognomonic of either this disease or diabetes. A cystoscopy is likely to show an indurated, inflamed area in the upper portion of the bladder. Occasionally fecal contamination can be seen coming from this region. A barium enema may be negative except for the presence of diverticulitis if the opening is small. However, in the presence of large lesions there will be reflux through the fistula into the bladder (Fig. 17.3).[10]

Operative treatment of sigmoidovesical fistulas consists of resection of the involved area of sigmoid and anastomosis and closure of the fistulous tract into the bladder. Closure of the opening in the bladder can usually be effected by two layers of catgut. Adequate drainage is maintained by means of an inlying Foley catheter, and a cystostomy tube is not necessary.

TABLE 17.1. Fistulas Secondary to
Diverticulitis[a]

	Number	Percent
Colovesical	131	53.3
Colocutaneous	77	31.3
Coloenteric	25	10.2
Colovaginal	4	1.6
Colocolonic	3	
Colouterine	2	
Colouterovesical	2	3.7
Coloureteral	1	
Coloperineal	1	
	246	

[a] Collected series (data from Colcock and Stahmann[2]).

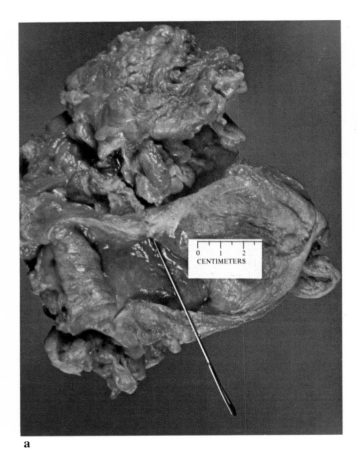

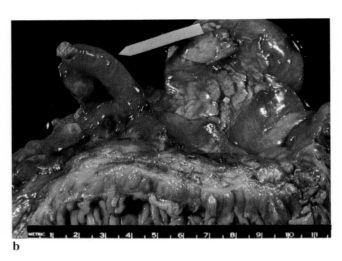

Fig. 17.2a and b. Sigmoidovesical fistulas. a. Autopsy specimen. b. Operative specimen.

a

b

The main controversy in the treatment of these fistulas is concerned with the necessity for a one-stage versus a staged procedure with a colostomy established either prior to or simultaneously with the resection. It is certain that most of these fistulas may be handled in a single stage, particularly if omentum is present that can be brought down to be interposed between the line of anastomosis of the colon and the closure of the bladder. In some patients who have had a fistula for a protracted period of time there may be an inordinate amount of fibrosis and pericolic inflammation. These conditions may predispose to breakdown of the suture line and refistulization. In advanced cases, therefore, we believe that it is wise to create a transverse colostomy at the time of the original resection and to maintain this for a period of months until it is proved by irrigations and barium enemas that the sigmoid has completely healed.

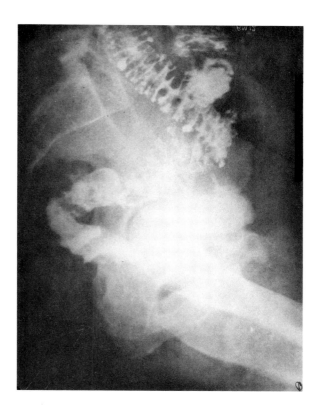

Fig. 17.3. Barium enema showing sigmoidovesical fistula.

Other fistulas usually can be treated by a one-stage resection and anastomosis. If the small bowel is involved, a concomitant resection and anastomosis of the segment is necessary. If the ureter is the site of fistulization, every attempt should be made to place the colon suture line well away from the ureter and protect the ureter as much as possible. A drain should be left in apposition with the ureter. When fistulas occur to the skin or vagina, no particular care of the fistulous tract is necessary. When the sigmoid is treated by resection and anastomosis the tract will heal.

Low Rectovaginal Fistulas

Fistulas from the rectum to the vagina that occur within 6 cm of the dentate line may be treated by either a rectal or vaginal approach. These fistulas generally follow childbirth or infection.

The rectal approach for fistulas that occur within 2 cm of the dentate line has been described by Russell and Gallagher.[9] An incision is made anteriorly a short distance below the mucocutaneous junction. The mucosa, the submucosa, and a portion of the internal sphincter are dissected upward past the fistula until normal tissue is reached. The fistula is excised and normal mucous membrane is overlapped, covering the defect. Russell and Gallagher do not perform a colostomy, and the majority of their patients have done well.

If the fistula is associated with disruption of the anal sphincter, repair is carried out as described in Chapter 22.[7]

For somewhat higher fistulas, Greenwald and Hoexter have employed a transanal approach for fistulas within 6 cm of the dentate line.[6] After careful preparation by mechanical means and antibiotics, the anal canal is dilated, the fistula is excised completely with surrounding tissues, and normal mucosa is brought down for repair of the defect by suture.

179

References

1. Aguirre A., Fischer J.E., Welch C.E. (1974) The role of surgery and hyperalimentation in therapy of gastrointestinal–cutaneous fistulae. Ann Surg 180: 393
2. Colcock B.P., Stahmann F.D. (1972) Fistulas complicating diverticular disease of the sigmoid colon. Ann Surg 175: 838
3. Dudrick S.I., Wilmore D.W., Vars H.M., Rhoads J.E. (1968) Long-term total parenteral nutrition with growth, development, and positive nitrogen balance. Surgery 64: 134
4. Edmunds I.H. Jr., Williams G.M., Welch C.E. (1960) External gastrointestinal fistulae arising from the gastrointestinal tract. Ann Surg 152: 445
5. Fischer J.E. (1976) Total parenteral nutrition. Little, Brown, Boston
6. Greenwald J.C., Hoexter B. (1978) Repair of rectovaginal fistulas. Surg Gynecol Obstet 146: 443
7. Henderson M.A., Small W.P. (1969) Vesico-colic fistula complicating diverticular disease. Br J Urol 41: 314
8. Roberts C., Reber H., Way L., et al (1978) External gastrointestinal fistulas. Ann Surg 188: 460
9. Russell T.R., Gallagher D.M. (1977) Low rectovaginal fistulas. Approach and treatment. Am J Surg 134: 13
10. Ward J.N., Lavengood R.W. Jr., Nay H.R., et al (1970) Diagnosis and treatment of colovesical fistulas. Surg Gynecol Obstet 130: 1082
11. Webster M.W. Jr., Carey L.C. (1976) Fistulae of the intestinal tract. Curr Probl Surg (June) 13: 1
12. Welch J.P. (1979) Internal and external gastric, duodenal and biliary fistulas. In: Maingot R. (ed) Abdominal operations, 7th edn. Appleton-Century-Crofts, New York
13. Welch, J.P., Warshaw A.L. (1977) Malignant duodenocolic fistulas. Am J Surg 133: 658

Prolapse of the Rectum 18

Although there is no standard terminology for the various lesions that are grouped together under this heading, most surgeons loosely define the term "prolapse" as the protrusion of either mucous membrane or the entire muscular wall of the rectum outside the anus. To be more specific, one should use the term "mucosal prolapse" or "procidentia," which is defined as the extrusion of the entire rectum including the muscular wall.

Quite similar changes may occur internally in the absence of the appearance of any external prolapse. Bacon et al. have called such changes "internal prolapses."[2,3] If only the mucous membrane of the rectum is involved, there may be symptoms of tenesmus due to the extraordinary amount of mucous membrane that may obstruct the upper portion of the anal canal; we believe that this change is more accurately called the "descending perineum syndrome," as described by Parks et al.[11] (see Chapter 21). Bacon et al. also use the term "internal procidentia," which is synonymous with intussusception in which the involved bowel does not project through the anal sphincters.

In this chapter the term "prolapse" will be used to describe the external manifestations of the disease. Minor degrees of prolapse that involve only the mucous membrane are usually accompanied by large prolapsing hemorrhoids. Consequently, the operative procedure for relief consists of a hemorrhoidectomy that is modified to carry the excision of mucous membrane higher than in ordinary hemorrhoidectomy. The usual care must be taken to be certain that mucosal bridges are left between the segments of hemorrhoids that are removed in order to avoid late stenosis.

The more advanced cases of true procidentia will be considered in the remainder of this chapter. These prolapses may occur at any time from childhood to old age. In childhood they are usually a result of constipation and the usual course ends in spontaneous relief by age 5. Operation is very rarely indicated in children; prolapse is reduced and the buttocks are strapped together after each defecation. The disease is relatively uncommon in youth and middle age but appears frequently in old age due to the increasing laxity of the sphincter muscles and the levator sling. There undoubtedly are other contributing causes. In nearly all instances there is an unusually long sigmoid, an elongated mesentery of the sigmoid and intraperitoneal rectum, and little intraperitoneal fixation of the rectum. The disease occurs somewhat more commonly in females; in Altemeier and Culbertson's series 60% of the patients were female.[1] Psychoses or neurological diseases are often present. The pathologic changes include a patulous external sphincter and a large defect in the pelvic diaphragm, allowing the pouch of Douglas to pass downward with the prolapsing bowel.

The symptoms are local pain, ulceration, and bleeding caused by contact of the mucous membrane with irritants such as clothes. Incontinence is extremely common and is difficult to relieve entirely by operative procedures.

There have been innumerable operations designed for the relief of complete prolapse.[4,5,9,10,12–14,16,17] In general they can be divided into two groups: first, the procedures that may be carried out through the perineum; and second, those that require an abdominal approach. A combined abdominoperineal procedure, described below, may also be used.

Perineal Operations

Probably the simplest procedure that has been devised consists of inserting a rather stiff rubber tube into the rectum, bringing the prolapse over it, and tying a necrosing ligature tightly about the prolapse just distal to the dentate line. Theoretically this will produce gradual necrosis and a spontaneous anastomosis. This operation, however, is not recommended. There may be loops of small bowel present in the hernia of the pouch of Douglas, and the possibility of sepsis cannot be minimized.

Thiersch was the first to insert a wire about the anal canal (Fig. 18.1a). This procedure has been advocated particularly in old patients. It is done very simply by Turell's technique (Fig. 18.1b).[15] A No. 20 wire is inserted subcutaneously at the posterior commissure and is advanced through a needle that has been inserted just lateral to the rectum. The wire is brought back through a second needle on the opposite side, and then the wire is snugged about the examining finger until the proper diameter of anal canal is achieved (Fig. 18.1c). This procedure requires only two small skin incisions and should minimize the problems of infection that may occur with this procedure. Silver wire has often been used since it is more resistant to infection.

While this method is comparatively simple, it is open to the complications of sepsis and wire breakage; thus the procedure is not a permanent one. Furthermore, the rectum may intussuscept above the wire and produce intestinal obstruction, requiring removal of the wire. On the other hand, it can be of value as a temporary measure in poor-risk patients or as an adjunct to some other operation, with the expectation that the wire will need to be removed in one-third of the patients.

The prototype of perineal operations was devised by Delorme.[4] It consisted of excision of the mucosa of the prolapsed segment, reefing of the underlying muscle, and reanastomosis of the mucosa to the anal skin at the level of the dentate line.

The perineal operation that has been used most frequently in recent years was developed by Altemeier and Culbertson.[1] Several important details must be observed in its proper execution. The excess colon and rectum are excised, and an anastomosis is made at the level of the dentate line. The pouch of Douglas is closed at a much higher level and the levator sling is tightened considerably.

The patient is placed in the lithotomy position. A circumferential incision is made about the prolapse just above the dentate line (Fig. 18.2a).

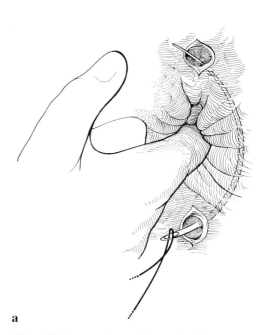

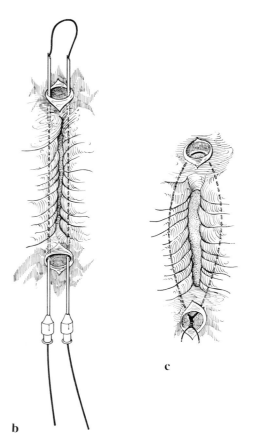

a

Fig. 18.1a–c. Insertion of Thiersch wire through a short posterior and anterior incision 1.5 cm from the anal verge. a. A No. 20 silver wire may be inserted by a Reverdin needle.

c

b

Fig. 18.1b and c. b. Long needles can be inserted lateral to the anus, which is stretched into essentially a straight line. The wire is then inserted through the needles and the needles are withdrawn (Turell's technique). c. The wire is tightened about the index finger of an assistant that is inserted as deeply as possible into the anal canal. The wire is tightened until it is comfortably snug on the finger.

Theoretically it is best to remove only the mucosa at this level in order to leave a cuff of sphincter muscles intact. This embodies the essentials of the Soave operation. However, Altemeier usually carries the incision through the outer layer of the entire rectal wall, dissociating the whole rectum, including the internal sphincter, from the anal canal. If the details of the Soave procedure are followed, the submucous dissection is carried up to approximately 5 cm above the dentate line, involving the entire circumference of the bowel, including the rectal wall, in the dissection.

Early in the dissection the base of the pouch of Douglas is identified anteriorly (Fig. 18.2b and c). It must be opened or retracted. It is generally better to open it so that at a later time the excess can be excised and the defect closed at a high level. The levator muscles then are identified on either side of the rectum. They will be found to be extremely lax. The dissection is carried up on the sigmoid as high as necessary to remove all of the redundant colon (Fig. 18.2d). At times this will be only 10 cm or so in length, but in some cases as much as 50 cm of redundant bowel will need to be excised. After complete mobilization of the redundant bowel the pouch of Douglas is obliterated by suture (Fig. 18.2e). The levators are sutured

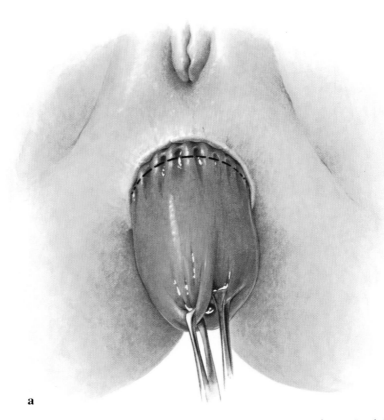

a

Fig. 18.2a–g.   Perineal resection and anastomosis. a. Incision of the rectal wall just above the dentate line (as shown by the broken line).

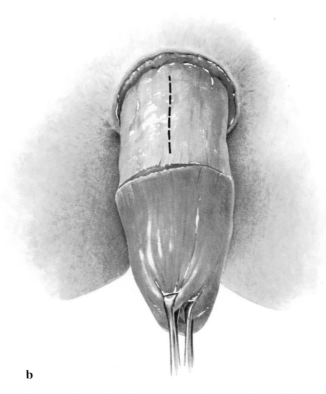

b

Fig. 18.2b.   The intussuscepting portion of the rectum is exposed. Traction displays the pouch of Douglas, which lies below the broken line.

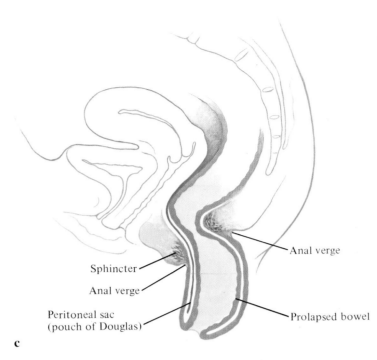

c

Sphincter

Anal verge

Peritoneal sac
(pouch of Douglas)

Anal verge

Prolapsed bowel

Fig. 18.2c. Sagittal section showing the relation of the prolapsed rectum and pouch of Douglas.

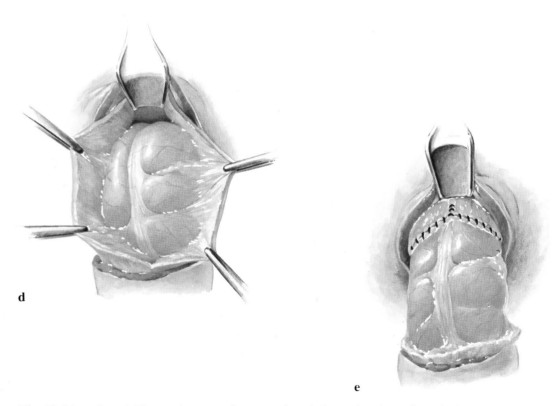

d

e

Fig. 18.2d and e. d. The peritoneum is opened and the redundant sigmoid is withdrawn. e. The excess peritoneal sac is excised and then the peritoneum is closed by suture.

185

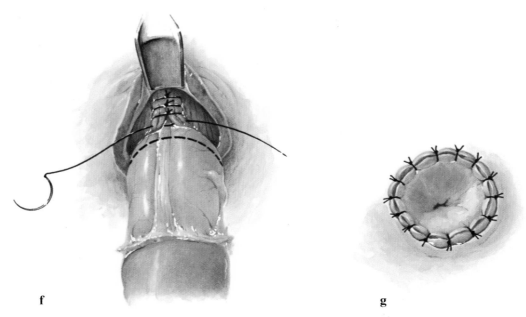

f   g

Fig. 18.2f and g.   f. The levators are plicated anterior to the rectum. Excess bowel is then resected along the broken line. g. Completion of a two-layer anastomosis of the intraperitoneal rectum or sigmoid to the dentate line.

together anterior to the rectum with several deep 0 chromic catgut sutures (Fig. 18.2f).

The sigmoid is amputated at a proper spot to secure an anastomosis at the level of the dentate line. A two-layer anastomosis is performed with absorbable sutures to reconstitute the continuity of the bowel and the anal canal (Fig. 18.2g). If there has been any persistent bleeding, a sump catheter may be inserted through a stab incision laterally into the operative field and left on suction for a few days.

Transabdominal Operations

The earliest transabdominal operation for prolapse was devised by Moschowitz.[9] This procedure essentially consisted of elevation of the rectum, suture to the uterus, and suspension of the uterus to the anterior abdominal wall. Recurrent prolapse was quite common. This problem led to the development of more extensive dissections and suspensions, such as those described by Pemberton et al.[12] Again, the incidence of recurrence tended to be high.

In order to hold the rectum and sigmoid in a more normal position, some surgeons then carried out a sigmoid colostomy with a secondary closure. It was hoped that in these instances a fixation of the sigmoid would prevent the recurrence of prolapse.

In our opinion by far the best results have been obtained with a low anterior resection combined with a fixation of the rectum to the posterior wall of the pelvis.[14] This procedure is carried out through a left paramedian incision. The rectum is first freed very widely (Fig. 18.3a). The inferior mesenteric vessels are divided below the left colic or upper sigmoid branches. The lateral hemorrhoidal vessels are then divided. The dissection is carried posteriorly as far as the coccyx and anteriorly downward on the posterior vagina or on the prostate. This part of the dissection is almost the same as it would be for a combined abdominoperineal resection of the rectum. The extremely redundant intraperitoneal rectum and sigmoid are then excised and an end-to-end anastomosis is carried out at a low level (Fig. 18.3b). Fixation of the colon is ensured by the dissection that has been carried out, but it may be made even more secure by the addition of sutures that attach the sigmoid mesentery to the presacral fascia or, if Bacon's technique is followed, to the tendons of the psoas minor muscles. Due care must be taken with these sutures to be certain that the sigmoid is not angulated severely. It may be impossible to place them after a wide dissection if the sigmoid is relatively free of appendices epiploicae.

Another procedure that has been used quite frequently in recent years involves the use of a cuff of plastic mesh about the rectum that retracts the rectum posteriorly and removes the straight course of the rectum and sigmoid, which is presumed to be one of the causes of the prolapse. Wells[16] has employed Ivalon and Ripstein and Lanter[13] have used a Teflon sling for this procedure. This is fitted into the pouch of Douglas and sutured in place

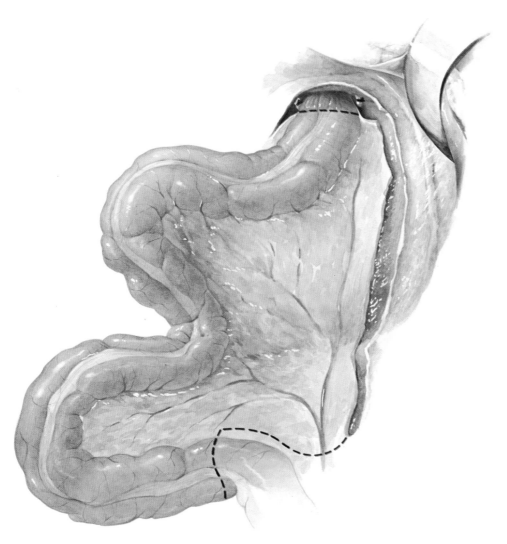

Fig. 18.3a and b.   Anterior resection and fixation of the rectum. a. Redundant sigmoid colon and intraperitoneal rectum have been mobilized widely and will be resected. The pelvic peritoneum is incised anterior to the rectum so that the extra-peritoneal rectum can be elevated. The broken line indicates the line of resection.

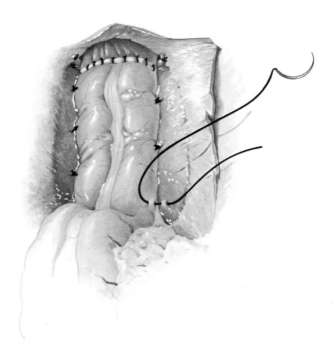

Fig. 18.3b. An end-to-end anastomosis is performed
in a fashion illustrated in Figure 3.1. The sigmoid is
anchored to the cut margin of the peritoneum and to
the posterior fascia overlying the sacrum.

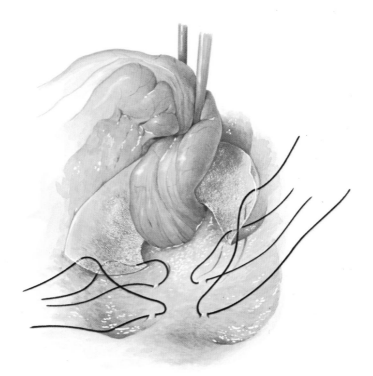

Fig. 18.4a.   The rectum is mobilized at the level of the
peritoneal floor and a sling of plastic mesh is passed
around the anterior surface. This will now be sutured
to the fascia overlying the sacrum with interrupted silk
sutures.

so that the rectum is angulated backward (Fig. 18.4). This operation has been approved by a number of eminent surgeons, including Sir Clifford Morgan.[8] However, it is not devoid of the possibility of recurrence. Another disadvantage is that afterward it is impossible to examine the rectum by sigmoidoscopy and even colonoscopy may be extremely difficult. In some instances, obstruction or infection has required removal of the mesh.

Combined Abdominoperineal Operations

Various combined procedures have been proposed. One is an anterior resection that could be combined at a later date with the insertion of a Thiersch wire to tighten the sphincters. Other more extensive perineal procedures have been employed. For example, Dunphy et al. have reefed the levator muscles anterior to the rectum through the perineum and carried out an anterior resection; this can be done in one or two stages.[5]

Complications

The most important postoperative complication is persistent fecal incontinence. The great majority of these patients were incontinent prior to operation and at least one-third of them continue to be incontinent postoperatively. However, Altemeier has reported nearly complete relief of this symptom after his operation. It is only fair to say that not all surgeons have attained similar success.

The second important complication is recurrent prolapse. In a summary of the innumerable operations that have been employed for prolapse Theuerkauf and co-workers reported the incidence of recurrence. The fig-

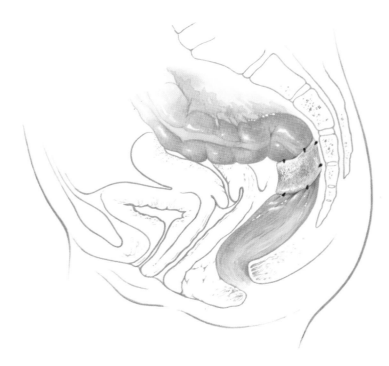

Fig. 18.4b. The completed sling angulates the rectum sharply posteriorly. Sutures are applied to hold the sling firmly in place on the rectal wall. Too tight a sling may obstruct the bowel.

189

ure for anterior resection is approximately 3.5%; with the old methods of Moschowitz and the less extensive resections the recurrence rate was over 40%.[14]

References

1. Altemeier W.A., Culbertson W.R. (1965) Technique for perineal repair of rectal prolapse. Surgery 58: 758
2. Bacon H.E. (1949) Anus–rectum–sigmoid colon, 3rd edn, Vols 1 and 2. Lippincott, Philadelphia, p 497
3. Bacon H.E., Arias E., Carroll P.T., et al (1956) Complete rectal prolapse or procidentia: Diagnosis and treatment. Geriatrics 11: 231
4. Delorme R. (1912) Sur le traitement des grands prolapsus du rectum. Bull Med Soc Chir Paris 38: 435
5. Dunphy J.E., Botsford T.W., Savlov E. (1953) Surgical treatment of procidentia of the rectum: An evaluation of combined abdominal and perineal repair. Am J Surg 86: 605
6. Ejaife J.A., Elias E.G. (1977) Delorme's repair for rectal prolapse. Surg Gynecol Obstet 144: 757
7. Frykman H.M., Goldberg S.M. (1969) The surgical treatment of rectal procidentia. Surg Gynecol Obstet 129: 1225
8. Morgan C.N. (1974) Operation for complete prolapse of the rectum. In: Maingot R. (ed) Abdominal operations, 6th edn, Vol 2. Appleton-Century-Crofts, New York, p 2157
9. Moschowitz A.V. (1912) The pathogenesis, anatomy and cure of prolapse of the rectum. Surg Gynecol Obstet 15: 7
10. Parks A.G. (1967) Post-anal perineorrhaphy for rectal prolapse. Proc R Soc Med 60: 920
11. Parks A.G., Porter N.H., Hardcastle J. (1966) The syndrome of the descending perineum. Proc R Soc Med 59: 477
12. Pemberton J. deJ., Kiernan P.C., Pemberton A.H. (1953) The results of the surgical treatment of complete rectal prolapse, with particular reference to suspension–fixation operation. Ann Surg 137: 478
13. Ripstein C.B., Lanter B. (1963) Etiology and surgical therapy of massive prolapse of the rectum. Ann Surg 157: 259
14. Theuerkauf F.J. Jr., Beahrs O.H., Hill J.R. (1970) Rectal prolapse: Causation and surgical treatment. Ann Surg 171: 819
15. Turell R. (ed) (1969) Diseases of the colon and anorectum, 2nd edn, Vol 2. Saunders, Philadelphia, p 1057
16. Wells C. (1959) New operation for rectal prolapse. Proc R Soc Med 52: 602
17. Woods J.H., DeCosse J.J. (1976) A parasacral approach to rectal prolapse. Arch Surg 111: 914

Vascular Lesions 19

Ischemic lesions of the colon may be divided into those that result from occlusion of a major vessel and those that occur in the absence of such blocks. Whatever the cause, however, the response of the bowel, and thus the clinical presentation and the course, are the same.[1–5,7,16,17]

The mucosa is the layer of the colon wall that is most susceptible to ischemic injury.[6] Mucosal slough and submucosal hemmorhage are responsible for the intraluminal bleeding characteristic of all such injuries. Ischemia to the muscle layers initially elicits spasm, and this may contribute to the pain that is almost always clinically observed in intestinal infarction. Ischemia itself also apparently elicits pain in that the pain persists even in the later stage of infarction when dilation rather than spasm characterizes the involved segment. When ischemia is severe enough, infarction and necrosis of the entire colon wall develops. It is associated with the formation of foul-smelling, bloody peritoneal fluid. Particularly on the left side of the colon, ischemia of the serosal layer is a strong stimulus to the formation of adhesions; this may lead to a delay of several days in the clinical presentation of perforations as the affected bowel becomes effectively sealed off until sepsis evolves.

The restoration of circulation to ischemic segments of colon, in the absence of full-thickness necrosis, is followed by a healing phase that may extend over several weeks. It is characterized by mucosal ulceration and bowel irritability. The former is usually associated with minor and sometimes major episodes of gastrointestinal bleeding. Diarrhea with minor degrees of malabsorption is also observed. Finally, delayed stricture formation may lead to continuing symptoms and even obstruction. Strictures appear as early as 6 weeks after the original ischemic injury, but they usually become apparent 2–4 months later.

Both digestive enzymes and the bacteria in the bowel lumen may alter the clinical presentation of ischemic injuries because the mucosal barriers to both are lost. Particularly in the colon, bacterial invasion disposes to the early appearance of sepsis and its complications.

Intestinal infarction is often (but not always) associated with leukocytosis and minimal elevations in serum amylase; other laboratory determinations are not helpful in establishing the diagnosis in any positive way. Early on, plain x-ray films of the abdomen sometimes show an absence of

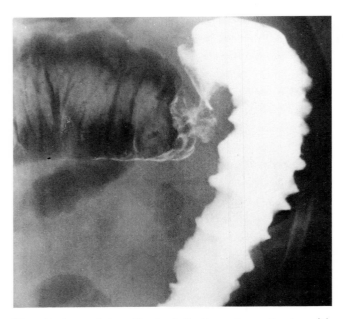

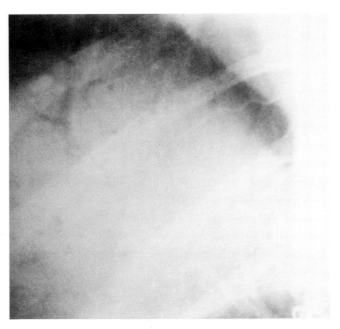

Fig. 19.1a and b. Typical findings in patients with diminished mesenteric circulation. a. Barium enema showing thumbprinting in the left colon.

Fig. 19.1b. Plain x-ray film showing air in the intrahepatic branches of the portal vein.

bowel gas, and later a pattern consistent with adynamic ileus or partial intestinal obstruction may be seen. Mucosal edema and hemorrhage, "thumbprinting," may be outlined by bowel gas but is better demonstrated by barium contrast studies (Fig. 19.1a). Gas in the portal venous system, seen on plain x-ray films, is a late sign (Fig. 19.1b). Angiography is very helpful in establishing a diagnosis and planning surgical management under some circumstances (Fig. 19.2).[20]

A knowledge of the arterial circulatory pattern to the colon and its variations is important in understanding and managing the various ischemic lesions. Primary arterial inflow is from the superior mesenteric artery (SMA) via the ileocolic and midcolic vessels as well as the right colic vessel when it is present, from the inferior mesenteric artery (IMA), and from the hypogastric arteries via the hemorrhoidals. The marginal arcades form an interconnection between these vessels and are the route of collateral flow when there is a central arterial occlusion. Although almost always present and complete, the arcades are variable in size and sometimes limited in their capability to furnish collateral inflow under acute circumstances. Thus, with occlusion of the SMA at its origin, the collateral inflow from the IMA almost always preserves viability of part of the transverse colon and in some instances will nourish the entire colon. With acute occlusion of the IMA, lateral flow usually protects the colon, but there is segmental infarction of the sigmoid colon in 3%–5% of cases. Collateral flow is also responsible for decreasing the extent of injury at the periphery of an infarct.

Prompt diagnosis is nowhere more important than in the management of intestinal infarction.[3] Because the signs and symptoms are nonspecific, this promptness is seldom achieved. Abdominal pain is the one symptom common to all cases. It is variable in location, may be crampy or steady, and is often very severe. Intestinal bleeding, vomiting, and diarrhea are variably present. Later, peritonitis supervenes, simplifying diagnosis. The infarction, however, is not reversible at this stage and the survival rate is very low.

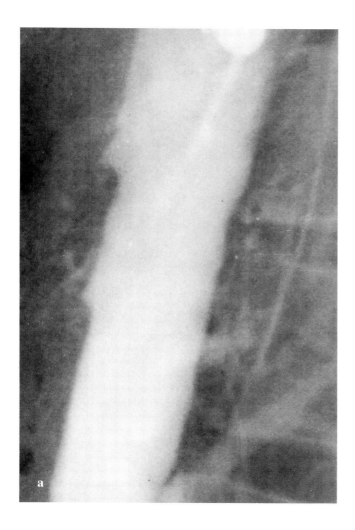
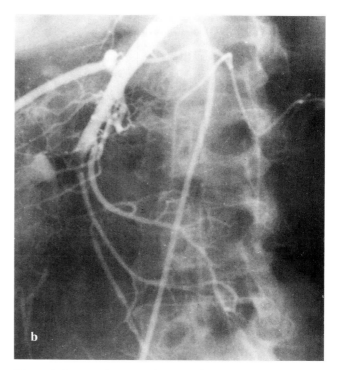

Fig. 19.2a and b.   Angiographic findings in acute occlusion of the superior mesenteric artery. a. Lateral view of acute thrombosis of the superior mesenteric artery in a patient with longstanding occlusion of the celiac axis. b. A superior mesenteric artery embolus lodged 2 cm beyond the origin of the middle colic artery.

Ischemic lesions of the colon fall into three major categories based on etiology[1,2,4,7,9]: (1) those associated with acute occlusion of the SMA and its branches; (2) those resulting from acute occlusion of the IMA; and (3) those that may be called nonocclusive ischemic lesions. The third group of lesions demonstrate the pathologic changes and follow the clinical course of ischemic injuries, but no occlusion of major vessels is found.

Lesions Associated with Arterial Occlusion

Acute occlusions of the SMA at its origin or in the segment between this point and the area beyond the origin of the middle colic artery and midjejunal branches invariably produce infarction. Sometimes the colon is uninvolved, but in more than half of these cases at least the cecum is injured. Depending on the patency of the IMA and adequacy of the marginal arcades, the infarction may extend to include the transverse, left, or even sigmoid colon segments. Acute occlusion of SMA branches (e.g., by an embolus) may be tolerated without infarction, but in some cases a segmental infarct will evolve. When the midcolic artery is occluded, an infarct of the transverse colon may follow.

When occlusion of an SMA branch results in segmental infarction of the small intestine or colon, resection without an attempt at revasculariza-

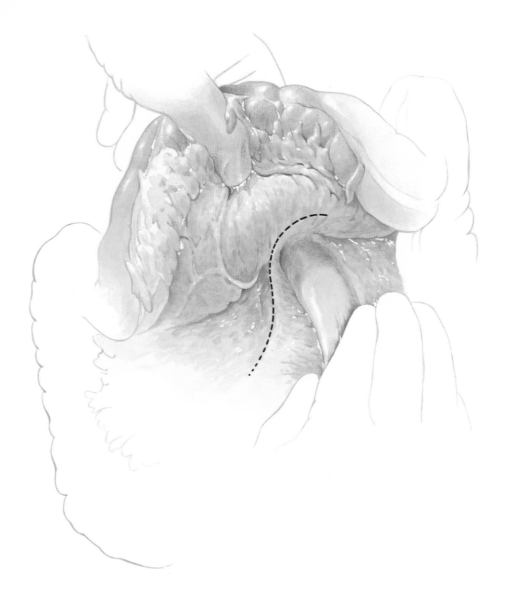

Fig. 19.3. Approach to the superior mesenteric artery, shown by the broken line. The jejunum is retracted downward and to the left, the transverse colon upward and to the right. The superior mesenteric artery lies immediately behind the ligament of Treitz.

tion is indicated. In these cases, normal pulses are present in the peripheral mesenteric vessels in the segments adjacent to the infarction. With a more central site of occlusion, a single segment, often in the distal small bowel, may appear to be the only portion severely affected. There will be an absence of pulses in the adjacent segments, however, and resection is almost invariably followed by further infarction, anastomotic leaks, and death. Extensive resections preserving only a few centimeters of proximal jejunum and the left colon are seldom an acceptable alternative.

The complexity and the outcome of the re-establishment of arterial flow in the SMA are related to the etiology of occlusion. Since thrombosis is a complication of arteriosclerotic occlusive disease, the block is usually located at the site of most common plaque formation, which is the origin of the SMA. Emboli, however, once they enter the SMA, tend to lodge at a major bifurcation either at the origin of the midcolic artery or beyond. The prognosis for successful revascularization and patient survival is much better with embolic than thrombotic occlusion.[7]

When the pattern of bowel involvement and the absence of normal pulses in the branches of the SMA suggest acute occlusion, the proximal

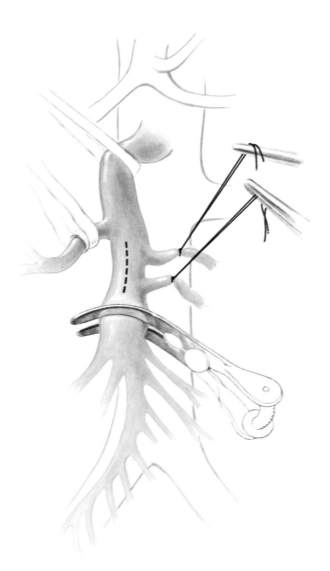

Fig. 19.4a and b. Embolectomy of the superior mesenteric artery. a. A vertical incision is made in the superior mesenteric artery. The two upper jejunal branches have been ligated and divided to provide exposure. The artery is opened along the broken line. A bulldog clamp has been placed on the distal artery to prevent further embolization. Flexible occluding tapes are passed around the midcolic artery and the proximal superior mesenteric artery.

vessels should be exposed. This may be done by dissecting the SMA out in the transverse mesocolon as it emerges from beneath the pancreas (Fig. 19.3). The vessel is controlled by suitable vascular clamps, it is opened, and the embolized material is removed with an embolectomy catheter (Fig. 19.4). In about 20% of cases a peripherally propagated thrombus must be similarly removed, but it is only rarely that the entire vessel cannot be cleared when an embolus is the cause of the occlusion. There may, however, be complications associated with revascularization (Fig. 19.5). With thrombosis proximal thromboendartectomy is sometimes possible; usually, however, the vessel cannot be satisfactorily cleared (Fig. 19.6). In some instances a bypass graft from the aorta or the iliac artery to the SMA is the only means of restoring arterial flow (Fig. 19.7). A fabric prosthesis may be used for this graft, but a reversed segment of saphenous vein is preferable because there is less risk of graft sepsis.

Following the restoration of arterial flow, irreversibly damaged segments of intestine should be resected. In some cases the surgeon cannot be certain of the extent of the resection that is needed. In these cases the questionable segments are left in and a "second-look" laparotomy is done.

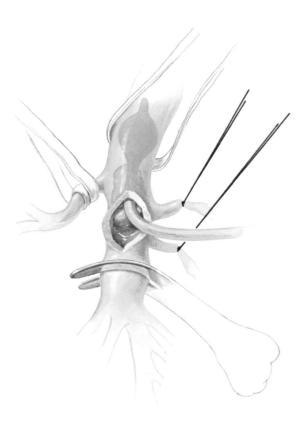

Fig. 19.4b. The superior mesenteric artery has been opened, demonstrating an embolus. The Fogarty catheter will be used for extraction.

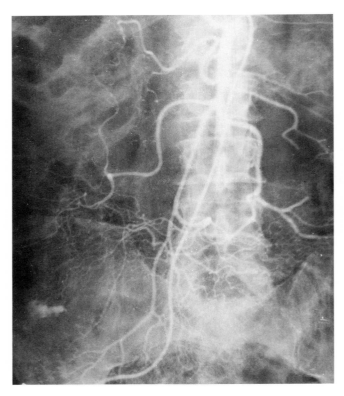

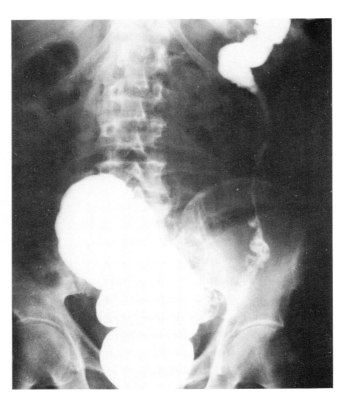

Fig. 19.5a and b. Complications of revascularization. a. Angiographic evidence of bleeding from the terminal ileum 8 days after a superior mesenteric artery embolectomy.

Fig. 19.5b. Barium enema showing stricture formation in the descending colon 8 weeks after superior mesenteric artery embolectomy in a patient with prior ligation of the inferior mesenteric artery.

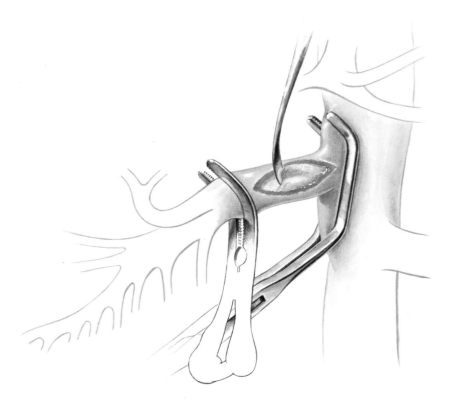

Fig. 19.6. Thrombectomy of the superior mesenteric artery. The aorta has been opened after the application of a Satinsky clamp.

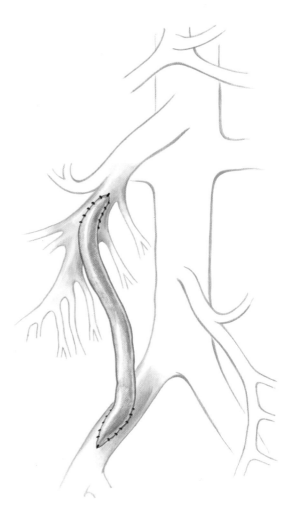

Fig. 19.7. Bypass from the iliac artery to the superior mesenteric artery distal to the thrombosis. Saphenous vein has been used for the bypass.

197

This may be carried out in 12–18 hr when the demarcation of nonviable intestine will be clear. The decision to perform such a re-exploration should be made at the time of closure; the clinical course over the next few hours will not provide a reliable indication of its necessity. In no case should clearly nonviable bowel be left behind, even if a second look is planned; the systemic effects of retained necrotic bowel may be unmanageable and fatal, even within a few hours.

Atherosclerotic involvement of the IMA is common, and in many older people this vessel will be found to have silently become occluded. Acute occlusion caused by either a thrombus or embolus nevertheless occasionally leads to infarction of the sigmoid colon. This sequence is, in fact, more commonly iatrogenic in origin, following ligation of the vessel during aortic resection and reconstruction.[8,18] The clinical course that follows is usually marked by left-sided abdominal pain and diarrhea, frequently bloody. Barium studies show mucosal changes characteristic of ischemic injuries. Sigmoidoscopy almost always allows visualization of the lower portion of the injured segment. The mucosa appears dusky and is found to be quite friable. Ulceration is sometimes observed.[6] Although re-establishment of the arterial flow may be feasible, especially when ischemic changes become apparent intraoperatively during aortic reconstruction, in every instance resection with re-establishment of colon continuity at a later stage is the best choice.

Infarction of the colon distal to the splenic flexure is better tolerated than that at a more proximal colonic site. As revascularization is not contemplated, operative intervention may be deferred until signs of perforation evolve. In a few patients a late stricture will necessitate subsequent resection. Most of these patients do not become asymptomatic after the initial episode of ischemia; severe diarrhea is the rule.[19] Even when the acute episode clearly seems to reflect vascular compromise, follow-up studies are important to rule out a malignancy or any other cause.

Lesions Not Associated with Arterial Occlusion

Intestinal infarction in the absence of major vascular occlusion is a poorly understood clinical entity. In some cases the infarction is precipitated by episodes of cardiac failure or impaired cardiac output, and arterial spasm has been assigned an important role in these instances. Others are associated with the use of oral contraceptive agents.[11] Many, however, present with no precipitating or causal factors. Any segments of small or large intestine, as well as other intra-abdominal organs, may be affected. Most cases of nonocclusive infarction are hopeless, but in a few resection combined with the reversal of underlying factors results in recovery.

One special form of nonocclusive infarction is termed "ischemic colitis" (Fig. 19.8).[9,13,14,21] Although this term has been used to describe all ischemic lesions of the colon, its use should be restricted to those cases that develop in the absence of major vascular occlusion and other known causes. In most such cases, it is the left side of the colon, especially in the region of the splenic flexure, that is involved. The usual presenting complaints are left-sided abdominal pain and bloody diarrhea. Tenderness over the involved segment is frequent. As the rectum is almost always spared, sigmoidoscopy will not disclose the mucosal changes seen with acute IMA occlusion. Barium studies of the colon will show mucosal edema and hemorrhage but they are often unnecessary.

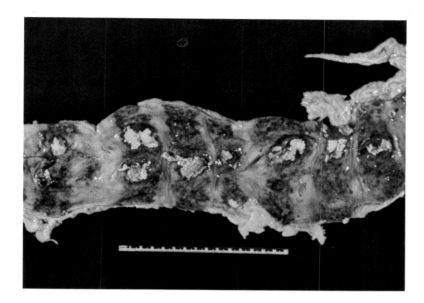

Fig. 19.8. Operative specimen of probable ischemic colitis.

Putting the colon at rest and administering systemic antibiotics may be helpful, but the most important element in management is close observation. Evidence of perforation is an indication for surgical intervention. Even when the patient recovers from the acute episode, there may be persistent diarrhea associated with mucosal ulceration and the later development of a stricture; either of these complications may sometimes require a resection.[10,15]

Vascular tumors rarely occur in the colon. Telangiectasis may involve the entire intestinal tract, such as in Osler-Weber-Rendu disease. Diffuse cavernous hemangiomas may involve the rectum. According to Jeffrey et al., only 75 have been described[12]; resection and colorectal anastomosis were employed in the last 5. We have observed 1 such case in the sigmoid that was associated with diffuse arteriovenous communication of the whole left lower extremity; segmental resection was required because of colonic bleeding.

References

1. Boley S.J., Brandt L.J., Veith F.J. (1978) Ischemic disorders of the intestines. Curr Probl Surg (April) 18: 1
2. Boley S.J., Gliedman M.L. (1971) Circulatory responses to mesenteric ischemia. In: Boley S.J., Schwartz S.S., Williams L.F. (eds) Vascular disorders of the intestine. Appleton-Century-Crofts, New York
3. Boley S.J., Krieger H., Schultz L., et al (1965) Experimental aspects of peripheral vascular occlusion of the intestine. Surg Gynecol Obstet 121: 789
4. Boley S.J., Schwartz S., Lash J., et al (1963) Reversible vascular occlusion of the colon. Surg Gynecol Obstet 116: 53
5. Boley S.J., Sprayregan S., Siegelman S.S., et al (1977) Initial results from an aggressive roentgenological and surgical approach to acute mesenteric ischemia. Surgery 82: 848
6. Carter R., Vannix R., Hinshaw D.B., et al (1959) Inferior mesenteric occlusion: Sigmoidoscopic diagnosis. Surgery 46: 845
7. Crawford E.S., Morris G.C. Jr., Myhre H.O., et al (1977) Celiac axis, superior mesenteric artery, and inferior mesenteric artery occlusion: Surgical considerations. Surgery 82: 856
8. Ernst C.B., Hagihara P.F., Daugherty M.E., et al (1976) Ischemic colitis incidence following abdominal aortic reconstruction: A prospective study. Surgery 80: 417

9. Hertzer N.R., Beven E.G., Humphries A.W. (1977) Colonic intestinal ischemia. Surgery 145: 321
10. Hunt D.R. (1977) Surgical management of gangrenous ischemic colitis: Report of five cases. Dis Colon Rectum 20: 36
11. Hurwitz R.L., Martin A.J., Grossman B.E., et al (1970) Oral contraceptives and gastrointestinal disorders. Ann Surg 172: 892
12. Jeffrey P.J., Hawley P.R., Parks A.G. (1976) Colo-anal sleeve anastomosis in the treatment of diffuse cavernous haemangioma involving the rectum. Br J Surg 63: 678
13. Marston A., Marcuson R.W., Chapmen M., et al (1969) Experimental study of devascularization of the colon. Gut 10: 121
14. Marston A., Pheils M.T., Thomas M.L., et al (1966) Ischaemic colitis. Gut 7: 1
15. Mozes M., Adar R., Tsur N., et al (1971) Intestinal obstruction due to mesenteric vascular occlusion. Surg Gynecol Obstet 133: 583
16. O'Connell T.X., Kadell B., Tompkins R.K. (1976) Ischemia of the colon. Surg Gynecol Obstet 142: 337
17. Ottinger L.W. (1978) The surgical management of acute occlusion of the superior mesenteric artery. Ann Surg 188: 721
18. Ottinger L.W., Darling R.C., Nathan M.J., et al (1972) Left colon ischemia complicating aorto-iliac reconstruction: Causes, diagnosis, management, and prevention. Arch Surg 105: 841
19. Shaw R.S., Maynard E.P. III (1958) Acute and chronic thrombosis of the mesenteric arteries associated with malabsorption: A report of two cases successfully treated by thromboendartectomy. N Engl J Med 258: 874
20. Tomchik F.S., Wittenberg J., Ottinger L.W. (1970) The roentgenographic spectrum of bowel infarction. Radiology 96: 249
21. Williams L.F. Jr., Bosniak M.A., Wittenberg J., et al (1969) Ischemic colitis. Am J Surg 117: 254

Hemorrhage from the Colon and Rectum

20

Bleeding from the rectum is recognized by the public as a very serious symptom. Consequently the surgeon will be required to examine many patients with this particular problem. Diagnosis and therapy must go hand in hand, particularly as the bleeding becomes more massive. In most instances a standard approach may be used. The causes of rectal bleeding are described below in order of increasing severity of bleeding:

1. *Bleeding manifested only in stools that are positive by the guaiac test:* Such patients are encountered if screening procedures are employed for possible colonic disease, and as a rule they are 50 years of age or over. The possibility of an occult carcinoma must always be entertained and further diagnostic measures are necessary.

2. *Small amounts of bright red bleeding encountered on the toilet paper or in the stool at the time of defecation:* This is the usual type of bleeding that is reported. In nearly all instances it is due to diseases of the anorectum. Hemorrhoids are the most common offender, but superficial fissures or traumatic excoriations from vigorous cleaning may also lead to bleeding. If the patient is examined almost immediately after a bloody bowel movement, the ulcerated area can be seen; but if a few hours elapse it may be almost impossible to find a local site of bleeding in the anorectal area.

3. *Continued small amounts of bleeding that persist over a period of several days in which the blood is noted mixed with the stool:* Such bleeding must always be regarded with great suspicion. In the adult the most common causes are cancer, polyps, or diverticular disease. In young adults this may be the first sign of idiopathic ulcerative colitis or Crohn's disease.

4. *Acute massive hemorrhage:* In this instance the patient will expel a large amount of either bright red or cherry red blood. Although the amount of blood is often alarming, these patients rarely develop shock, and the total amount of blood loss will average considerably less than when bleeding comes from the upper gastrointestinal tract. However, this is the one group of patients in whom immediate therapy may be required; in all the preceding groups the treatment of the hemorrhage will be that of the underlying disease.

If the patient is bleeding massively at the time of entry to the hospital, some clue may be gained from the consideration of his age. In a child or an

201

early adolescent the possibility of a Meckel's diverticulum is very high; the bleeding arises from an adjacent ulcer in the ileum. Teenagers and young adults may bleed massively from ulcerative colitis; massive hemorrhage, on the other hand, is rare with Crohn's disease. In adults, the common lesions are diverticular disease[2] and angiodysplasia.[7–10,12]

The term "angiodysplasia" has been given to single or multiple tiny localized submucosal areas of dilated veins 1–5 mm in diameter by Galdabini; superficial ulcerations can lead to serious hemorrhage. The cause of these lesions is not known.[3] They nearly always occur near the ileocecal valve. Because pressure in the colon is highest in the cecum, Boley et al. believe that compression by the muscular wall may lead to venous dilatation and may cause these lesions.[3] Special injection techniques are necessary for the pathologist to detect these tiny lesions.

The diagnosis of angiodysplasia is made by arteriography, as will be described below. In a few instances it has been possible to demonstrate bleeding by means of the colonoscope. If a lesion can be found by colonoscopy in a well-prepared bowel, electrocoagulation has been suggested as a possible method of therapy; however, follow-up studies are not yet available showing whether this will ultimately be satisfactory. The inability to clean the colon well under emergency conditions suggests that this will not become a popular method of therapy.

After entry the patient with acute massive hemorrhage is examined in the usual fashion. Anoscopy will eliminate the possibility that bleeding from internal hemorrhoids has filled the rectum above a competent sphincter, and proctosigmoidoscopy can eliminate any other lesion in the lower part of the bowel. If the results of these examinations are negative and the patient continues to bleed vigorously, emergency angiography is indicated. This is very likely to demonstrate the site of bleeding provided that the loss of blood is greater than 0.5 ml/min. Furthermore, if a bleeding point can be identified, at least temporary control of bleeding can usually be secured by injection of Pitressin into the catheter.

Bleeding from diverticular disease or angiodysplasia is most common in the eighth decade. In our experience the best method of differentiation is selective arteriography. Athanasoulis has found that with diverticular bleeding the arterial phase has shown intraluminal extravasation of dye in three-quarters of the cases, and the venous phase is normal[12] (Fig. 20.1). With angiodysplasia the arterial phase is normal, intraluminal extravasation is rare, and vascular tufts are occasionally seen in the capillary phase. However, the cardinal finding is the presence of an early filling, dilated tortuous vein in the ileocecal area (Fig. 20.2). A barium enema will show diverticula in all cases of diverticular bleeding and in 25% of cases of angiodysplasia. Angiodysplasia probably exists in some normal persons and may be present in patients with a bleeding diverticulum in another section of the colon.

Massive bleeding may originate at any site in the colon but in two-thirds of the cases it arises proximal to the splenic flexure.[4] In our experience bleeding from diverticula is controlled in nearly three-quarters of the cases by the injection of vasopressin (Pitressin) into the corresponding mesenteric artery.[12] If no lesion can be found and the patient continues to bleed vigorously, or if vasopressin injection is not successful in stilling the hemorrhage, then an immediate operation will be necessary. Transcatheter embolization, advised by Goldberger and Bookstein,[7] may be hazardous in the colon.

If the site of bleeding is demonstrated and bleeding is controlled by angiography, there is no need for immediate surgery and the surgeon must

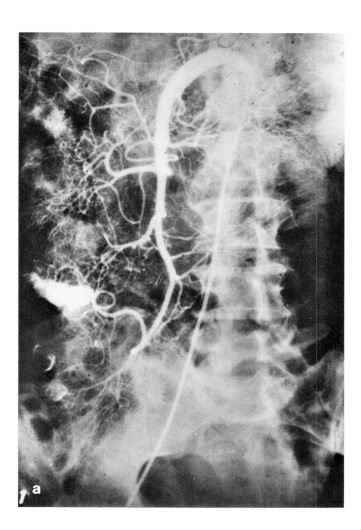

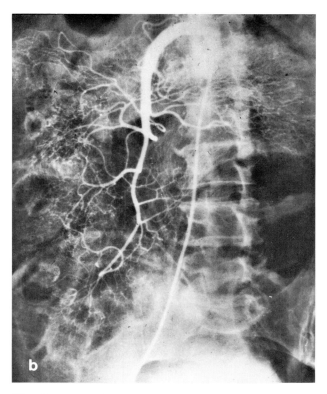

Fig. 20.1a and b. Selective arteriography showing bleeding from a diverticulum. a. Arterial phase. b. After injection of vasopressin into superior mesenteric artery.

decide whether or not to carry out a semielective operation within a day or two or whether to attempt continued control by the same method. It is possible to leave the catheter in place and administer additional injections within the course of the next few days in the poor-risk patient. If the patient is known to have widespread diverticular disease or has bled previously, it often seems wisest to proceed with an operation within a few days.

If a diagnosis of angiodysplasia has been made by arteriography, and the patient has bled, operation is indicated; even though angiodysplasia may occur in the absence of bleeding, once bleeding starts it is almost certain to continue. On the other hand, bleeding from diverticular disease does not always mean an operation is indicated. Nearly half of our patients have left the hospital without surgery and have done well. Surgery is indicated for continuing or repeated hemorrhage or other concomitant symptoms of diverticular disease.

The choice of operations must depend upon whether or not the site of bleeding has been determined, the age and condition of the patient, and the possibility of future bleeding.[12] At the present time it seems justified to suggest the following procedures for bleeding from either angiodysplasia or diverticular disease. For angiodysplasia a right colectomy extending to the midtransverse colon is recommended, assuming that the typical findings of angiodysplasia have been noted in the area by angiography. This has proved curative in 27 of 31 cases we have followed. For diverticular bleeding from a known source, a segmental resection can be used in poor-risk

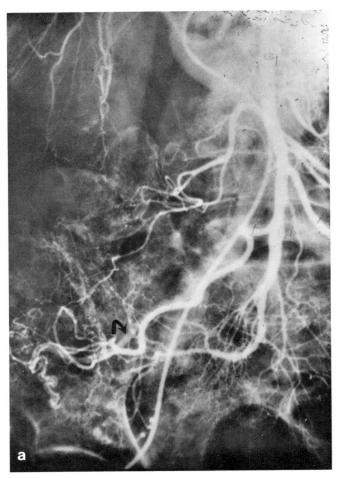

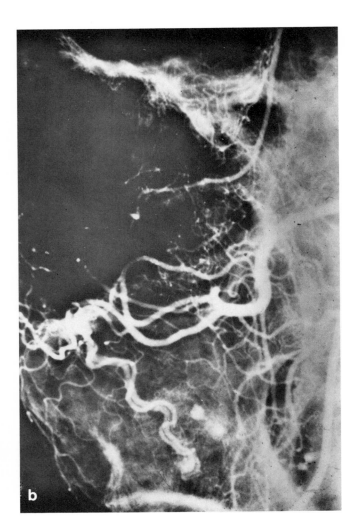

Fig. 20.2a and b. Selective arteriography showing angiodysplasia. a. Arterial phase; arrow points to premature filling of tortuous vein. b. Venous phase.

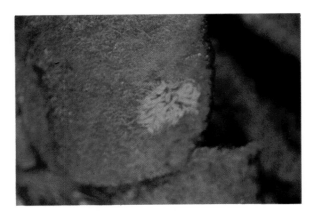

Fig. 20.3. Injected specimen showing angiodysplasia.

patients. Subtotal colectomy is recommended for (1) diverticular bleeding in which diverticula are scattered throughout the colon, (2) angiodysplasia on the right side and extensive diverticulosis on the left, and (3) massive bleeding from an undetermined site.

The arguments in favor of a segmental resection rather than a subtotal colectomy are that if the bleeding is coming from the one known site and can be handled in that fashion, the mortality of the operation will be less and postoperative sequelae such as severe diarrhea (which occurs in one-sixth of the patients) will be avoided.[11] The mortality of subtotal colectomy for cancer has proved to be at least four times that of segmental resection in our cases at Massachusetts General Hospital, and it seems reasonable to expect that the same ratio would hold for bleeding from diverticula or angiodysplasia. Drapanas et al. reported a mortality of 11% in a follow-up of 33 patients with massive rectal bleeding treated by subtotal colectomy.[6]

Regardless of the type of operation employed, the chances of postoperative complications are higher than after the usual resection of the colon because the colon is full of blood that is often badly infected. Complications are more likely to occur if there is any leakage from the contaminated colon contents at the time of anastomosis. Adequate blood replacement and pre- and postoperative antibiotic therapy are indicated in these patients.

Cecal ulcers have been cited as sources of bleeding. They were originally described by Wilkie[13] and have been listed as a reason for right colectomy by several authors since that time.[5]

However, it is important to note that since the diagnosis of angiodysplasia has been made in the past few years, essentially no cases of cecal ulcers have been reported. These lesions can be distinguished microscopically by injection techniques (Fig. 20.3). Therapeutically, if hemorrhage results from either one of them, the proper operation is a segmental colectomy. It is our belief that the old diagnosis of cecal ulcer usually represented angiodysplasia or rare stercoral ulcers. One of the recent Massachusetts General Hospital patients bled massively from a granuloma of the ileocecal valve.

It is important to emphasize that the angiographic diagnosis of angiodysplasia does not mean that the lesion is causing the hemorrhage. A barium enema or colonoscopy should be obtained as well. Several cancers of the cecum have been associated with the findings of angiodysplasia. A recent patient had angiodysplasia demonstrated by superior mesenteric angiography, and a simultaneous bleeding diverticulum in the splenic flexure on inferior mesenteric injection. Adams has suggested that the barium enema also has a therapeutic effect and may stop bleeding from diverticula.[1] Our radiologists have not confirmed this observation.

References

1. Adams J.T. (1970) Therapeutic barium enema for massive diverticular bleeding. Arch Surg 101: 547
2. Behringer G.E., Albright N.L. (1973) Diverticular disease of the colon. A frequent cause of massive rectal bleeding. Am J Surg 125: 419
3. Boley S.J., Sammartano R., Adams A., et al (1977) On the nature and etiology of vascular ectasias of the colon: Degenerative lesions of aging. Gastroenterology 72: 650
4. Casarella W.J., Kanter I.E., Seaman W.B. (1972) Right-sided colonic diverticula as a cause of acute rectal hemorrhage. N Engl J Med 286: 450
5. Corry R.J., Bartlett M.K., Cohen R.B. (1970) Erosions of the cecum. A cause of massive hemorrhage. Am J Surg 119: 106
6. Drapanas T., Pennington D.G., Kappelman M., et al (1973) Emergency subtotal colectomy: Preferred approach to management of massively bleeding diverticular disease. Ann Surg 177: 519
7. Goldberger L.E., Bookstein J.J. (1977) Transcatheter embolization for treatment of diverticular hemorrhage. Radiology 122: 613

8. Klein R.R., Gallagher D.M. (1969) Massive colonic bleeding from diverticular disease. Am J Surg 118: 553
9. Marx F.W. Jr., Gray R.K., Duncan A.M., et al (1977) Angiodysplasia as a source of intestinal bleeding. Am J Surg 134: 125
10. McGuire H.H. Jr., Haynes B. W. Jr., (1972) Massive hemorrhage from diverticulosis of the colon: Guidelines for therapy based on bleeding patterns observed in fifty cases. Ann Surg 175: 847
11. Ottinger L.W. (1978) Frequency of bowel movements with ileorectal anastomosis. Arch Surg 115: 1048
12. Welch C.E., Athanasoulis C.A., Galdabini J.J. (1978) Hemorrhage from the large bowel with special reference to angiodysplasia and diverticular disease. World J Surg 2: 73
13. Wilkie D. (1937) Simple ulcer of the ascending colon and its complications. Surgery 1: 655

Hemorrhoids

21

Hemorrhoids are symptomatic, conglomerate masses composed of arteries, arterioles, veins, and surrounding soft tissues. There is evidence that in the normal person erectile tissues are found in the anorectum that are very similar to those in the corpora cavernosa of the penis.[13] There is free communication between arteries and veins in these areas. Congestion and/or inflammation can lead to symptoms of bleeding, protrusion, or thrombosis; when these symptoms appear the diagnosis of hemorrhoids is made.[11,12] With increasing size and protrusion, mucous membrane of the rectum may be extruded to form a true prolapse. After prolonged periods of time secondary hemorrhoids may develop between the primary hemorrhoids.

Hemorrhoidectomy

We believe that hemorrhoidectomy furnishes the most effective treatment of all types of hemorrhoidal disease, particularly when there is both an internal and external component or there is moderate prolapse. The internal hemorrhoids are those that arise above the anorectal line and the external hemorrhoids are the components that are located inferior to this line.

The operation of hemorrhoidectomy has undergone many minor modifications. Essentially it consists of the excision of the three primary hemorrhoids with the closure of the defect that has been produced. Operative techniques vary depending upon whether a section of mucous membrane overlying the hemorrhoid is removed together with the underlying mass, or whether the mucous membrane is merely opened, the mass dissected out from beneath, and the mucous membrane resutured. The method that we have employed consists of the removal of the overlying mucosa together with the hemorrhoidal mass, as described by Ferguson et al.[4] This decision is based on the fact that there is usually a great deal of redundancy of the mucous membrane by the time the hemorrhoid becomes symptomatic.

Hemorrhoidectomy may be carried out in either of two positions. We prefer the lithotomy position. In this position the hemorrhoidal veins fill well, allowing their exact size to be easily determined. The position is somewhat more uncomfortable for the assistant but this is essentially the

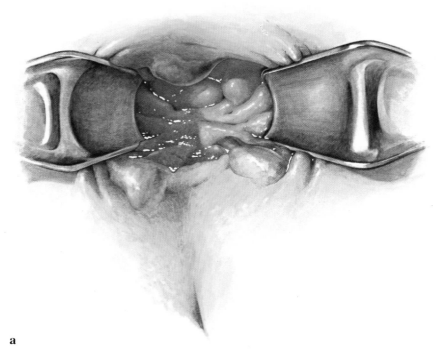

a

Fig. 21.1a–e. Hemorrhoidectomy. a. The first step is dilatation of the anal canal. This demonstrates the three major hemorrhoids in the usual positions at 4, 7, and 11 o'clock when the patient is in the lithotomy position.

only disadvantage. In the Buie position the patient is prone on the table with the head and legs lower than the buttocks. This affords an excellent view for both the surgeon and assistants but has the disadvantage that the hemorrhoids are collapsed at the time the procedure is carried out.

After the patient has been placed in position, a total of 25 cc of long-lasting local anesthetic is injected in four areas around the anal verge, putting the injection close to the area of the internal sphincter. A mixture of equal parts of 1% lidocaine (Xylocaine) and 0.5% bupivocaine (Marcaine) is preferred. Local infiltration will be sufficient for the operation in the poor-risk, elderly patient. The anal canal is then thoroughly dilated to approximately four fingers. Two Richardson retractors are used to expose the circumference of the anal canal and lower rectum. Usually the three main hemorrhoids are very prominent (Fig. 21.1a). Fibrous polyps may be seen at the upper end of the hemorrhoids. There may be an extremely lax mucous membrane, particularly on the anterior wall; in this setting the dissection should be carried higher than usual. The redundancy may cause tenesmus when the patient attempts to excrete this hypertrophied mucous membrane.

By rotating the two retractors, excellent exposure of each hemorrhoid may be obtained in turn. The hemorrhoid is then elevated with two Allis clamps (Fig. 21.1b). A short V of skin is excised to include the external hemorrhoid. The hemorrhoidal mass is elevated and grasped firmly with a curved Kelly clamp. (Fig. 21.1c). A 0 plain catgut suture is then placed above the clamp and tied. The hemorrhoid is then excised. An over-and-over suture is carried down along the clamp and the clamp is removed. The suture is tightened, locked at the outer end at the anal verge by a lock

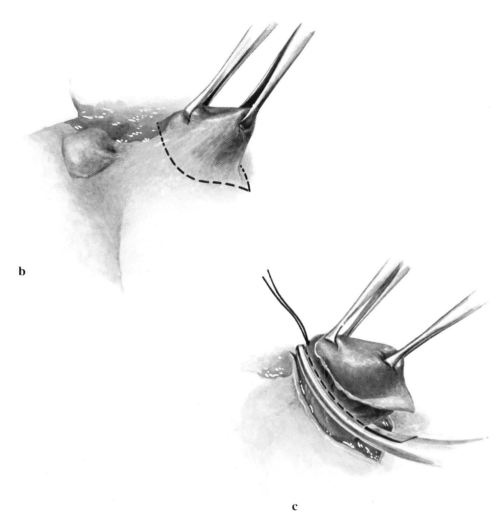

b

c

Fig. 21.1b and c. b. The hemorrhoid is grasped with Allis forceps. An incision is made through the skin surrounding the external component. c. A curved clamp is applied superficial to the sphincters but beneath the hemorrhoidal mass. Prior to excision of the hemorrhoidal mass a 0 catgut suture will be placed above the clamp and tied. The hemorrhoid is then excised.

stitch, and the same stitch is carried back as a second row and then tied to the original standing suture (Fig. 21.1d). No attempt is made to close the portion of the incision external to the anal verge because this could lead to a hematoma. The wound should be dry at the completion. It is important that the clamp be applied exactly in a vertical direction since the formation of scar tissue at a later date will help relieve any prolapse. Bridges of mucous membrane and skin should be left between the points of excision of the hemorrhoids, particularly between those at 4 and 7 o'clock, to avoid later stricture formation (Fig. 21.1e). The excised hemorrhoids must be examined by the pathologist to eliminate the possibility of an unexpected cancer.

Hemorrhage may occur early if hemostasis has not been complete. Small amounts of bleeding may occur as the sutures dissolve at the end of a week. Infection is uncommon unless the patient has had diarrhea at the time of the operation and it continues afterward. In rare instances an abscess forms beneath the mucosal stitch and requires drainage.

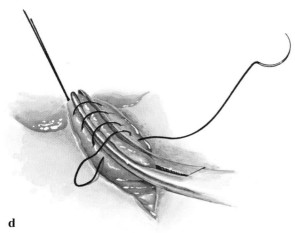

d

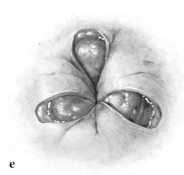

Fig. 21.1d and e. d. Hemostasis is accomplished by running the suture over the clamp, locking it at the outer end, and then continuing back as a second suture, which will close the mucous membrane. e. The final appearance. The site of excision of the external portion of the hemorrhoidal complex is left open. Care must be taken to excise as little skin as necessary in order to prevent redundancy. There should be wide skin and mucous membrane flaps between the sites of the three excisions.

e

If the method described above is used, it is unusual for a person to bleed postoperatively unless he is on anticoagulants or has a bleeding dyscrasia. If bleeding occurs, tamponade with a small pack usually will be sufficient. If bleeding is severe, the operative field should be explored with the patient under anesthesia and the bleeding point should be ligated.

Some surgeons have advocated the division of the pectinate band (the lowermost portion of the internal sphincter) at the time of hemorrhoidectomy. Minor degress of incontinence may follow this procedure, and we do not think it should be done except in unusual cases of severe stenosis in which a lateral sphincterotomy may be indicated.

Minor degrees of incontinence may occur if too wide an excision, particularly of skin, is carried out. Under these circumstances mucous membrane may be everted and give rise to mucous discharge and a moist perineum.

Late stricture should never occur if the proper precautions are taken and the excisions are not too radical. On the other hand, late stricture has been a frequent complication of the Whitehead technique.

A second method of hemorrhoidectomy may be illustrated by the technique used by Parks.[9] The essential features of his operation include the submucous dissection of each of the three hemorrhoids separate from the underlying internal sphincter muscle, a high ligation of the hemorrhoidal mass, conservation of the squamous epithelium of the lower portion of the anal canal, excision of redundant mucous membrane, and elevation of the squamous epithelium to a higher level. Necrosis of skin flaps is prevented by maintaining a 1-cm bridge of undissected mucous membrane between each of the hemorrhoids.

The Whitehead technique for hemorrhoidectomy consists of an incision at the mucocutaneous junction circumferentially about the anal canal and submucous dissection of the hemorrhoids and mucous membrane upward for a distance of approximately 4 cm, so that the entire hemorrhoidal area is excised. Continuity is restored by anastomosis of the mucous membrane to the skin with a series of 00 interrupted catgut sutures. This technique is still indicated for low-lying villous adenomas that surround the entire rectum but extend upward for only a short distance. Because no bridges of mucous membrane and skin are left, the incidence of stricture has been high. It is necessary to carry out dilatations regularly during the process of healing.[14] Therefore, the technique has been abandoned for hemmorrhoidectomy.

Postoperative anal stenosis is uncommon except after the Whitehead operation. In minor degrees it may be relieved by generous dilatation, with care being taken not to rupture the external sphincter. When this is impossible a plastic repair may be carried out. An incision is made posteriorly at the mucocutaneous margin and the mucosa is freed. The anal sphincter is thoroughly dilated and, if necessary, the superficial portion of the external sphincter is divided and the mucous membrane is cut vertically at the posterior commissure. A skin flap is developed and sutured into the defect that is produced in such a way as to enlarge the external opening of the anal canal.

Thrombosed Hemorrhoids

The term "thrombosed hemorrhoid" refers to a sudden, painful, purple swelling that appears in the hemorrhoidal area. The etiology is assumed to be a hematoma produced by a rupture of one of the small arterioles in the hemorrhoidal complex or a thrombosis in a hemorrhoidal vein. If the "thrombosis" is exterior to the dentate line, it can be relieved easily, but if it involves the internal hemorrhoid, severe pain and edema of the tissues about the entire anal canal can result. If the hematoma is extensive it may

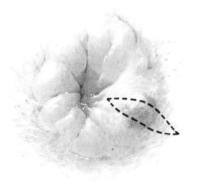
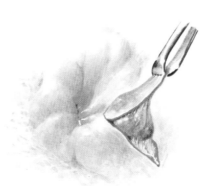

Fig. 21.2. Excision of thrombosed hemorrhoid. Under local anesthesia a section of mucous membrane and skin is excised over the clot and the clot is extracted. Since the hematoma may extend around several septa, they should be broken up in order to prevent recurrence.

be associated with prolapse of the entire hemorrhoidal mass and surrounding mucous membrane. This may be followed by necrosis and gangrene of this area. Septic thrombosis of hemorrhoidal veins does occur but it is rare; extension to the portal system has been known to result in mesenteric thrombosis.

If the thrombosis is only in the external area, prompt evacuation of the clot is recommended. This may be done with the patient under local infiltration anesthesia. An incision is made over the mass and the clot is extruded by pressure. A section of mucous membrane should also be excised since secondary bleeding may occur, and unless the opening is wide the clot may recur (Fig. 21.2). At the time of removal it is important to palpate with the finger in the anal canal to be sure that all clot has been removed, since it tends to accumulate in various loculated compartments. The incision is left open. The patient is allowed warm baths within a few hours. Prompt relief of pain and resolution of the tumor is to be expected.

If the patient delays, the clot may become organized and densely adherent. It still may be possible to remove it a few days after onset, but under these circumstances, if the mass is showing spontaneous improvement it is usually as satisfactory to leave it alone as to interfere at a late stage.

If the thrombosis involves one or more internal hemorrhoids, severe swelling occurs that may even lead to prolapse and gangrene. Under these circumstances it is advisable to attempt to treat the patient conservatively with bed rest, warm compresses, and antibiotics. If possible, any operative procedure should be delayed until the acute symptoms subside. However, sometimes it will be necessary to operate upon the patient in an emergency. Because there is a danger of sepsis, the procedure should be minimized to relieve only the areas of thrombosis.

Other Methods of Treatment

Other methods of treatment include manual dilatation of the anal canal, necrosis by rubber band, injection of sclerosing solutions, and cryotherapy.

Lord Technique

The Lord technique is based upon the fact that many of the symptoms of hemorrhoids are due to spasm of the sphincters or a tight pectinate band, making it difficult for venous return to occur from the tissues in the hemorrhoidal mass external to the sphincter. He advised a very thorough dilatation of the anus under anesthesia.[7] The dilatation is carried up to approximately 8 fingers. A pack is put in to be left over night.

Reports indicate that relief is obtained in approximately 80% of patients who undergo this procedure.[3,8] The remainder require operation at a later date. We have been somewhat concerned about the dangers of incontinence after this operation and have not used it as a definitive treatment for hemorrhoids. However, anal dilatation under anesthesia is a very effective procedure for patients with a tight sphincter. It may also aid bowel function after a laparotomy.

Barron Rubber Band Technique

The rubber band technique of Barron has been used by many surgeons.[1,2,6] This consists of the application of a rubber band ligature about an internal hemorrhoid. It is done as an office procedure by means of a special applica-

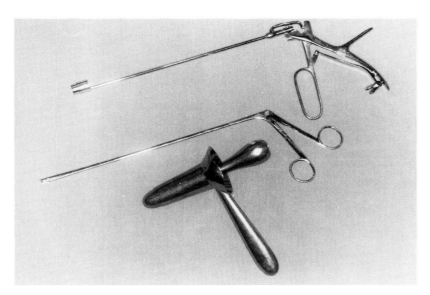

Fig. 21.3. Rubber band applicator for internal hemorrhoids. The rubber band is applied over the special conelike tip, which is then removed. The photograph shows, from below upward, (1) the anal speculum employed for exposure; (2) special clamp for seizing the internal hemorrhoid, which is passed through the head of (3), the applicator. As the handles of the applicator are closed, the rubber band is pushed over the hemorrhoid.

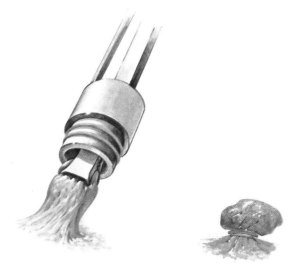

Fig. 21.4. Rubber band technique for removal of internal hemorrhoids. The hemorrhoid can be elevated with a special clamp that is passed through the head of the instrument and the rubber band is applied by pushing the handles. Care must be taken to see that the lower end of the band is several millimeters above the pectinate line.

tor (Fig. 21.3). It may be expected that the hemorrhoids will necrose and undergo self-amputation within the course of a few days (Fig. 21.4).

This method is applicable to internal hemorrhoids. Bands cannot be placed below the pectinate line because severe pain will follow. If the hemorrhoids are combined in type this is not a satisfactory method. Several complications may follow its use. The application may be very painful if the rubber band approaches within 5 mm above the dentate line. There may be thrombosis of the external hemorrhoids. There may be bleeding, particularly around the seventh day, at the time the necrotic hemorrhoid is extruded. Another disadvantage is that pathological examination of the tissue is not available; it is conceivable that an early carcinoma could be missed.

213

Injection Therapy

Injection treatment is frequently used for hemorrhoids. In certain instances the hemorrhoids may be comparatively small and only internal in type. If such patients bleed it is often expeditious to treat them with injections: 2 cc 5% quinine urethane is injected into the internal hemorrhoid. This is extremely painful if not done above the dentate line. Bleeding is usually controlled by one injection. Prolapse also may be aided, although the results are not as satisfactory. Injection therapy may be done as an ambulatory procedure and is painless.

The problems associated with it include the very rare case of idiosyncrasy to quinine. Furthermore, most hemorrhoids of the size that produce symptoms are combined in type, and this procedure cannot be expected to aid any external components. Several years after injection therapy the main hemorrhoidal masses tend to have been obliterated but secondary hemorrhoids may occur at other areas around the periphery of the anus. In our experience they have been more difficult to handle than they would have been if injection therapy had not been employed.

Cryosurgical Techniques

Cryosurgical techniques may be suitable for the treatment of external and internal hemorrhoids on an ambulatory basis. As a single hemorrhoid is treated at each visit, several applications may be needed. The results have been held to be excellent by some, although other proctologists have noted recurrence after such treatment as well as a prolonged period of anal discharge and slow healing. This technique does offer an alternative in those patients who would usually be treated by hemorrhoidectomy but cannot or will not undergo the procedure.

Descending Perineum Syndrome

The "descending perineum syndrome," described by Parks et al., is an entity that is rarely recognized but may produce severe symptoms and may be cured by surgery.[5,10] Patients complain of the desire to move their bowels frequently. Attempts often produce only small amounts of stool, though sometimes a small amount of mucus or blood appears. The symptoms return a short time later and again lead to further ineffectual attempts at evacuation. Meanwhile, there is no evidence of obstruction and on palpation the rectum is found to be free of feces.

The symptoms are due to very loose, lax folds of rectal mucosa located just above the hemorrhoidal area. They can be observed on sigmoidoscopy or even better at the time of hemorrhoidectomy when the patient is under anesthesia. Since this mucosa is congested and perhaps, in common with hemorrhoids, is the site of arteriovenous anastomoses, it is easy to see why the sensation of need for defecation could easily arise.

The operative procedure for correction consists of the excision of a section of this extremely redundant mucosa. The operation is an extensive hemorrhoidectomy in which the removal of the usual three hemorrhoids is carried up several centimeters higher than it would be for the normal hemorrhoids and all of the redundant tissue is removed. This lesion is rarely encountered, and this procedure will give remarkable relief in properly selected cases.

References

1. Barron J. (1963) Office ligation of internal hemorrhoids. Am J Surg 105: 563
2. Bartizal J., Slosberg P.A. (1977) An alternative to hemorrhoidectomy. Arch Surg 112: 534
3. Chant A.D.B., May A., Wilken B.J. (1972) Haemorrhoidectomy versus manual dilatation of the anus. Lancet 2: 398
4. Ferguson J.A., Mazier W.P., Ganchrow M.I., et al (1971) The closed technique of hemorrhoidectomy. Surgery 70: 480
5. Hardcastle J.D. (1969) The descending perineum syndrome. Practitioner 203: 612
6. Hood T.R., Williams J.A. (1971) Anal dilatation versus rubber band ligation for internal hemorrhoids: Method of treatment in outpatients. Am J Surg 122: 545
7. Lord P.H. (1969) A day-case procedure for the cure of third-degree hemorrhoids. Br J Surg 56: 747
8. MacIntyre I.M.C., Balfour T.W. (1972) Results of the Lord non-operative treatment for haemorrhoids. Lancet 1: 1094
9. Parks A.G. (1971) Hemorrhoidectomy. Adv Surg 5: 1
10. Parks A.G., Porter N.H., Hardcastle J. (1966) The syndrome of the descending perineum. Proc R Soc Med 59: 477
11. Thulesius O., Gjöres J.R. (1973) Arterio-venous anastomoses in the anal region with reference to the pathogenesis and treatment of hemorrhoids. Acta Chir Scand 139: 476
12. Turell R. (1972) A modern look at the problem of hemorrhoids. Am J Surg 123: 245
13. Stelzner F. (1976) Die Anorectalen Fisteln (English translation), 2nd edn. Springer, New York, p 20
14. Whitehead W. (1882) The surgical treatment of haemorrhoids. Br Med J 1: 148

22 Other Anorectal Diseases

Fissure-in-Ano

Fissures are usually due to inordinate stretching of the anal canal by hard fecal concretions but may occur with tuberculosis, Crohn's disease, or ulcerative colitis. They are almost always located posteriorly in the midline and may vary from superficial cracks to very deep, heavily scarred lacerations that extend as deep as the internal sphincter and may be 2–3 cm in length. A papilla at the upper end of the fissure may hypertrophy, and, in the same fashion, skin at the outer edge may become edematous and form a "sentinel pile."[10] The treatment depends entirely upon the severity of the process.

Superficial fissures occur rather frequently in infants and children and are the commonest cause of bright red rectal bleeding in this population. Nearly all of them will heal spontaneously. Healing may be aided by the application of bland ointments such as Vaseline. Ellison reported that only 1 of 117 patients in this age group required operation.[3]

In adults the symptoms include severe pain that appears a few minutes after a bowel movement and persists for 10–15 min thereafter. A few drops of blood are often noted with bowel movements. Many adult superficial fissures will respond to the application of over-the-counter anorectal products and the use of a bland diet.

More advanced fissures require dilatation of the anus for relief because the very tight, spastic lower portion of the internal sphincter is causing the pain. After dilatation, spasm and pain disappear and the fissure has a chance to heal. Dilatation may be performed as an office procedure after the introduction of a local anesthetic such as lidocaine by perianal injection, but usually it is done in the hospital so that other anal pathology can be corrected.

Deep fissures with a great deal of fibrosis must be treated under regional or general anesthesia in a hospital. The anal canal is gently but thoroughly dilated. The fissure together with papilla and sentinel pile are excised with a scalpel, the margins of mucosa are removed, and the lower portion of the internal sphincter which forms the base of the fissure is curetted (Fig. 22.1). Any bleeding is stopped by catgut ligatures. The surgeon then has the option of leaving the incision wide open, as we prefer, or closing the mucosa over the defect. In recent years some surgeons have

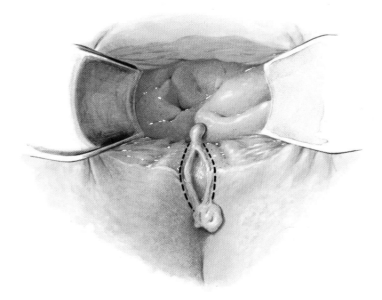

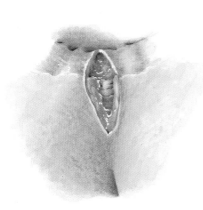

Fig. 22.1a and b. Excision of fissure-in-ano. a. The anal canal has been thoroughly dilated. The fissure in the posterior commissure is excised totally with a small margin of mucous membrane. The sentinel pile is included in the excision.

Fig. 22.1b. After excision, the circular muscle of the internal sphincter is seen at the base of the excision. The sphincter is not cut.

advised closure of the mucosa over the defect in the belief that this produces more rapid healing.

Dilatation for the mild cases or excision, either with or without suture of the mucous membrane, may be depended upon to give excellent results without any complications. Nonetheless, many proctologists have preferred a somewhat more radical procedure. They advise a division of the lower portion of the internal sphincter as well, by a sphincterotomy in the bed of the fissure in the posterior commissure.[11–15] The disadvantage of this procedure is that a minor degree of incontinence may result.

Notaras found that anal stretching led to minor defects of anal control in 25% of patients and posterior internal sphincterotomy led to defects in 43%. He therefore uses a lateral internal sphincterotomy.[11–13] The fissure itself is not touched unless a sentinel pile needs removal. The section between the internal and external sphincters is identified at 3 or 9 o'clock, a scalpel is inserted in the groove, and the lower portion of the internal sphincter is cut. This technique of lateral sphincterotomy has attained a great deal of popularity in recent years.

Perianal Infections and Fistulas

There are many causes of infection in the perianal area. The most important is presumed to be infection in one of the perianal glands that are located at the level of the pectinate line between the internal and external sphincter muscles. If suppuration occurs it tends to rupture through the capsule of the gland and then penetrate externally; meanwhile, the communication with the rectal lumen is maintained by the anal duct. In these instances a fistula often results after an incision and drainage of an abscess. Infections can also begin in the crypts; cryptitis is presumed to be one of the instigating causes of hemorrhoids. In rare instances infections may be

217

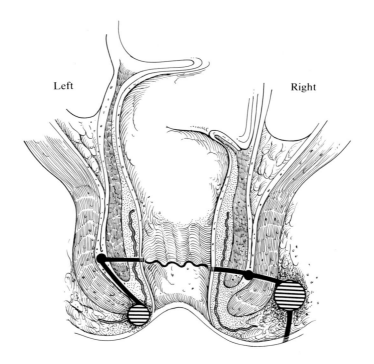

Left

Right

Fig. 22.2. Intra- and transsphincteric infections and fistulas. Ninety-five percent of all abscesses and fistulas are one of these two types. Left. Perianal abscess and fistula. The location of an anal gland is shown by the black dot. The internal opening has tracked via a duct through the internal sphincter to an anal crypt. The external tract has dissected within the external sphincter to form an abscess in the perianal area. A fistula forms after drainage of the abscess. Right. Ischiorectal abscess and fistula. The abscess has dissected through the internal sphincter and formed an abscess deep in the ischiorectal fossa. [Adapted from Parks A.G., Thomson J. P. S. (1977) The rectum and anal canal. In: Sabiston D. C. Jr. (ed.) Davis-Christopher textbook of surgery, 11th edition. Saunders, Philadelphia, p. 1134.]

secondary to perforations of the rectum by foreign bodies. Infection can also follow operative procedures such as hemorrhoidectomy.

Perianal and ischiorectal abscesses are the two most important manifestations of perianal infections. Parks has studied the mechanism of their formation.[15] It is assumed that they begin from infection in the perianal glands. From the perianal glands the infection may burrow in either a vertical or a lateral direction. In this way several distinct types of infections and fistulas are produced. Parks et al. have divided them into four groups as follows[17]:

Intrasphincteric
Infection that begins in a perianal gland usually proceeds downward between the sphincters and then, after passing below the lower end of the internal sphincter, presents as a perianal abscess, usually in the posterior commissure (Fig. 22.2, left). Meanwhile, there is a tendency for pus to discharge via the duct of the anal gland directly through the internal sphincter into the lumen of the rectum at the level of the pectinate line. When the abscess is opened by a perineal incision, a fistula will follow if the tract through the internal sphincter is still present.

Under unusual circumstances the infection tracks upward rather than downward and remains trapped between the sphincters. A tender submucosal swelling can be noted that may be 2–3 cm above the dentate line. This unusual type of abscess is best approached by incision through the mucosa and internal sphincter, allowing internal drainage.

Transsphincteric

The abscess can track directly through the external sphincter and into the ischiorectal fossa, forming an ischiorectal abscess (Fig. 22.2, right). Difficult to diagnose in its early stages, this type of abscess is accompanied by a great deal of pain and later swelling. As soon as a probable diagnosis is made, the ischiorectal abscess should be evacuated by incision and drainage. It is best to make an incision in a radial direction in case a fistula is encountered. The abscess cavity should be entered, all fibrous bands broken up, and drainage maintained by means of stuffed Penrose drains.

If the abscess has also tracked internally through the internal sphincter, a fistula will be noted at the time of this operation or will develop at a later date.

Suprasphincteric

The abscess may track upward and then pass either above the external sphincter or through the uppermost portion of it, later proceeding downward through the ischiorectal fossa and the skin (Fig. 22.3, left). Fortunately this is an unusual type of presentation. The initial symptoms are due to an ischiorectal abscess, which is drained as described above. If a fistula forms later the problem will be much more difficult.

Extrasphincteric

This is another very rare type. The infection may begin from a perforation of the rectum above the levator ani or as an infection of the perianal glands that tracks through the levator ani into the rectum and outward through the perineum (Fig. 22.3, right). The presence of other diseases such as Crohn's disease must always be considered with such fistulas. The treatment involves identification of the causative lesion and appropriate therapy either by bowel resection or colostomy combined with opening of the tract.

Treatment of Fistulas

The ordinary mode of presentation of an infection is either as a perianal abscess or an ischiorectal abscess. The usual plan is to drain these abscesses widely. If a fistula can be identified easily at the same time it is opened as well, provided that it involves only the lowermost portion of the sphincters. No attempt should be made to divide the sphincters to a high level.

Unusual fistulas may appear about the rectum. Some run into the pilonidal sinus area and involve multiple tracts in the buttocks with one or more entries in the rectum. They require wide opening and sometimes colostomy to allow healing of the very wide incisions. Other fistulas may appear in the presence of an inflammatory disease, such as Crohn's disease,[9] tuberculosis, or lymphogranuloma, or they may be secondary to perforation caused by a foreign body or cancer. Excised tissue should always be examined by the pathologist to rule out one of these underlying diseases. The treatment of these unusual fistulas is much more difficult because there is a tendency for recurrence even when the fistulous tract is opened

219

Left   Right

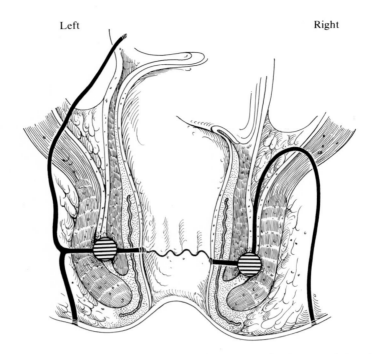

Fig. 22.3. Supra- and extrasphincteric infections and fistulas. Left. Ischiorectal abscess with suprasphincteric fistula. A submucosal abscess may be palpable through the wall of the rectum before an external fistula forms; it can be drained by a transrectal incision. If a fistula develops and the tract involves a substantial portion of the external sphincter (as shown in this diagram), the use of a seton should be considered rather than a long incision through the entire tract. If one tract extends into the peritoneal cavity, the possibility of diverticulitis or Crohn's disease should be considered; laparotomy and/or colostomy may be necessary. Right. Ischiorectal abscess with extrasphincteric fistula. The tract runs through the internal sphincter and then above the puborectalis segment of the levator ani. This rare fistula cannot be treated by long incision because incontinence will result. A seton or a colostomy is indicated for therapy. [Adapted from Parks A.G., Thomson J.P.S. (1977) The rectum and anal canal. In: Sabiston D.C. Jr. (ed) Davis-Christopher textbook of surgery, 11th edn. Saunders, Philadelphia, p 1134.]

widely. Fortunately, some of the fistulas about the anus that occur in association with Crohn's disease may subside after resection of an involved terminal ileum and/or right colon.

Some fistulas may appear a slight distance away from the anus and actually are due to diverticulitis or Crohn's disease that has penetrated through the levator ani. Whenever one of these diseases is suspected, an injection of the fistula should be carried out to determine by x-ray, barium enema, and sigmoidoscopy whether or not there is an opening into the rectum, sigmoid colon, or small bowel at a higher level.

In the treatment of anal fistulas it is first necessary to identify the fistulous tract (Fig. 22.4). The outer opening is usually easy to find but may at times be temporarily occluded by partial healing. The internal opening may be extremely difficult to locate. Fistulas that are located anterior to the anterior half of the anus track directly into the anus, while those that are located posterior to this line nearly always enter at the posterior commissure. Fistulas in the posterior portion may be quite extensive and may extend laterally onto both buttocks in the configuration of a horseshoe.

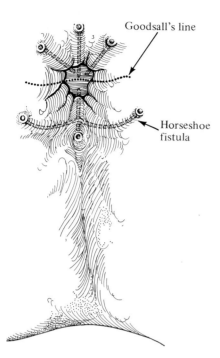

Fig. 22.4. Fistulous tracts. Note the relationship to Goodsall's line. Anterior fistulas run directly into the rectum; posterior fistulas run through the midline.

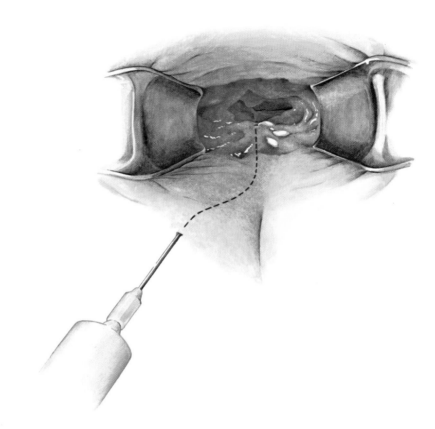

Fig. 22.5. Injection of milk through a fistulous tract (broken line) to identify the internal opening. This method was described by Houston over 2 centuries ago.

When the patient is in lithotomy position, the line running from 3 to 9 o'clock is known as "Goodsall's line."[4]

In order to identify the internal opening the surgeon should probe it very gently, being careful not to produce false passages. If this is not possible, milk may be injected into the outer opening through a blunt needle (Fig. 22.5). The internal opening can often be easily identified in this way. Next a probe and then a grooved director is passed entirely through the tract and the tract is opened widely. The scar tissue about it is excised and submitted for study by the pathologist. The whole area is packed open and allowed to granulate.

A special problem exists when the fistulas are of either the supra-sphincteric or extrasphincteric type. If one attempts a wide opening of the fistula, either the external sphincter or both the internal and external sphincters may be sacrificed. Incontinence is sure to follow because the wound has to be packed open during the period of healing. If an internal opening can be identified and it is found at the level of the dentate line, it may be possible to divide the lowermost portion of the sphincters and provide external drainage, leaving the major portion of the external sphincter intact. Likewise, the fistulous tract lateral to the external sphincter can be opened and drained. However, extensive section of the external sphincter is dangerous.

An alternative technique consists of the passage of a thread or rubber band entirely through the fistulous tract as a seton. The seton is gradually

221

tightened and allowed to cut through the sphincters so that healing occurs behind it as it passes downward and then finally cuts through the perineum. We have had no experience with this method, but it has been recommended by Hanley and others.[7,8]

Rectovaginal fistulas secondary to obstetric injuries now are rare. They may be repaired by excision and closure in layers; the approach may be through the vagina or through the rectum.[5]

Condylomata

Condylomata acuminata are caused by a virus. They consist of numerous wartlike growths that extend widely around the anus, in the perineum, and occasionally into the anal canal and vagina (Fig. 22.6). They may be destroyed by various methods.[22] There is, however, a tendency for them to recur and it may be necessary to carry out the procedure on two or three occasions before they are finally eliminated.

We prefer to destroy these lesions by electrodesiccation. With the patient under regional or general anesthesia, the Bovie unit is used to destroy all lesions. This procedure involves careful observation of the anal canal and the destruction of any lesions that are found within it.

Postoperatively there is a moderate amount of discomfort, particularly if wide destruction of the outer layers of the skin has been incurred by electrocoagulation. This is treated by the application of ointments and healing may be expected within 2 weeks.

Another method of therapy is to apply an extract of podophyllin. This substance apparently has a specific effect upon the cells of the condyloma. It is, however, intensely irritating and may be quite painful. It may be applied as an office procedure, but it is better to err on the side of conservatism and to use repeated applications rather than to produce a wide burn that will be exceedingly uncomfortable for the patient. A 25% solution is applied directly to the condylomata for 1 hr. The surrounding skin is protected with mineral oil.

Since the electrodesiccating unit is easy to use in treating these lesions, we have preferred to use it rather than the more protracted and painful method of podophyllin application. Cryosurgical removal should also be satisfactory, although we have had no experience with this method.

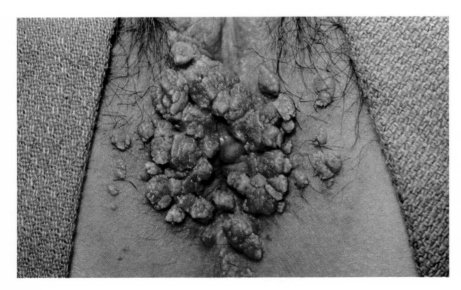

Fig. 22.6. Condylomata acuminata. These lesions were successfully destroyed by electrodesiccation.

Condylomata lata, or flat anal warts, are a manifestation of secondary syphillis and are rarely seen. The treatment is that of the underlying disease.

Cryptitis and Papillitis

Cryptitis may be diagnosed by the presence of localized pain and tenderness in the area of one or more of the anal crypts. Minor infections that originate in the crypts of Morgagni are believed to be one reason that hemorrhoids may become symptomatic; that is, the hemorrhoids are exacerbated by the edema that follows the infection in the region of the anal canal. Cryptitis may originate in the anal glands and may occur preliminary to the development of an anal fistula. Unless further complications develop, cryptitis is usually self-limited and will not require any treatment other than diagnosis, warm sitz baths, and perhaps, if there is rather severe spasm, a dilatation of the anal canal.

Hypertrophied papillae often accompany cryptitis. The end stage of papillitis is a fibroepithelial polyp that may be palpated by the patient when it is extruded from the anus. With the patient under local or general anesthesia, one or more prolapsing papillae may either be removed by suture of the base and excision, or be destroyed by electrodesiccation.

Anal Stenosis (Pectenosis) and Rectal Stricture

There are several causes of anal stenosis. Frequently the lower portion of the internal sphincter tends to thicken and stenose in later life. A ring is formed about 1 cm in width that is called the "pecten band"; this band can be palpated by the examining finger. This disease, sometimes known as "pectenosis," is the most important cause of senile anal stenosis. Anal stenosis secondary to scarring may be very severe after a Whitehead type of hemorrhoidectomy.

Usually a simple dilatation will relieve the symptoms and in many older people it will provide a great deal of relief from annoying constipation

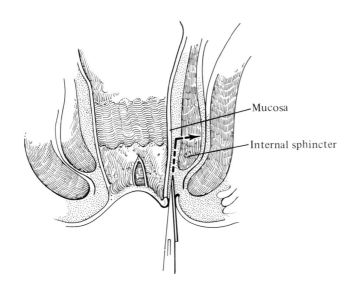

Mucosa

Internal sphincter

Fig. 22.7. Lateral sphincterotomy (closed method). This can be accomplished at the 3 o'clock or 9 o'clock position, or in both areas. A scalpel is inserted between the mucous membrane and the internal sphincter, and the pecten band (the lower tight section of the internal sphincter) is divided by a lateral cut through the sphincter (method of Notaras).

223

or incontinence. The use of rectal dilators by the patient at home later on may also be helpful. If simple dilatation under anesthesia is not sufficient, the lower portion of the internal sphincter may have to be divided. Internal sphincterotomy incisions should be placed lateral to the posterior commissure at 3 and, if necessary, 9 o'clock when the patient is in the lithotomy position. The method of internal sphincterotomy as described by Notaras is shown in Fig. 22.7.[11-13] According to him, postoperative incontinence is only seen in 5% of patients and is never severe; this contrasts with a 20% incidence after forceful dilatation. Open incision techniques have been described by Parks and by Oh[14] (Fig. 22.8).

Severe strictures that follow hemorrhoidectomy in which a large area of skin has been removed will require some type of a plastic operation in order to provide more skin for the anal canal. Incisions may be made according to the lines in Figure 22.9 and a skin flap may be raised and sutured within the anal canal. Provided the sphincter mechanism is intact this procedure should give good results. It obviously only rarely needs to be used.

Strictures may occur in the rectum at any point above the anal canal. They are quite rare, but there are several possible causes. A postanastomotic stricture after a very low anastomosis is one of the more common types. Lymphogranuloma venereum must always be considered a possible cause. Crohn's disease may lead to a tight stricture just above the anal ring. A submucous infiltrating carcinoma can cause extensive narrowing of the rectal lumen. Extrinsic pressure from tumors in the perirectal tissues is also possible. Stricture may follow radiation therapy of pelvic organs. Rectal strictures lead to constipation and fecal incontinence.

When the stricture is associated with an anastomotic procedure, it may be possible to divide it either by direct exposure through the dilated anus or at a higher level by electrocoagulation through an appropriate endoscope. If there is no underlying inflammatory disease or tumor this procedure can give good results. If there is a question as to the cause of the process, deep biopsies may be necessary to rule out stricture due to intramural tumor.

Fecal Incontinence

Fecal incontinence is a serious problem, especially in older patients. The success of any operative procedure depends more upon the cause than upon any other feature.

Fecal incontinence is often caused by intrinsic anorectal diseases such as the following: prolapsing hemorrhoids, ulcerative colitis, or Crohn's disease with damage to the sphincter; stenosis of the anus with secondary fecal impaction and fecal overflow; cancer of the anal canal or lower rectum; infections due to amoebae or lymphogranuloma; Hirschsprung's disease; and rectal prolapse. Specific therapy is possible for nearly all of these diseases. Injuries from accidents or foreign bodies and obstetrical injuries involving tears of the sphincters likewise have a high probability of successful treatment.

After certain surgical procedures incontinence may be a major problem. For example, after many of the pull-through operations for cancer or inflammatory disease in which the sphincters have been sacrificed, patients are likely to be completely incontinent; they must rely upon regular irrigations to clean the bowel and must continue on a highly constipating diet. Incontinence has followed many operations for rectal prolapse, particularly when the anorectal mucosa and sphincters have been sacrificed.

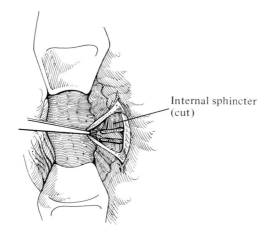

Internal sphincter
(cut)

Fig. 22.8. Lateral sphincterotomy (open incision). An incision is made along the mucocutaneous margin. The mucosa is dissected upward above the dentate line. The lower portion of the internal sphincter is divided under direct vision (Park's method). A small portion of the sphincter can be excised under direct vision (Oh's method).

Forceful dilatation of the anal canal with rupture of the sphincters is dangerous. The excessive dilatation of the anal canal by the Lord technique for hemorrhoids, hemorrhoidectomy that is accompanied by division of the sphincter, or division of the sphincter secondary to operations for anal fissure or fistula are other causes. Neurological conditions, such as spina bifida or spinal cord tumors, may also contribute.[16,19]

Unfortunately, at the present time many of the more serious problems are caused by old age or invalidism. In some of these unfortunate patients there will be little success with any local surgical measures and the patient will be condemned to either a diaper life or a colostomy.

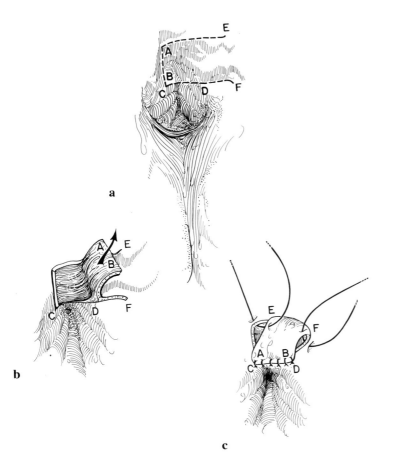

Fig. 22.9a–c. Development of perianal skin flaps for relief of stricture. a. Incisions are made along the broken line. The innermost portion of the incision must be made at the line of stricture but as much mucous membrane as possible must be conserved. b. The skin flap is raised and will be repositioned. c. Closure is made with the skin flaps sutured in the new position.

225

In mild cases the patient is usually placed on sphincter-tightening exercises and urged to maintain a low-residue, constipating diet. Anal cleansing, occasional small enemas, and the use of diphenoxylate hydrochloride with atropine sulfate (Lomotil) or the temporary administration of deodorized tincture of opium are helpful. These measures will relieve many mild cases.

Severe incontinence that is so bothersome that the patient's perineum is eroded by feces may require other measures. If some other disease of the colon is found, such as diverticulitis, proper surgical treatment of the underlying disease may improve the situation.

Many methods of surgical repair have been attempted. The usual procedure has been to identify the transected ends of the sphincter muscles and approximate them end to end. Other surgeons have reefed the sphincter muscles through a posterior incision. Unfortunately, the results are not extremely good. In a series of 133 cases collected by Blaisdell in 1940 only 42% of the surgical results were classified as good.[2] The results range from good, for the treatment of incontinence caused by obstetric injuries, to poor, for incontinence due to old age.

If the patient has not responded to conservative measures or to the relief of other diseases of the colon by appropriate measures, a surgical repair is indicated. If there is any hope that the repair will hold, a preliminary colostomy is done. The operative procedure then consists of a wide excision of all scar tissue around the anus and identification of the transsected muscles (Fig. 22.10a). The site of the incision necessary for this purpose will be determined by the underlying cause. An incision is made at the anal verge and dissection is carried outside the sphincter muscles. It is important to look for the sphincters, but do not separate them widely from their surrounding scar tissue. The muscular tube of the mucosa must be reconstructed. The sphincters are then overlapped and sutured in position

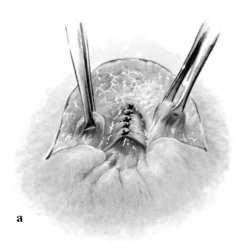

a

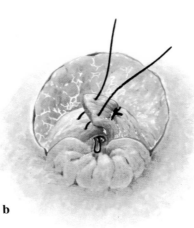

b

Fig. 22.10a and b. Sphincteroplasty for fecal incontinence. a. The area of scar has been excised. The mucous membrane is freed and the torn sphincters are identified. The mucous membrane of the anal canal is reconstituted by several sutures. b. The muscle bundles and surrounding scar tissues are overlapped and pleated with interrupted 30 wire sutures. A complementary colostomy is advised.

with wire (Fig. 22.10b). This method has led to success in the hands of Parks and McPartlin[16,18] and also in seven patients reported by Hagihara and Griffen.[6]

Other methods that have been suggested are the insertion of a Thiersch wire, a fascial strip, or muscle from the gracilis or transverse perineal muscles.[1,20,21,23] Although success has been reported after each of these procedures, in general there is not a great deal of enthusiasm about their use.

In the unfortunate, old patient who has lost anal sensation a colostomy may prove to be tolerated much better than any other procedure. This is particularly true of invalids who must lie in bed.

Pruritus Ani

Pruritus can almost always be controlled by a judicious combination of good hygiene, dietary measures, the omission of irritating clothes (particularly nylons), and the application of cortisone-containing ointments. In few instances, however, a surgical attack will be necessary.

At times pruritus is associated with significant hemorrhoidal disease, with prolapse and perhaps secondary discharge of either mucus or feces on the perienum. A hemorrhoidectomy combined with other local measures can be curative.

Exceedingly severe pruritus may be alleviated by the subcutaneous injection of 95% alcohol. This technique may introduce infection and sloughing of the skin. It should therefore be used only in intractable cases. The injection of 1 cc 95% alcohol in five or six different areas may be sufficient to alleviate the symptoms of the disease. The effect will persist for at

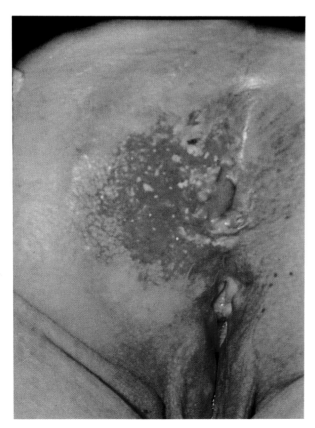

Fig. 22.11. Paget's disease of the perianal skin. This is a rare lesion that preferably is treated by wide local excision.

least a matter of several months and the absence of scratching will allow further healing to occur.

The wide excision of involved skin has been described by Turell.[24] We have never used this method.

Paget's Disease of the Perianal Skin

Paget's disease of the perianal skin is marked by a thin, irritated epithelium that becomes dry, scaling and itching, and later becomes ulcerated (Fig. 22.11). The typical Paget's cells are seen on the biopsy specimen.

This is a premalignant disease and its cure requires a wide excision of perianal skin. Even after wide excision, however, the disease may develop in other areas.

References

1. Birnbaum W. (1969) Fecal incontinence. In: Turell R. (ed) Diseases of the colon and anorectum, 2nd edn, Vol 2. Saunders, Philadelphia, p 1029
2. Blaisdell P.D. (1940) Repair of incontinent sphincter ani. Surg Gynecol Obstet 70: 692
3. Ellison F.S. (1960) Anal fissure occurring in infants and children. Dis Colon Rectum 3: 161
4. Goodsall D.H., Miles W.E. (1900) Diseases of the anus and rectum, Part I. Longmans, Green, London
5. Greenwald J.C., Hoexter B. (1978) Repair of rectovaginal fistulas. Surg Gynecol Obstet 146: 443
6. Hagihara P.F., Griffen W.O. Jr. (1976) Delayed correction of anorectal incontinence due to anal sphincteral injury. Arch Surg 111: 63
7. Hanley P.H. (1977) Anorectum. In: Hardy J.D. (ed) Rhoads textbook of surgery, 5th edn. Lippincott, Philadelphia, p 1259
8. Hanley P.H. (1978) Rubber band seton in the management of abscess–anal fistula. Ann Surg 187: 435
9. Homan W.P., Tang C., Thorbjarnason B. (1976) Anal lesions complicating Crohn's disease. Arch Surg 111: 1333
10. Miles W.E. (1939) Anal fissure. In: Rectal surgery: A practical guide to the modern surgical treatment of rectal diseases. Cassell, London, p 147
11. Notaras M.J. (1969) Lateral subcutaneous sphincterotomy for anal fissure— A new technique. Proc R Soc Med 62: 713
12. Notaras M.J. (1971) The treatment of anal fissure by lateral subcutaneous internal sphincterotomy—A technique and results. Br J Surg 58: 96
13. Notaras M.J. (1974) Some nonmalignant lesions of the ano-rectal region. In: Maingot R. (ed) Abdominal operations, 6th edn, Vol 2. Appleton-Century-Crofts, New York, p 2140
14. Oh C. (1978) A modified technique for lateral internal sphincterotomy. Surg Gynecol Obstet 146: 623
15. Parks A.G. (1961) Pathenogenesis and treatment of fistula-in-ano. Br Med J 1: 463
16. Parks A.G. (1975) Anorectal incontinence. Proc R Soc Med 68: 681
17. Parks A.G., Gordon P.H., Hardcastle J.D. (1976) A classification of fistula-in-ano. Br J Surg 63: 1
18. Parks A.G., McPartlin J.F. (1971) Late repair of injuries of the anal sphincter. Proc R Soc Med 64: 1187
19. Parks A.G., Porter N.H., Hardcastle J. (1966) The syndrome of the descending perineum. Proc R Soc Med 59: 477

20. Pickrell K.L., Boradbent T.R., Masters F.W., et al (1952) Construction of a rectal sphincter and restoration of anal continence by transplanting the gracilis muscle. Ann Surg 135: 853
21. State D., Katz A. (1955) The use of superficial transverse perineal muscles in the treatment of post-surgical anal incontinence. Ann Surg 142: 262
22. Thomson J.P.S., Grace R.H. (1978) The treatment of perianal and anal condylomata acuminata: A new operative technique. J R Soc Med 71: 180
23. Turell R. (1954) The Thiersch operation for rectal prolapse and anal incontinence. N Y State J Med 54: 791
24. Turell R. (1969) Treatment of intractable anal pruritus. In: Turell R. (ed) Diseases of the colon and anorectum, 2nd edn, Vol 2. Saunders, Philadelphia, p 1007

23 Other Colorectal Diseases

Operations Related to Cancer

Combination Therapy

Numerous combinations of radiation therapy and chemotherapy with surgery for cancer of the colorectum have been proposed.[1,12,17,23,28,29] No clear protocol has evolved at the present time; the remarks presented here undoubtedly will have to be modified after further investigations.

The use of radiation therapy has essentially been limited to patients with cancer of the rectum.[3,28,35,36,46,52] There is no doubt that large, questionably removable tumors may at times be reduced in size by radiation therapy, allowing subsequent radical excision. The role of preoperative or postoperative radiotherapy in operable rectal cancers is controversial. The greatest interest at present is centered on preoperative therapy. Published reports indicate a wide range in the amount of radiation and the time span over which it has been given. Very heavy doses, in the neighborhood of 5000 rads, reported by Allen et al., have in their experience been associated with a lower incidence of involved lymph nodes at the time of resection than would have been expected, and also are followed by almost complete elimination of late recurrence in the perineum.[3] Whether the life span of these patients has been increased is questionable; distal recurrences seem to cause death in these patients almost as rapidly as in patients who did not receive radiation. Most radiotherapists have used a lower dose of approximately 2500–3000 rads given approximately 2 weeks prior to operation.

The surgical procedures following radiation remain the same as those that would be used without it. There has been no apparent increase in the technical difficulties of such operations.

In Massachusetts General Hospital a trial series is being run by Gunderson in which postoperative radiotherapy is being used for patients with Dukes type C colorectal tumors. This method has the advantage that patients who have had excision of a tumor that has not extended through the bowel wall or to lymph nodes do not require therapy. Whether it will result in a higher incidence of late survivals is not yet clear.

The use of chemotherapy has been reduced essentially to postoperative treatment of metastatic cancer in the liver or to patients with Dukes C cancers of the colorectum.[11,19,22,39] Even here there have been serious doubts as to whether or not the present use of 5-fluorouracil (5-FU, which is known to be the most potent drug) is actually of any value; combined with chloroethylcyclohexylnitrosourea (CCNU) there is hope that better results may be obtained. At any rate, there is at the present time no enthusiasm about the use of chemotherapy at the time of operation either by intravenous injection or by instillation into the colon itself. Some studies are under way to determine whether or not patients with Dukes C tumors in the absence of demonstrated metastases should have a prophylactic trial with chemotherapy. This will require further investigation.

Intraluminal injection of 5-FU at the time of resection was advocated by Rousselot et al.[48] Although the statistics appeared favorable, a prospective study by Lawrence et al. indicated the method has no value.[39] A further study by the followers of Rousselot (Grossi et al.) may revive interest in the method since their recent series show better, though not statistically significant results in patients receiving the 5-FU in addition to resection.[22]

In Massachusetts General Hospital metastatic cancer of the liver (except in unusual cases of single metastases) is treated with 5-FU, at times in combination with other chemotherapeutic agents such as methyl CCNU. The 5-FU is usually given intravenously; it may also be administered by mouth, in which instance it is absorbed almost quantitatively into the portal vein, or by intra-arterial injection, either through a Seldinger catheter introduced through the brachial or femoral arteries or through a catheter introduced directly into the hepatic artery by laparotomy. Occasional long-term survivors after the institution of such therapy have led to continued hope that more effective agents will be found.

Carcinoembryonic antigen determinations may be used to measure the progression of a tumor; they are particularly of value when no other clinical manifestations of disease are apparent.[18,27,41,47]

Surgical Treatment of Metastatic Cancer

A secondary operation for known local or metastatic recurrence of a cancer of the colorectum is required in a number of instances.

Suture-line recurrence after a sphincter-saving procedure for cancer of the rectum is the most common reason for secondary operation. A secondary Miles resection may turn out to be curative in some of these cases. Usually the suture-line recurrence is secondary to recurrence outside the rectal wall, making the possibility of total excision of a tumor at the second operation quite unlikely. Nevertheless, this possibility should be entertained since otherwise the patient will have no chance of relief.

Perineal recurrences after a Miles procedure may occasionally be excised. In our experience this treatment has essentially never been curative and recurrence must be expected. For this reason it is wise to consider radiation therapy prior to or after a secondary surgical excision has been carried out.

Metastatic disease to the liver is encountered very frequently. While there is generally little enthusiasm for the resection of multiple metastatic liver masses, it can be of value in cases of a single metastatic lesion from a cancer of the colorectum or in cases of extensive metastases of carcinoid tumors, for excision of as much of the bulk of tumor as possible may relieve carcinoid symptoms. Wanebo et al. excised synchronous liver metastases in 28 patients and had a 5-year survival rate of 28%.[57] Wilson and Adson reported 60 patients who had resection of hepatic metastases; 15 of 36 with single metastases who were followed were alive 5 years later.[64]

Single metastatic masses can be excised either by a deep wedge resection or by a formal lobectomy.[16] Some of the most optimistic figures have been reported by Fortner et al. from Memorial Hospital, New York City; 18% of such patients survived 5 years after this radical surgery.[15]

When a single metastasis is encountered at the time of a colon resection for cancer of the colon, the question arises as to how it should be treated. In the light of our present knowledge it is probably better to plan the resection of the liver mass at a second stage rather than at the time of the original colon resection unless the tumor extends directly into the liver, in which case it would be necessary to excise a large section of liver along with the primary tumor. The reason for this is that the resection of the liver may carry many complications in its wake, and furthermore it would be wise to precede the resection by a liver scan to be certain that there are not numerous other nodules scattered deep within the liver. On the other hand, a scan could be done prior to the bowel resection, and if a single metastasis is confirmed at the time of laparotomy, both the tumor and the metastatic mass could be resected simultaneously.

Occasionally there are single metastatic lesions to the lung; they may be removed by lobectomy. In a study at Memorial Hospital, New York City, approximately half of the single nodules that appeared in the lung fields within a few years after resection of a cancer of the colorectum were due to metastatic cancer; the other half were due to primary cancer of the lung.[5] The end results after resection of this metastatic lesion have been quite satisfactory and the procedure is recommended. Wilkins et al. have reported 35 cases from Massachusetts General Hospital.[63]

Second-Look Operations

"Second-look" operations were instituted by Wangensteen.[59,60] He theorized that if any residual cancer is left after a presumably curative operation for a cancer of the colon, at a second look 6 months after any new areas of cancer could be recognized and excised. The important feature distinguishing his concept is that the second-look procedure is done even when the patient has no symptoms of recurrent disease.

Most surgeons would have very little argument with the point of view that a second-look procedure is advisable under certain circumstances, for example, if the primary operation is known to have been inadequate from the point of view of wide resection of the bowel or mesentery, or if the patient has recurrent symptoms indicating the possibility of recurrent cancer. It is an entirely different matter, however, to consider a secondary operation in a patient who has presumably had an adequate cancer operation and is now asymptomatic.

The early enthusiasm generated by Wangensteen and his associates has diminished in recent years. The dangers of such second-look operations should not be minimized. The postoperative complications include intestinal obstruction and fistula formation from extensive dissections. The possibility of the presence of a suture-line recurrence would need to be eliminated prior to operation, not only by barium studies but also by colonoscopy, since this theoretically could be a site of origin of secondary carcinoma.

It has been suggested that patients who have had a negative carcinoembryonic antigen test immediately after a colon resection and later show a rising titer are the ones in whom a second look would be desirable.[58] Such a guideline could eliminate unnecessary procedures. The possibility of the presence of diffuse metastasis is eliminated prior to the second laparotomy as far as possible by x-rays of chest and bone, and liver and bone scans. If these studies all show negative results and the serum carcinoembryonic antigen levels are elevated, a second look should lead to the discovery of some removable masses of recurrent tumor.

The value of secondary procedures for patients who are symptomatic after operations for the cure of colorectal cancer is emphasized by the studies of Welch and Donaldson.[61] They found that a substantial number of patients were cured in this fashion.

Electrocoagulation Treatment for Cancer of the Rectum

Electrocoagulation of polypoid tumors of the rectum that contain cancer in the tip of the polyp but show no invasion of the muscular wall at the base of the polyp is accepted as a curative procedure by the majority of surgeons. However, there is a great deal of argument about the wisdom of the electrocoagulation treatment of a florid carcinoma of the rectum that invades the muscular wall.[8,37,49,54]

This method is mentioned here although it must be said that we personally are not enthusiastic about it. Madden and Kandalaft suggest that it can be done by the induction of full anesthesia, wide dilatation of the anal canal, and deep electrocoagulation of the tumor.[42] This may require repetitive desiccations until the entire tumor is destroyed; an average of four sessions were used in their cases. In order to be eligible for such treatment the tumor should be located below the peritoneal reflection and preferably on the posterior wall so that there will not be any perforation of the urinary tracts in the male or the vagina in the female. They have reported 5-year survival results in a small group of patients that are equivalent to those achieved with the Miles resection.

Our objections are raised on both theoretical and practical grounds. Studies have shown that approximately 40%–50% of ulcerating carcinomas of the rectum already have established lymph node metastases. Local coagulation cannot influence these metastases unless one invokes the unproved possibility that there may be spontaneous regression of such metastases after destruction of the primary tumor. When a tumor is coagulated deeply the protective barrier of the wall of the rectum is broken and the perirectal tissues are invaded. This not only means that if the tumor recurs that it will then recur outside the rectum, but it also introduces the possibility of extensive sepsis in the retroperitoneal tissues and the possibility of secondary hemorrhage. Many patients who have been regarded as "inoperable" because of age actually can tolerate a curative resection far better than is indicated by the protagonists of electrodesiccation. Thus in Massachusetts General Hospital the operability rate of cancer of the rectum is over 90%, compared with 70% in Madden's series; the Massachusetts General Hospital postoperative mortality was 2%. Finally, when tumors are treated in this fashion the one chance for cure that a patient may have may be lost.

There are no figures available that document the frequency of recurrence after this procedure, though Madden's figures indicate a survival rate comparable to that after the standard abdominoperineal resection. Wanebo and Quan from Memorial Hospital, New York City, have seen many recurrences and have had more since their paper was published; only about 10% of these patients have been cured once recurrence has appeared after primary electrodesiccation.[56]

233

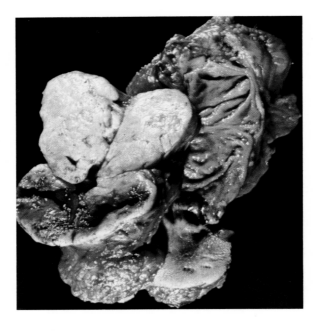

Fig. 23.1. Operative specimen of leiomyosarcoma of the rectum.

It is quite possible that the published series that show excellent results[8,37,42,53] include a high percentage of favorable cases, making the patients and results not comparable. Thus for "ulcerating cancers" treated by Madden and Kandalaft the 5-year survival rate was 30%, and for encircling tumors it was 0%.[43]

Other Tumors of the Colorectum

There are many other relatively rare tumors of the colon and rectum that should be mentioned. They are all treated by the standard techniques but the prognosis may be quite variable.

Primary melanomas of the anus are manifested by fungating, black tumors near the anal canal. These tumors are very highly malignant and despite combined abdominoperineal resection there are nearly always rapid metastases of the generalized type; cure is very rare.

Malignant melanoma likewise may metastasize to any part of the gastrointestinal tract. Typically it will produce either intussusception or bleeding.

Carcinoids are comparatively common in the rectum.[62] In approximately 90% of the cases carcinoids in this area are polypoid and relatively small. If they are under 2 cm in diameter, a local excision is advised. Unless there is widespread involvement of the lymphatics this procedure is nearly always curative. The other 10% of the carcinoids of the rectum tend to be very highly malignant. They are characterized by large tumors with widespread lymphatic metastases and metastatic nodes. They are generally incurable despite radical excisions.

Carcinoids are much less common in other portions of the colon. The treatment is the same as that of any other malignant tumor of that section of the colon. Lymphosarcomas, leiomyosarcomas, and fibrosarcomas all may occur in the colon and the rectum but again are quite rare (Fig. 23.1).

Benign tumors include lipomas, hemangiomas, and leiomyomas. Submucous lipomas may become polypoid; they may reach a large size in the right colon and are apt to be manifested by intussusception. By far the most common benign tumors are adenomas (see Chapters 5 and 7).

Retrorectal Tumors

Tumors can be found in the retrorectal space lying immediately behind the rectum and in front of the coccyx or sacrum. In a series of such tumors collected by Jackman et al., dermoid cysts were the most common. In addition there were entities such as fibromas and leiomyomas.[31] A meningomyelocele should be suspected if there is a high lesion. Teratomas are the most common tumors encountered in infancy.

The proper treatment of all such tumors is by excision. If the lesion is malignant it is usually necessary to carry out a combined abdominoperineal resection as well in order to secure a wide area about the tumor.

Retrorectal cysts have been misdiagnosed as perirectal abscesses and have been incised and drained. After this procedure they tend to persist, and unless the true nature of the cyst is recognized and the whole area is excised, healing will not occur. Some of these "cysts" may represent duplications of the rectum.

Hernias Containing Colon

Sliding hernias contain the sigmoid colon on the left side and the cecum and appendix on the right side. They almost always occur in males. Unless the presence of a sliding hernia is considered by the surgeon, it is easy to damage the colon at the time of dissection because there is no true sac; consequently the peritoneum must be opened gingerly on the anterior surface of the hernia. The presence of the loop of colon can then be determined and the whole colon together with its mesentery that is splayed out on the posterior surface can be dissected free from the spermatic cord.

Repair of these hernias is more difficult than the ordinary indirect hernia. The whole mass must be pushed back in an extraperitoneal fashion and the muscular wall closed very tightly. If the surgeon wishes to be more certain of the repair it is wise to cut the cord either with or without an orchiectomy.

The colon also may be trapped in a hiatus hernia or in the chest after traumatic rupture of the diaphragm.[21] The colon also may be involved or obstructed in spigelian or ventral hernias.

Constipation

Surgeons have dealt with chronic constipation for centuries. The enthusiasm for extensive colon resections was great several decades ago but fortunately has subsided. Nevertheless, there are certain instances in which the symptom of constipation is important for the surgeon.

Obviously, if it is a new development, it may be the symptom of some other disease, and should be considered seriously. Cancer or diverticulitis are the two most common causes in adults. In infants Hirschsprung's disease is a relatively common cause and in neglected cases this may persist into adolescence without a diagnosis having been made. Attempts have been made by pediatric surgeons to change the anorectal angle in some constipated children. The rationale behind this procedure is that sometimes the anus is placed abnormally forward, and in an attempt to defecate in the erect position the anterior wall of the rectum is pressed down against the posterior one, providing a valve that prevents defecation; if this concept is correct, displacement of the anus to a more posterior position

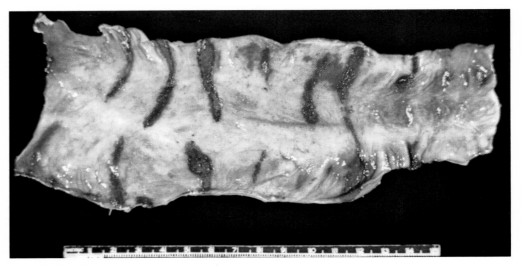

Fig. 23.2. Fecal ulcerations of the colon.

should correct the problem.[25] Somewhat similar conditions are encountered in the descending perineum syndrome in adults. In patients with volvulus of the colon, constipation may be an important factor, and wide resections of the colon may be curative in these cases.

Chronic constipation may prove so serious that an operation is required for it.[6] For example, after the ingestion of barium a rocklike scybala may be produced that may be caught in the sigmoid colon and lead to perforation. Particularly when such a rock is encountered above an area of diverticular disease, it should be removed surgically if it persists over a matter of several days, since the risk of perforation is high. Ulcerations of the colon caused by impacted feces may also be considered an indication for surgery (Fig. 23.2).

The problem remains, however, as to whether there are any instances in which the patient complains of constipation and an operation may be of value even though the bowel is apparently normal by all methods of investigation. There is a tendency to downgrade any surgical attacks on such colons. Nevertheless, in some refractory cases continued abdominal distention, localized left lower quadrant discomfort, and severe cramps may be combined with nausea and vomiting, and the gastroenterologist finally asks the surgeon for help. The cause of such symptoms is not apparent since studies of the ganglion cells in excised segments usually show them to be normal. We have encountered a few patients in whom an eventual ileostomy or transverse colostomy has provided complete relief of symptoms. Sometimes a subtotal colectomy in which the dissection is carried down to a point about 20 cm above the anal verge has provided relief.[51]

Such operative procedures are always regarded with skepticism. It is clear that they should only be used as measures of last resort. It is our purpose here merely to point out that occasionally they can be of value.

Infectious Diseases of the Colon

In this section several complications of infectious diseases of the colon that require treatment by surgery will be mentioned. It is recognized that they are all extremely rare.

Tuberculosis of the lower bowel may be accompanied by hypertrophic changes in the cecum that lead to intestinal obstruction. A right colec-

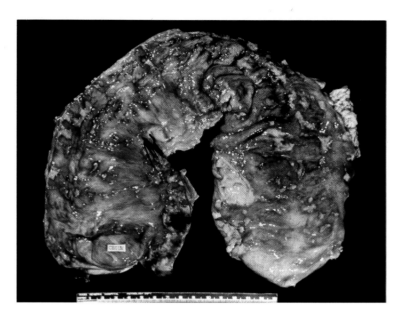

Fig. 23.3.   Autopsy specimen of amoebic ulcers of the colon.

tomy may be necessary. These lesions, formerly thought to be entirely the result of tuberculosis, are now known to be usually caused by Crohn's disease. Widespread colorectal tuberculosis may lead to the formation of fistulas that prove to be very difficult to cure. Fistulas-in-ano that occur in a patient with active tuberculosis may show acid-fast bacilli on smear and also prove to be difficult to cure by ordinary surgical methods. Chemotherapy for all such manifestations of tuberculosis is obviously important in conjunction with any appropriate surgical therapy.

Actinomycosis may lead to a low-grade perforation and fistulas from any area in the colon.[32] The appendix or cecum appears to be the more likely site of such infections.

Schistosomiasis, a very common disease in tropical countries, may lead to the formation of numerous pseudopolyps in the colon and rectum. Rectal bleeding is the major symptom of such polyps. The treatment is that of the underlying disease. Any attempt to remove the polyps in the absence of successful medical treatment will lead to their re-formation.

Lymphogranuloma venereum is caused by an infection arising from *Chlamydia trachomatis*.[50] The chlamydiae are obligatory intracellular parasites that are similar in some respects to gram-negative bacteria. Organisms of the same species are a major cause of nongonoccal urethritis. Inguinal lymphadenopathy, accompanied by chills and fever, is an early symptom. Serologic tests—either complement fixation or microimmunofluorescence—for antibody are necessary to make the diagnosis. Treatment involves one or more 21-day courses of tetracycline or sulfonamides. Chronic symptoms are most likely to be noted by females; rectal stricture is the most prominent.[44] Squamous cell carcinoma may develop at the site of a stricture.

Amebiasis is common in tropical countries. It is first manifested by involvement of the colon and colitis (Fig. 23.3). The drug of choice for treatment is metronidazole and prompt resolution is expected, as shown by the report of 5087 cases by Adams and MacLeod.[2] The most important complication is perforation of the colon. This usually occurs slowly by seepage rather than by acute perforation. A toxic megacolon may develop

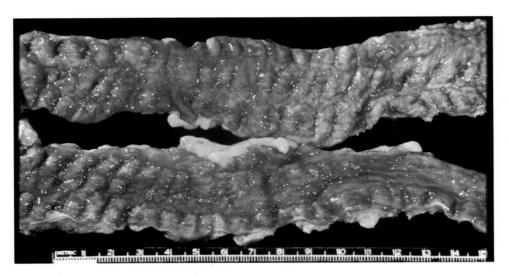

Fig. 23.4. Autopsy specimen of pseudomembranous enterocolitis.

and is noted at times in pregnancy; the mortality is extremely high, but immediate colectomy can save approximately half of the patients.

Chronic infection with amebae may lead to hypertrophic changes in the colon that produce amebomas almost indistinguishable from carcinomas. Resection will be necessary to treat obstruction.

The most common complication of amebiasis is liver abscess.[55] Adams and MacLeod recommend aspiration and metronidazole.[2] Death occurred in only 13 of their 1859 patients with uncomplicated amebic abscess. Perforation of an amebic abscess into the peritoneal cavity requires drainage. Emetine and chloroquine are other drugs that have been used in the treatment of amebic liver abscess with satisfactory results. Peritonitis also may follow migration of amebae through the wall of the colon. Despite attempts at drainage or colectomy, mortality is high for amebic peritonitis.

Pseudomembranous enterocolitis follows wide-spectrum antibiotic therapy and may be caused by a staphylococcal or gram-negative infection (Fig. 23.4; see also Chapter 24).[40] Rectal gonorrhea may simulate proctitis or cryptitis. It should be confirmed by cultures and treated by antibiotics.

Pneumatosis

Pneumatosis may occur anywhere in the colon or in the small intestine (Fig. 23.5). It may be entirely asymptomatic or may lead to episodes of subacute obstruction depending upon the size of the blebs. Rupture of one of the blebs may produce a pneumoperitoneum. The cause is unknown, and consequently it is difficult to be certain that any operative procedure can be instituted that is certain to be helpful. However, if acute obstructive symptoms arise in the presence of pneumatosis, a localized resection and anastomosis of the involved area of colon or small intestine may be necessary. Several cases have been reported in which this was done and there was permanent relief of symptoms.

Foreign Bodies

Foreign bodies may be inserted into the rectum or directly into the colon through a colostomy. The greatest dangers occur from perforation. Some

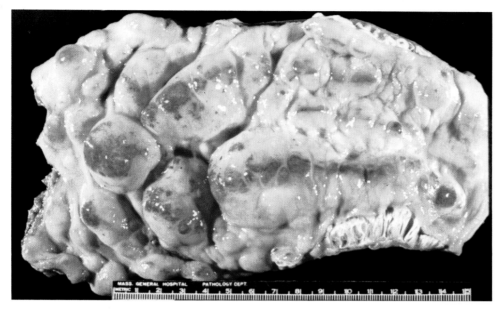

Fig. 23.5. Operative specimen of pneumatosis coli involving the entire sigmoid.

foreign bodies may remain for a long period of time without symptoms; but if they are large they may produce edema and obstruction, or if they are sharp, lacerations may produce bleeding as well as perforation.

A summary of the treatment of 31 foreign bodies by Eftaiha et al. contains some interesting technical suggestions.[13] They grouped the foreign bodies according to cause of introduction: (1) diagnostic or therapeutic maneuvers (e.g., thermometer, barium, rectal tube, disposable rectal enema tip, or irrigation catheter), (2) self-administered treatment to alleviate symptoms of anorectal disease, (3) criminal assault, (4) autoeroticism, and (5) accidental introduction.

Every attempt should be made to bring the foreign body down low into the rectum and to remove it after dilatation of the anal sphincters under adequate anesthesia. If the foreign body nearly fills the rectum, a helpful trick they recommend is to pass one or more Foley catheters past the foreign body and blow up the balloons so that any suction effect that would draw mucosa downward with the attempted extraction of the foreign body is eliminated. In some instances abdominal manipulation will aid the movement of a foreign body down from the high rectum into a position near the anus where it can be grasped with forceps and removed. At times the colonoscope and the snare may be employed to reach the foreign body.[4]

A laparotomy may be necessary if the foreign body cannot be removed from below. At this time it may be possible to manipulate it farther down into the rectum and to remove it transanally.

If there is any perforation of the bowel, obviously a laparotomy is indicated. When this occurs in the rectum the opening should be closed. Whether or not a transverse colostomy is required depends upon the circumstances. An early sharp perforation probably can be closed safely, but delay introduces the danger of sepsis and a colostomy will provide protection.

After the foreign body has been removed, complete sigmoidoscopy is carried out to be certain that there is no uncontrolled bleeding and no evidence of perforation. Enemas and catheters are contraindicated prior to extraction because they may increase edema or the danger of perforation. Perforations of stomas are discussed in Chapter 24.

Endometriosis of the Colon

Endometriosis of the colon may occur either before or after the menopause. Usually it occurs prior to the menopause and produces obstruction that is more likely to be symptomatic during menstruation. However, after the menopause fibrosis may ensue and lead to a secondary contraction of the colon.

Since these endometrial nodules are located extrinsic to the mucosa, the surgeon may have several options.[20,33,38] In general he must consider a resection and anastomosis of the involved bowel or a salpingo-oophorectomy, since the onset of surgical menopause may diminish the activity of the endometrial nodules on the colon. The decision will depend upon the age of the patient and various other individual factors. Usually a sigmoid resection and anastomosis will be considered to be the wisest choice. If these lesions are encountered at the time of a pelvic laparotomy in the relatively unprepared bowel, the surgeon must determine whether or not a concomitant transverse colostomy should be performed.

Colitis Cystica Profunda

This disease is characterized by cysts containing mucus located beneath the colonic or rectal mucosa. The areas may be localized, segmental, or diffuse.[14,26,30]

The proper treatment, when possible, is excision of the localized area. In the diffuse cases this may be impossible, but in localized cases there may be a soft submucosal tumor that is available for complete removal. There is essentially no treatment for the other types of the disease.

Pregnancy

Several colorectal diseases have a definite relationship to pregnancy. For example, ulcerative colitis may have its onset during the course of a pregnancy. At times this course may be progressive and extremely severe. In other instances pregnancy may supervene upon an established colitis that has been treated medically. The course is quite variable. At times the colitis may be better during pregnancy; at times there may be exacerbations.

Acute toxic megacolon may supervene in patients with known ulcerative colitis. In Mexico pregnant patients with amoebiasis of the colon may develop a peculiarly lethal type of toxic megacolon. It has been stated that unless radical surgical therapy is carried out, the mortality is nearly 100%. This can be approximately halved by a colectomy. We fortunately have had no experience with this particular problem.

Pregnancy in a patient who has undergone a total proctocolectomy for ulcerative colitis or Crohn's disease is somewhat more hazardous than in the normal person because there is an increased possibility of intestinal obstruction from previously established adhesions. However, in general, pregnancy has been well tolerated after this procedure.

Pregnancy almost always leads to the formation of hemorrhoids that may be exceedingly symptomatic during the later stages. Fortunately, conservative therapy almost always suffices and remarkable improvement can be expected after the pregnancy is completed.

As a consequence of delivery, tears of the sphincter or rectovaginal fistulas may occur (see Chapters 17 and 22).[24]

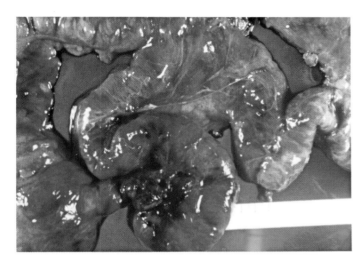

Fig. 23.6. Operative specimen of radiation injury of the colon.

Radiation Injury

Radiation injuries of the colon and small bowel are not uncommon after heavy therapy for diseases such as carcinoma of the cervix or the fundus uteri (Fig. 23.6). Fixation of the bowel in the pelvis tends to increase the possibility of such damage, and thus the sigmoid and upper rectum are particularly vulnerable.[7,10,45,51]

The symptoms are those of inflammation at an early stage. Later on bleeding may develop secondary to telangiectasia. Further fibrosis may lead to angulation and obstruction. In some instances breakdown of a tumor that has not been cured will lead to fistula formation between the colon and the adjacent viscera such as the vagina or bladder.

It is obvious that all of the problems posed by these changes can be very difficult. Usually mild degrees of damage are treated expectantly. However, if some of the major complications such as bleeding, obstruction, or fistulization occur, a diverting colostomy will be necessary. If the small bowel is found to be involved as well, it must be recognized that any anastomoses that are performed within the peritoneal cavity are likely to do much more poorly than in normal bowel. Dehiscence of the anastomosis is not uncommon.[48a]

It is very uncommon to be able to consider a resection and re-establishment of intestinal continuity after extensive radiation damage to the colon. It is conceivable that after a diverting colostomy in some instances a resection of the involved sigmoid colon and upper rectum could be carried out combined with a low anastomosis such as the D'Allaines type. However, this procedure would be performed with a great deal of hazard and must be undertaken only if the individual appears to be cured of the underlying cancer and the life expectancy is reasonably good.

Malakoplakia of the Colon and Rectum

Malakoplakia is a rare disease that may involve the colon and produce a diffuse inflammatory reaction that may simulate carcinoma.[9] The disease typically occurs in debilitated persons and may involve a wide variety of viscera, including the bladder and the retroperitoneal tissue. Microscopically, atypical submucous and intramural infiltration with histiocytes is

241

found; the histiocytes contain Michaelis-Gutmann bodies. Intestinal obstruction and fistulas have been reported.

Joyeuse et al. have collected a series of 21 cases from the literature.[34] The course in most cases proved to be fatal, although there were a few survivors after segmental resections of the colon.

Diseases of the Appendices Epiploicae

The appendices epiploicae are often attached to the colon by a very narrow pedicle. Consequently, they are subject to twisting and, later, necrosis and self-amputation. The symptoms of such torsion usually are subclinical. The occasional finding of a free, beanlike structure in the peritoneal cavity is probably a result of this problem. Occasionally the symptoms of pain and local tenderness are severe enough to lead to laparotomy. The affected epiploic appendix is excised.

Intraoperative Radiation Therapy for Cancer

The use of radiation therapy for cancer of the colorectum has been limited in many instances by the presence of other abdominal viscera that will not tolerate a cancercidal dose. The small bowel is particularly vulnerable to excessive doses of radiation. It has been postulated that an operative procedure that is combined with radiation therapy could be effective. If areas of removable disease or potential recurrence could be treated vigorously at the time of operation, cancercidal doses of radiation theoretically could be delivered safely. This type of combination therapy was first used in Japan.[1] It is now under study in a number of institutions in the United States.

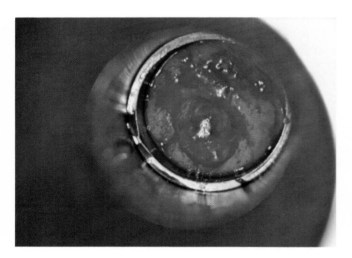

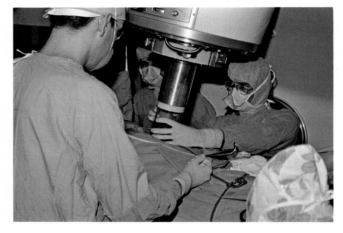

Fig. 23.7a and b. Intraoperative radiation therapy for recurrent cancer of the sigmoid and rectum. a. A cone approximately 10 cm in diameter is placed against the posterior wall after the abdominal dissection and prior to the perineal excision. This view shows the inner surface of the cone. The left iliac artery and sacral prominence can be observed behind the perivascular tissues, which are exceedingly hyperemic due to previous radiation.

Fig. 23.7b. Attachment of the linear accelerator cone to the plastic cone. A dose of 1500 rads will be delivered to the tumor bed in approximately 5 min.

A patient treated in this fashion is shown in Figure 23.7. This patient had had three previous operations for cancer of the intraperitoneal rectum and had developed a local recurrence without any evidence of metastasis to the liver. She was referred to Massachusetts General Hospital for radiation therapy. Approximately 5000 rads was administered to the pelvis at the site of the recurrence by external beam. It was clear, however, from barium studies of the small intestine that the small bowel lay exactly in the field of radiation and further radiation in this area would not be tolerated.

At her fourth operation a combined abdominoperineal resection was carried out and as far as could be determined all gross disease was removed at the time of this "fourth look." After the resection the small bowel and left ureter were packed away from the field, which was maintained by means of a large plastic cone to which the linear accelerator was attached. The tumor bed located near the bifurcation of the aorta was then treated intraoperatively with an additional 1500 rads delivered by the linear accelerator within a 5-min period. The remainder of the operation was carried out in the usual fashion after the radiation therapy was completed.

References

1. Abe M., Takahashi M., Yabumoto E., et al (1975) Techniques, indications and results of intraoperative radiotherapy of advanced cancers. Radiology 116: 693
2. Adams E.B., MacLeod I.H. (1977) Invasive amebiasis. Medicine 56: 315
3. Allen C.V., Fletcher W.S. (1970) Observations on preoperative irradiation of rectosigmoid carcinoma. Am J Roentgenol Radium Ther Nucl Med 108: 136
4. Barone J.E., Sohn N., Nealon T.F. Jr. (1976) Perforations and foreign bodies of the rectum: Report of 28 cases. Ann Surg 184: 601
5. Cahan W.G., Castro E.B., Hajdu S.I. (1974) The significance of a solitary lung shadow in patients with colon carcinoma. Cancer 33: 414
6. Childress M.H., Martel W. (1976) Fecaloma simulating colonic neoplasm. Surg Gynecol Obstet 142: 664
7. Cram A.E., Pearlman N.W., Jochimsen P.R. (1977) Surgical management of complications of radiation-injured gut. Am J Surg 133: 551
8. Crile G. Jr., Turnbull R.B. Jr. (1972) The role of electrocoagulation in the treatment of carcinoma of the rectum. Surg Gynecol Obstet 135: 391
9. De LaGarza T., Nuñéz-Rasilla V., Alegre-Palafox R., et al (1973) Malakoplakia of the colon: Report of a case with a review of eight previous case reports. Dis Colon Rectum 16: 216
10. Deveney C.W., Lewis F.R. Jr., Schrock T.R. (1976) Surgical management of radiation injury of the small and large intestine. Dis Colon Rectum 19: 25
11. Duschinsky R., Pleven H., Heidelberger C. (1957) The synthesis of 5-fluoropyrimidines. J Am Chem Soc 79: 4559
12. Dwight R.W., Humphrey E.W., Higgins G.A., et al (1973) FUDR as an adjuvant to surgery in cancer of the large bowel. J Surg Oncol 5: 243
13. Eftaiha M., Hambrick E., Abcarian H (1977) Principles of management of colorectal foreign bodies. Arch Surg 112: 691
14. Farman J., Dallemand S., Robinson T., et al (1974) Colitis cystica profunda, an unusual solitary tumor: Report of three cases. Dis Colon Rectum 17: 565
15. Fortner J.G., Shiu M.H., Kinne D.W., et al (1974) Major hepatic resection using vascular isolation and hypothermic perfusion. Ann Surg 180: 644
16. Foster J.H., Berman M.M. (1977) Solid liver tumors. Saunders, Philadelphia
17. Friedmann P., Park W.C., Afonya I.I., et al (1978) Adjuvant radiation therapy in colorectal carcinoma. Am J Surg 135: 512
18. Gold P., Freedman S.O. (1965) Demonstration of tumor-specific antigens in human colonic carcinomata by immunological tolerance and absorption techniques. J Exp Med 121: 439

19. Grace T.B., Metter G.E., Cornell G.N. (1977) Adjuvant chemotherapy with 5-fluorouracil after surgical resection of colorectal carcinoma (COG protocol 7041). Am J Surg 133: 59

20. Gray L.A. (1973) Endometriosis of the bowel: Role of bowel resection, superficial excision and oophorectomy in treatment. Ann Surg 177: 580

21. Grodsinsky C., Ponka J.L. (1975) Entrapment of colon following diaphragmatic injuries: Report of eight cases. Dis Colon Rectum 18: 72

22. Grossi C.E., Wolff W.I., Nealon T.F. Jr. (1977) Intraluminal fluorouracil chemotherapy adjunct to surgical procedures for resectable carcinoma of the colon and rectum. Surg Gynecol Obstet 145: 549

23. Gunderson L.L., Sosin H. (1974) Areas of failure found at reoperation (second or symptomatic look) following "curative surgery" for adenocarcinoma of the rectum. Clinicopathologic correlation and implications for adjuvant therapy. Cancer 34: 1278

24. Hagihara P.F., Griffen W.O. Jr. (1976) Delayed correction of anorectal incontinence due to anal sphincteral injury. Arch Surg 111: 63

25. Hendren W.H. (1978) Constipation caused by anterior location of the anus and its surgical correction. J Ped Surg 13: 1505

26. Herman A.H., Nabseth D.C. (1973) Colitis cystica profunda: Localized, segmental, and diffuse. Arch Surg 106: 337

27. Herrera M.A., Chu T.M., Holyoke E.D., et al (1977) CEA monitoring of palliative treatment for colorectal carcinoma. Ann Surg 185: 23

28. Higgins G.A. Jr., Conn J.H., Jordan P.H. Jr., et al (1975) Preoperative radiotherapy for colorectal cancer. Ann Surg 181: 624

29. Hill G.J. II, Johnson R.O., Metter G., et al (1976) Multimodal surgical adjuvant therapy for a broad spectrum of tumors in humans. Surg Gynecol Obstet 142: 882

30. Howard R.J., Mannax S.J., Eusebio E.B., et al (1971) Colitis cystica profunda. Surgery 69: 306

31. Jackman R.J., Clark P.L. III, Smith N.D. (1951) Retrorectal tumors. JAMA 145: 956

32. James A.W., Phelps A.H. (1977) Actinomycosis of the colon. Can J Surg 20: 150

33. Jenkinson E.L., Brown W.H. (1943) Endometriosis. A study of 117 cases with special reference to constricting lesions of rectum and sigmoid colon. JAMA 122: 349

34. Joyeuse R., Lott J.V., Michaelis M., et al (1977) Malakoplakia of the colon and rectum: Report of a case and review of the literature. Surgery 81: 189

35. Kligerman M.M. (1975) Irradiation of the primary lesion of the rectum and rectosigmoid. JAMA 231: 1381

36. Kligerman M.M. (1977) Radiotherapy and rectal cancer. Cancer 39: 896

37. Kratzer G.L. (1973) Technique in fulguration of carcinoma of the rectum. Surg Gynecol Obstet 137: 673

38. Kratzer G.L., Salvati E. (1955) Collective review of endometriosis of the colon. Am J Surg 90: 866

39. Lawrence W. Jr., Terz J.J., Horsley S. III, et al (1975) Chemotherapy as an adjuvant to surgery for colorectal cancer. Ann Surg 181: 616

40. Levine B., Peskin G.W., Saik R.P. (1976) Drug-induced colitis as a surgical disease. Arch Surg 111: 987

41. Livingstone A.S., Hampson L.G., Shuster J., et al (1974) Carcinoembryonic antigen in the diagnosis and management of colorectal carcinoma. Arch Surg 109: 259

42. Madden J.L., Kandalaft S. (1971) Electrocoagulation in the treatment of cancer of the rectum: A continuing study. Ann Surg 174: 530

43. Madden J.L., Kandalhaft S. (1974) In: Maingot R. (ed) Abdominal operations, 6th edn. Appleton-Century-Crofts, New York, p 2135

44. Miles R.P.M. (1972) Benign strictures of the rectum. Ann R Coll Surg Engl 59: 310

45. Palmer J.A., Bush R.S. (1976) Radiation injuries to the bowel associated with the treatment of carcinoma of the cervix. Surgery 80: 458

46. Papillon J. (1975) Resectable rectal cancers: Treatment by curative endocavitary irradiation. JAMA 231: 1385

47. Proceedings of the First International Conference on the Clinical Uses of Carcinoembryonic Antigen, June 1–3, 1977, Lexington, Kentucky. Cancer 42: 1397 (1978)

48. Rousselot L.M., Cole D.R., Grossi C.E., et al (1968) A 5 year progress report on the effectiveness of intraluminal chemotherapy (5-fluorouracil) adjuvant to surgery for colorectal cancer. Am J Surg 115: 140

48a. Russell J.C., Welch J.P. (1979) Operative management of radiation injuries of the intestinal tract. Am J Surg 137: 433

49. Salvati E.P., Rubin R.J. (1976) Electrocoagulation as primary therapy for rectal carcinoma. Am J Surg 132: 583

50. Schachter J. (1978) Chlamydial infections. N Engl J Med 298: 490

51. Smith B., Grace R.H., Todd I.P. (1977) Organic constipation in adults. Br J Surg 64: 313

52. Stearns M.W. Jr., Deddish M.R., Quan S.H.Q., et al (1974) Preoperative roentgen therapy for cancer of the rectum and rectosigmoid. Surg Gynecol Obstet 138: 584

53. Strauss, A.A., Strauss, S.F., Crawford R.A., et al (1935) Surgical diathermy of carcinoma of the rectum: Its clinical end results. JAMA 104: 1480

54. Turell R. (1977) Electrocoagulation of carcinoma of the rectum. Surg Gynecol Obstet 144: 918

55. Wallace R.J. Jr., Greenberg S.B., Lau J.M., et al (1978) Amebic peritonitis following rupture of an amebic liver abscess. Arch Surg 113: 322

56. Wanebo H.J., Quan S.H.Q. (1974) Failures of electrocoagulation of primary carcinoma of the rectum. Surg Gynecol Obstet 138: 174

57. Wanebo H.J., Semoglou C., Attiyeh F., et al (1978) Surgical management of patients with primary operable colorectal cancer and synchronous liver metastases. Am J Surg 135: 81

58. Wanebo H.J., Stearns M., Schwartz M. (1978) The use of CEA as an indicator of early recurrence and as a guide to selected second-look procedure in patients with colorectal cancer. Ann Surg 188: 481

59. Wangensteen O.H. (1949) Cancer of the colon and rectum. Wis Med J 48: 591

60. Wangensteen O.H., Lewis F.J., Arhelger S.W., et al (1954) An interim report upon the "second look" procedure for cancer of the stomach, colon, and rectum and for "limited intraperitoneal carcinosis." Surg Gynecol Obstet 99: 257

61. Welch J.P., Donaldson G.A. (1978) Detection and treatment of recurrent cancer of the colon and rectum. Am J Surg 135: 505

62. Welch J.P., Malt R.A. (1977) Management of carcinoid tumors of the gastrointestinal tract. Surg Gynecol Obstet 145: 223

63. Wilkins E.W. Jr., Head J.M., Burke J.F. (1978) Pulmonary resection for metastatic neoplasms in the lung. Experience at the Massachusetts General Hospital. Am J Surg 135: 480

64. Wilson S.M., Adson M.A. (1976) Surgical treatment of hepatic metastases from colorectal cancers. Arch Surg 111: 330

24 Complications of Colorectal Surgery

The complications following specific operations for colorectal disease have been discussed in previous chapters. In this section all the major complications will be summarized.

Early Complications

The early complications after an operation on the colorectum include bleeding, sepsis, suture-line perforation, intestinal obstruction, and urinary tract infections. In addition to these problems, which are peculiar to these operations, there are, of course, all of the usual complications that can follow any operation.[10]

Bleeding
Bleeding within 24 hr after surgery is not uncommon after Miles resections for a cancer of the rectum. Persistent bleeding, demonstrated by profuse hemorrhage from the perineum, may require revision of the posterior wound within a matter of a few hours or within the first day.

Identification of the bleeding vessel may at times be very difficult. In our experience the most likely site is in the region of the middle hemorrhoidal vessels. The ligation of individual bleeders or the use of clips or the Bovie unit may be helpful. In some instances no bleeding point can be found and large gauze packs must be inserted tightly into the cavity.

Postanastomotic suture-line bleeding may at times be controlled by vasopressin (Pitressin) introduced through an arterial catheter; vasopressin given through a peripheral vein (0.2–0.4 unit/min) may also be effective. Re-exploration is advised unless there is prompt control. Intraperitoneal hemorrhage may be excessive before there are obvious abdominal signs; a falling hematocrit despite transfusions should alert the surgeon, and a laparotomy should be done. Anastomotic line bleeding also can occur 7–8 days after the operation. This type of bleeding is usually not serious but may require one or two transfusions.

Sepsis
Sepsis may occur at any level of dissection. Wound infection is noted in about 20% of patients who have not had any preliminary treatment with

antibiotics. When prophylactic antibiotics are used according to the recommended methods this figure is reduced to below 5%. Fortunately, synergistic gangrene of a portion of the abdominal wall or gas gangrene infection of the abdominal wall are very rare. They require wide excision of all involved tissues and later reconstruction of the abdominal wall.

A much more common complication is the formation of an intraperitoneal abscess. The most common site is deep in the pelvis after an anterior resection and anastomosis. The insertion of a suction catheter at the time of the original operation to remove loculated blood is an excellent prophylactic measure. The development of peritonitis at a later date is usually caused by perforation at a suture line.

Subdiaphragmatic abscesses are rare but do occur after operations on the colon. After a resection of the splenic flexure they are more likely to occur in the region of the left diaphragm, where undetected bleeding can eventually result in an abscess.

Perforation

The incidence of perforation after anastomosis will vary depending upon the method of investigation.[8,9,10,13] It could be assumed that if barium enemas were given almost immediately after every colonic anastomosis, 100% of them would show some leakage. Goligher et al. found that approximately 16% of anastomoses show some evidence of leakage.[2] Minor dehiscences are subclinical and are of little import; major leaks, however, occur in approximately 5% of all anastomoses. The reasons this leakage occurs have been elucidated by Schrock et al.[8] Peritonitis, debilitating diseases, tension, inadequate blood supply, and the administration of such drugs as cortisone may all be contributing factors.[3–5] A leaking anastomosis is usually attended by more pain than the patient normally should exhibit after an intraperitoneal procedure. The presence of fever or tenderness at the site of anastomosis also should alert the surgeon. In rare instances the convalescence may be very smooth until the seventh or eigth day, when a sudden perforation occurs.

The best method of handling a perforation, if possible, is to exteriorize the anastomosis and form a proximal and distal stoma. If the anastomosis is low in the pelvis, as is often the case, this will be impossible. In that event the best method is to drain the local area and perform a transverse colostomy.

Intestinal Obstruction

Intestinal obstruction is a very serious and common complication after colectomy for ulcerative colitis or cancer of the rectum. Adhesions, volvulus about a stoma, or strangulation of a loop of small intestine through a pelvic floor defect are all possible; early reoperation is advised rather than a protracted period of nasogastric or intestinal tube drainage because of the danger of strangulation.

Obstruction of the stoma is usually caused by mechanical problems: the lumen was too small initially, adhesions have formed very close to the anastomosis, or there is a localized perforation. Usually an anastomosis that is 1 cm or more in diameter in the colon will be functional; it is unusual for one that is smaller than this to function well. In order to avoid this complication, some surgeons have introduced a long tube through the rectum running upward past the suture line of a low anterior resection; this tube is left in place for several days until the patient deflates.

Pseudomembranous Enterocolitis

Pseudomembranous enterocolitis is a complication of antibotic therapy.[1] It has followed the use of aminoglycosides. In particular, the use of clindamycin and lincomycin has been associated with this lesion. The antibiotic may have been given by mouth or it may have been used parentally. Sigmoidoscopy shows a highly irritated mucosa with numerous elevations, scattered ulcerations, and a free mucous discharge. The differentiation between pseudomembranous enterocolitis and acute ulcerative colitis may be difficult or impossible except on the basis of history. Several decades ago the usual causative agent of this type of enterocolitis was the *Staphylococcus*. At that time adequate antibiotic coverage was not available and the death rate was very high. At the present time any staphylococcal infection can be controlled satisfactorily by antibiotics. This disease is now usually associated with gram-negative infections and is much less virulent than it was.

The therapy consists of discontinuance of the offending antibiotic, immediate smears and cultures of the bowel to determine the predominant organisms, and the institution of some other type of antibiotic therapy that will provide proper coverage. Severe cases will require large amounts of fluid. In the past corticosteroids were found to be helpful in management.

The surgical therapy of this disease has been hampered by the fact that the small intestine may be involved as well as the colon. If the disease is localized to the colon, ileostomy, as a method of fecal diversion, or total colectomy can be considered. Success after ileostomy alone has been reported by Saylor et al.[7] and success after subtotal colectomy has been reported by Levine et al.[6]

Urinary Tract Infections

Urinary tract dysfunction and infection are common after colorectal operations, particularly in the male. In order to prevent undue distention of the bladder the Foley catheter is routinely inserted at the time of operation and kept in place for several days until the patient is passing gas by the rectum. If there is a history of prostatic disease the catheter may be left in for a longer time. The objective is to avoid repeated catheterizations and to insert the initial catheter in as aseptic a fashion as possible. If symptoms persist after removal of the catheter, a transurethral resection may be performed. Another option is to discharge the patient on catheter drainage and have him return to the urologist's office 2 weeks later, when function may have been regained; if it has not, he is readmitted for a transurethral resection. Bethanechol chloride (Urecholine; 10 mg, p.o., t.i.d.) is often helpful for the sluggish bladder.

Late Complications

Catheter Perforation of a Colostomy Stoma

The diagnosis of a catheter perforation of a colostomy stoma is easily made because the symptoms of acute pain and often localized peritoneal signs immediately follow colostomy irrigation. Some conception of the site of the perforation may be gained by considering the depth to which the catheter was inserted. When only a short catheter is used and compression is maintained with a nipple on the stoma, perforation is uncommon; if it does occur it will be near the entrance to the peritoneal cavity. If a long catheter has been used, the perforation may be more proximal.

248

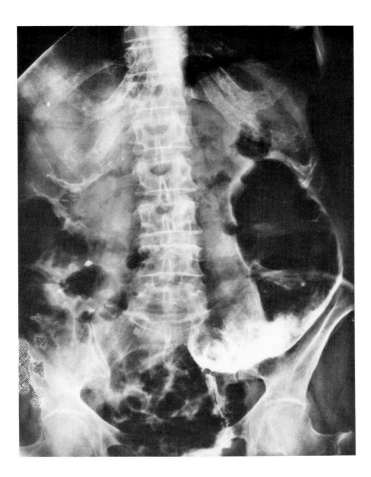

Fig. 24.1. Plain x-ray film of anastomotic stricture 7 years after colon resection for Crohn's disease.

Any doubt about the diagnosis may be resolved if a Gastrografin injection of the stoma shows a perforation; however, this is not a totally reliable method of determination of injury because the opening may seal off rather rapidly.

Laparotomy is necessary if the symptoms suggest perforation. It is often difficult to find the site of the laceration during the operation. For this reason the usual method of treatment is to resect a further length of colon and fashion a new stoma. This procedure is necessarily accompanied by careful inspection of the excised specimen and of all colon that is left in situ to be certain that there has been no more proximal peforation. It may be necessary to transplant the stoma from the left lower quadrant into the left upper quadrant, bringing out the left transverse colon if the perforation has been high.

Anastomotic Stricture

Anastomotic strictures are more likely to occur after operations for inflammatory diseases of the bowel than after operations for cancer (Fig. 24.1). They may also arise from constriction of an original anastomosis that was made too narrow.

The minimum diameter of anastomosis in the colon that is presumed to work satisfactorily is 1 cm. Although it is possible for feces to pass through an even smaller lumen, it is unlikely that patients with a smaller lumen will be free of obstructive symptoms.

Once an anastomotic stricture has occurred any attempts to dilate with either the sigmoidoscope or the colonoscope will not be effective. Reoperation and the formation of a new anastomosis is the proper method of therapy.

Hernia Through the Mesenteric Trap

Whenever possible mesenteric traps are closed very carefully. This is always possible after a right colectomy and after a low sigmoid resection. However, after a left colectomy this may be an extremely difficult matter, and if the mesentery has been excised widely it may be impossible to effect such a closure. Under such circumstances the trap should be left wide open because a small opening is more serious than a large one. At times even a well-closed trap may open, allowing a loop of bowel to prolapse through.

Similarly, after a side-to-side anastomosis of the ileum to the colon or the colon to the colon, a trap is left behind the anastomosis and a loop of bowel may herniate through it. This can progress to strangulation of the bowel; a second laparotomy and repair are necessary. Other, more unusual herniations also occur. For example, after a left colectomy in which the trap has been wide open, if the lesser omental sac has been opened, a loop of intestine may herniate into it and then pass from left to right behind the portal triad. The signs of strangulating intestinal obstruction soon after an operation should alert the surgeon to the possibility of an internal hernia of this type.

Persistent Diarrhea

This symptom may be very troublesome after subtotal colectomy or total colectomy in an older patient even though the remaining section of the bowel is entirely normal. In our experience, about one patient out of six will have severe diarrhea after such operations. The therapy consists of diphenoxylate hydrochloride with atropine sulfate (Lomotil) or tincture of opium in severe cases. Dietary measures include the omission of milk and the use of constipating foods such as cheese.

After some resections of the right colon diarrhea may be extremely persistent and severe, amounting to 12–30 movements a day. It is speculated that this type of diarrhea is caused by irritation of the colon by bile salts, and hence the use of cholestyramine (Questran) may be quite effective. This type of diarrhea differs from the diarrhea that occurs after total colectomy; in the latter, the substantial reduction of the absorbing mucous membrane of the colon plays a role. The absorption of water, which characteristically is carried out almost entirely in the cecum and ascending colon, can occur through the lower portions of the colon after a period of adaptation.

Persistent Fistulas

Fistulas may follow anastomotic leaks, drains, or epithelialized or mucous membrane–lined tracts (Fig. 24.2) (see Chapter 17).

Suture-Line Implantation of Cancer

This complication is rare, except in the rectum or low sigmoid, where some surgeons estimate it occurs in 10% of cases.[11,12] We doubt that the incidence is that high. It is the result of inadequate margins about the tumor or,

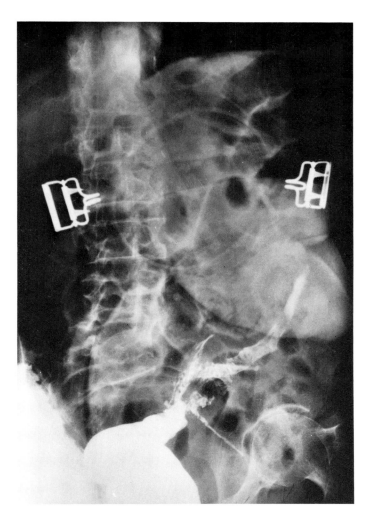

Fig. 24.2. Plain x-ray film of multiple fistulas from the anastomotic line after sigmoid resection for diverticulitis.

in many instances, retrorectal recurrence with secondary involvement of bowel.

References

1. Fee H.J., Ament M.E., Holmes E.C. (1977) Pseudomembranous colitis associated with cephalozin therapy. Am J Surg 133: 247
2. Goligher J.C., Graham N.G., De Dombal F.T. (1970) Anastomotic dehiscence after anterior resection of rectum and sigmoid. Br J Surg 57: 109
3. Irvin R.R., Hunt T.K. (1974) Reappraisal of the healing process of anastomosis of the colon. Surg Gynecol Obstet 138: 741
4. Irvin T.T. (1976) Collagen metabolism in infected colonic anastomoses. Surg Gynecol Obstet 143: 220
5. LeVeen H.H., Wapnick S., Falk G., et al (1976) Effects of prophylactic antibiotics on colonic healing. Am J Surg 131: 47
6. Levine B., Peskin G.W., Saik R.P. (1976) Drug-induced colitis as a surgical disease. Arch Surg 111: 987
7. Saylor J.L., Anderson C.B., Tedesco F.J. (1976) Pseudomembranous colitis treated with completely diverting ileostomy. Arch Surg 111: 596
8. Schrock T.R., Deveney C.W., Dunphy J.E. (1973) Factors contributing to leakage of colonic anastomoses. Ann Surg 177: 513

9. Sharefkin J., Joffe N., Silen W., et al (1978) Anastomotic dehiscence after low anterior resection of the rectum. Am J Surg 135: 519
10. Welch C.E., Hedberg S.E. (1975) Complications in surgery of the colon and rectum. In: Artz C.P., Hardy J.D. (eds) Management of surgical complications, 3rd edn. Saunders, Philadelphia, p 600
11. Wheelock F.C. Jr., Toll G., McKittrick L.S. (1959) Evaluation of anterior resection of rectum and low sigmoid. N Engl J Med 260: 526
12. Wright H.K., Thomas W.H., Cleveland J.C. (1969) The low recurrence rate of colonic carcinoma in ileocolic anastomoses. Surg Gynecol Obstet 129: 960
13. Yamakawa T., Patin C.S., Sobel S., et al (1971) Healing of colonic anastomoses following resection for experimental "diverticulitis." Arch Surg 103: 17

Pilonidal Sinus

25

Pilonidal cysts and sinuses usually become manifest in the late teens. They are much more common in males than in females. While some are asymptomatic, many will harbor repeated infections until surgical ablation is carried out. Acute abscesses require drainage under local anesthesia.

Operative Procedures

Numerous operations have been proposed for the removal of these sinuses. The risk of recurrence has been high under nearly all circumstances. The senior author has obtained uniform success by the somewhat protracted but certain method of healing that is afforded by excision of the tract and healing by secondary intention. This is the operation that will be described as the preferential one. Two other methods—simple unroofing of the sinus tract and excision with primary or delayed closure—will also be discussed. In any event, the patient is placed face down on the operating table. The buttocks are elevated and the sinus that overlies the sacrum is exposed. Adhesive tapes are used to spread the buttocks (Fig. 25.1).

Open Excision and Packing
The tract is probed and opened throughout its full extent with the Bovie unit (Fig. 25.2a). The Bovie unit is then used for the excision of the entire tract. As small an area of skin as possible is removed; it is not necessary to remove an excessive amount of fat around the sinus tract. It is important to be certain that all ramifications of the tract are excised. With the Bovie unit it is very easy to identify any tract and to carry out the excision in an entirely bloodless field. It may be necessary to resect as deep as the presacral fascia. The presacral fascia, however, should not be disturbed, and it is preferable to leave some fat on the anterior surface of the fascia (Fig. 25.2b).

After removal of the tract the wound is packed open with either plain or iodoform gauze. If bleeding is not satisfactorily controlled by the electrocoagulation, a few bleeders may require catgut ties.

The operation can be done under either general or local infiltration anesthesia. In the latter event the whole procedure can be done on an ambulatory basis and the patient can be discharged after the operation. Usually,

253

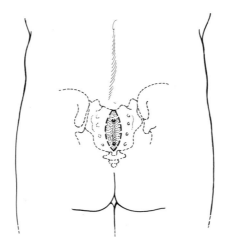

Fig. 25.1. Orientation. Patient lies on abdomen, buttocks strapped apart. The openings of the sinus and surrounding induration are shown in the typical area overlying the sacrum. The sinuses may extend caudally down to or even beyond the anus.

however, it is better to have the patient remain in the hospital overnight to be certain that there is no bleeding.

The incision will remain essentially painless for the first few days. The packing is changed approximately 4 days after the original operation. Then repacking is carried out every 1–2 days thereafter until healing results.

The postoperative care is extremely important. The skin surrounding the incision should be kept free of hair either by depilatory or by shaving. It is essential to be certain that the granulation tissue is solid at the base and that the skin does not seal over the top, since if this happens a new sinus tract may form. The patient is ambulatory the day after the operation and can resume ordinary activities within a few days.

The postoperative dressings may require a variety of local applications. Secondary fungal infection is common and Mycolog ointment may be helpful. If granulation tissue becomes spongy and infected, curettage or cauterization with silver nitrate, application of a strong astringent such as tincture of myrrh solution, or the use of scarlet red ointment is recommended. Sitz baths may be employed after 1 week from the date of operation. Healing is usually complete within 6 weeks, though it may be more prolonged.

Unroofing of the Sinus Tract
This has been proposed as a simple method for the treatment of pilonidal sinuses. The Bovie unit is employed to open the tract widely. It is presumed that epithelialization will occur over the granulating tract and that healing will follow.[2] We have had little experience with this method but doubt that it will be satisfactory. Epithelium usually has been destroyed by inflammation, and the scar is likely to be thin and wide.

Cryosurgery
Gage and Dutta have reported 29 cases treated by cryosurgery with only 1 recurrence. They froze the entire sinus tract to a depth of 5 mm. Healing required an average of 15.5 weeks.[3]

Primary Closure
The essential feature of this operation is that after the excision of the sinus tract the fat anterior to the sacral fascia is undermined for a short distance

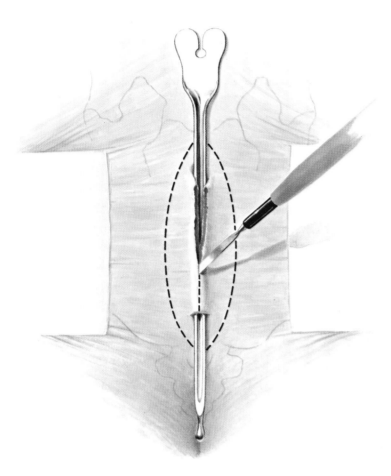

Fig. 25.2a and b.   Open excision of pilonidal sinuses. a. A probe is inserted into the sinus. The Bovie unit is used to open the entire tract and any extensions.

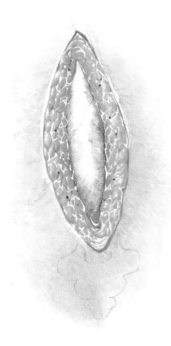

Fig. 25.2b.   Appearance after excision of entire tract. A relatively small amount of surrounding skin and fatty tissue has been removed. The presacral tissue is exposed at the base of the wound. Hemostasis is secured by either electrocoagulation or ligature.

255

so that the wound can be brought together with interrupted wire sutures. Dead space must be completely eliminated because if a hematoma forms there is always the chance of a recurrence of the sinus tract. The patient must be kept in the hospital for several days after this procedure with activity relatively limited lest the skin flaps pull apart.[4-7]

Abramson described a method of excision and delayed closure.[1] This can be done as an outpatient procedure. Sutures placed at the time of the excision were tightened on the fourth postoperative day and removed 12 days later. Healing time averaged 23.6 days. There were 3 recurrences in 46 patients. Primary excision and partial closure also has been employed.[1,5]

While these operations can result in more rapid healing than the open method, the period of hospitalization is longer and the incidence of recurrence is definitely higher.

Complicated Fistulas

Sometimes very extensive fistulas may form from the pilonidal area and extend down to the anal canal or even beyond it on the perineum. The etiology of these fistulas is not clear. At times they may represent typical pilonidal disease. They may be unusual fistulas-in-ano or perhaps complications of Crohn's disease. They furnish very difficult problems in management. Essentially the only method that can be used to cure them is to open every tract very widely. If the tract runs into the rectum as a fistula, it will be necessary to treat it as a rectal fistula as well. A temporary transverse colostomy may be required.

References

1. Abramson D.J. (1977) Excision and delayed closure of pilonidal sinus. Surg Gynecol Obstet 144: 205
2. Buie L.A., Curtiss R.K. (1952) Pilonidal disease. Surg Clin North Am 32: 1247
3. Gage A.A., Dutta P. (1977) Cryosurgery for pilonidal disease. Am J Surg 133: 249
4. Healy M.J. Jr., Hoffert P.W. (1954) Pilonidal sinus and cyst. A comparative evaluation of various surgical methods in 229 consecutive cases. Am J Surg 87: 578
5. Healy M.J., Hoffert P.W. (1969) Pilonidal disease. In: Turell R. (ed) Diseases of the colon and rectum, 2nd edn, Vol 2. Saunders, Philadelphia, p 1248
6. Lamke L.L., Larsson J., Nylen B. (1974) Results of different types of operation for pilonidal sinus. Acta Chir Scand 140: 321
7. Monro R.S., McDermott F.T. (1965) The elimination of causal factors in pilonidal sinus treated by Z-plasty. Br J Surg 52: 177

Surgery of the Appendix

26

Appendectomy for Acute Appendicitis

The removal of an appendix can range from a very simple to a very complicated procedure depending upon the state of inflammation and the location of the appendix. The same principles, however, are followed in all cases. The important features are an adequate exposure, complete hemostasis, removal of the entire appendix whenever possible, and a firm closure of the appendiceal stump. Antibiotic therapy is not indicated for early, acute appendicitis but with any purulent exudate it should be used preoperatively and postoperatively to reduce the incidence of complications.

Adequate preoperative preparation includes antibiotic therapy, fluid replacement, and fever reduction by cooling. Early operation after such preparation can be done safely and has replaced the conservative therapy that previously was used in cases of perforation with general peritonitis.[4] This method has reduced the mortality of acute appendicitis essentially to zero in many series.[5] Appendicitis in pregnancy still carries an appreciable mortality.[3]

The incision to be used will depend upon the location of the appendix (Fig. 26.1a). The surgeon usually can be guided by the exact location of the maximum point of tenderness and an incision can be centered over that point. If the diagnosis is not clear, a paramedian incision is the most advantageous.

The most commonly used incision is centered over McBurney's point (Fig. 26.1b). An oblique incision is made in the direction of the external oblique fibers. The external oblique is exposed and split just lateral to the rectus sheath. The internal oblique is then separated at a right angle in the direction of its fibers. The transversalis muscle is usually small and runs horizontally; it can be separated in the same fashion. The peritoneum is then opened and the cecum and appendix are exposed.

At times the cecum and appendix cannot be delivered through this incision and it is necessary to extend it. If a more medial exposure is necessary the anterior rectus sheath can be opened by the Weir extension in an oblique direction along the course of the skin incision; the rectus is retracted and the posterior sheath of the rectus is divided in the same direction. Care must be taken to avoid any nerve that may be encountered

257

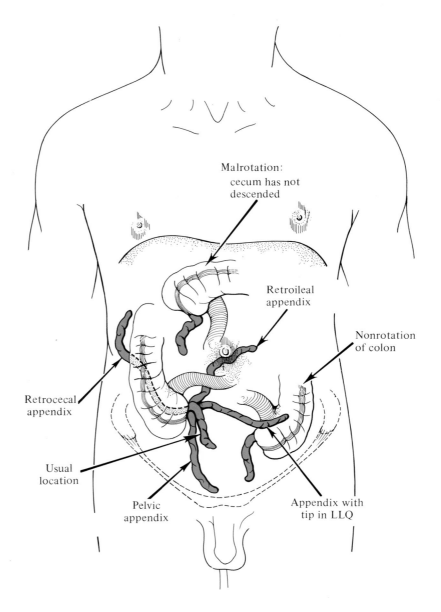

Malrotation:
cecum has not
descended

Retroileal
appendix

Nonrotation
of colon

Retrocecal
appendix

Usual
location

Pelvic
appendix

Appendix with
tip in LLQ

Fig. 26.1a and b.   Incisions for surgery of the appendix. The type of incision to be used depends upon the location of the appendix. a. Location of the appendix. The appendix may lie in many different areas. In the presence of nonrotation of the colon it may be found in the lower midline, or if rotation is incomplete, in the right upper quadrant. In the rare cases of situs inversus it is in the left lower quadrant. Even when the cecum is in its normal position, the location of the appendix may vary greatly. Usually it is found in the ileocecal fossa, but it may be retrocecal or extend to the left of the midline or deep into the pelvis. One of the most unusual and difficult locations is behind the mesentery of the terminal ileum; this will require mobilization of the right colon for exposure.

in the lateral margin of the sheath. If the appendix is long and retrocecal, an extension of the lateral end of the incision may be necessary. This may have to be done by dividing the internal oblique rather than splitting it.

The right pararectus or Battle incision also is used frequently. The skin incision is either oblique, as described above, or more vertical. In many patients the rectus muscle is wide, and what is proposed to be a McBurney incision actually turns out to be centered over the rectus. In

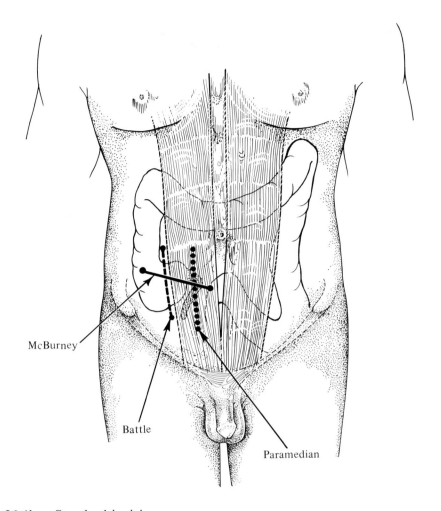

Fig. 26.1b. Standard incisions.

these instances the rectus sheath may be divided vertically close to the lateral margin. The rectus muscle is mobilized and retracted medially. Care is taken to preserve the intercostal nerves that will run posterior to the muscle on the peritoneum. The deep epigastric vessels also lie beneath the muscle and may be injured unless care is taken. The peritoneum is then opened in a vertical direction. It is possible, if necessary, to cut one nerve without causing any weakness in the abdominal incision, but if more than one is cut, later weakness of the rectus may result.

The right paramedian incision is very helpful if the diagnosis is in doubt or if a long retrocecal appendix is suspected. It can be extended upward if unexpected pathology is found in the region of the gallbladder or the duodenum; also a long retrocecal appendix can be exposed by mobilization of the right colon. In very rare instances the appendix lies behind the mesentery of the ileum; a paramedian incision provides the best exposure.

At times the surgeon will have made a McBurney incision in the belief that he was dealing with an acute appendix but find a normal appendix and exudate that suggests a process somewhere else in the abdomen. Under these circumstances we believe it wise to make a second incision of the paramedian type immediately in order to carry out adequate exploration.

The acutely inflamed appendix must be handled with great care. Perforation by rough dissection on the operating table can be very serious and

259

should never occur. In early cases the cecum can usually be withdrawn through the incision and the appendix will follow. In later cases, however, this will be impossible and the appendix must be exposed by retraction of small bowel and cecum and then dissection with great care. In general, the appendix can be removed in one of two ways. The usual method is to begin the dissection near the distal end and carry it down to the base of the cecum. The mesentery of the appendix is clamped and sectioned as the dissection progresses (Fig. 26.2a). As the base is neared, the appendix usually becomes relatively normal. It is grasped at the base with three straight clamps (Fig. 26.2b). A 000 chromic tie is then placed in the crush produced by the clamp closest to the cecum and tied. As this is being done the second clamp is removed (Fig. 26.2c). The third clamp prevents the extrusion of any fecal matter during the course of the dissection. The appendix is then divided through the crush of the second clamp. The short stump of the appendix distal to the tie may then be treated by the application of a neomycin solution or by a drop of carbolic acid followed by alcohol—essentially the only obeisance that modern surgery pays to Lister in these days. The appendiceal stump is then buried by means of purse-string or Z suture of 00 chromic catgut (Fig. 26.2d). The purse-string must be placed relatively close to the appendiceal stump but far enough away to allow adequate inversion. Too wide an inversion will produce a polypoid defect in the cecum that may be mistaken for a polyp at a later date.

In some instances the appendix is so immobilized by adhesions that it is unsafe to attempt dissection in this fashion. In such cases the base of the appendix is identified. It is divided using the same three-clamp technique and the stump is ligated and inverted. The dissection is then carried out in a

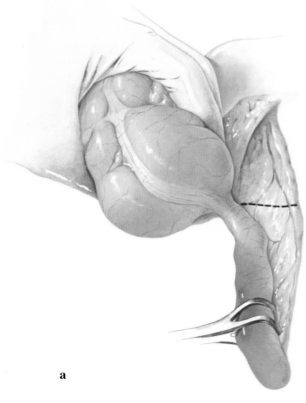

a

Fig. 26.2a–d. Appendectomy. a. The inflamed appendix is grasped with a Babcock forceps. The mesentery will be divided along the broken line.

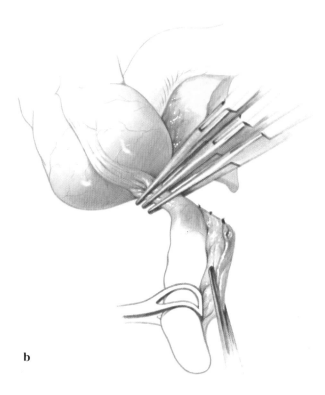

b

Fig. 26.2b. The appendix is freed down to its base and three clamps are applied.

retrograde fashion (Fig. 26.3). This method is advantageous if the appendix is very adherent, acutely inflamed, and apparently ready to burst.

There are several variations in technique that require discussion. If the appendix is retrocecal it tends to have a segmental blood supply and numerous small vessels may be encountered rather than the typical one large vessel that appears in the normal appendiceal mesentery. Meticulous control of these vessels is necessary to prevent postoperative bleeding or hematoma.

The method of treatment of the appendiceal stump has been argued for many years. We firmly believe that it is essential to invert the appendiceal stump with a second layer of sutures. There have been numerous reports of catastrophes involving noninverted appendiceal stumps, which may perforate a few days later and lead to fatal peritonitis.

It has been suggested that it would be better not to ligate the stump of the appendix but merely to invert it within the cecum so that there will be no opportunity for an abscess to arise between the proximal tie on the base of the appendix and the purse-string suture of the turn-in. We believe this risk has been greatly exaggerated and have never seen an abscess in this location using the technique described.

At times the appendix may be so inflamed that the entire base is involved and it may be impossible to ligate the stump. This is particularly true when the inflammation extends onto the wall of the cecum. Usually the cecum can be turned in by two layers of running catgut sutures that catch the cecum in a relatively normal area. Hemostasis should be complete before this turn-in is carried out. If a closure is believed to be hazardous, a catheter may be inserted through the open area into the cecum and brought out through the abdominal wall. This will create a temporary fecal

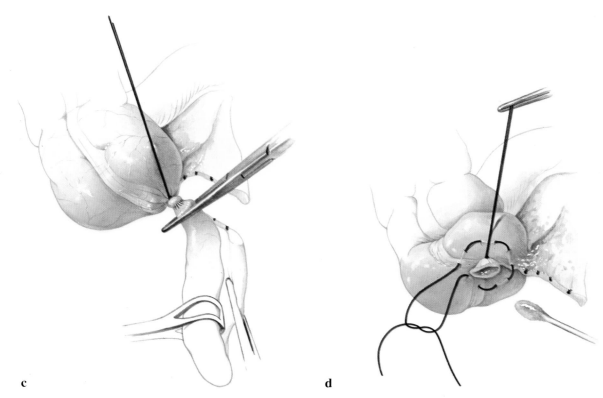

c   d

Fig. 26.2c and d.   c. The base of the appendix is tied through the crush of the proximal clamp with 00 chromic catgut. As the tie is tightened the middle clamp is removed. d. The lumen of the appendix is sterilized by a drop of carbolic acid followed by a pledget of 95% alcohol. The stump is then inverted by means of a purse-string suture.

fistula that will close spontaneously unless the colon is involved by inflammatory disease.

Double appendixes are pathologic rarities. Some two dozen cases have been reported in the literature. Occasionally, a patient will enter the hospital with all of the signs of acute appendicitis but with a history of a previous appendectomy. While it is more likely that some other lesion such as Crohn's disease is producing the symptoms, it must be remembered that if the first appendectomy did not remove the entire base of the appendix, appendicitis can recur in the appendiceal stump. This danger emphasizes the importance of the accurate dissection of the entire appendix at the time of the original operation.

Other diseases are often confused with appendicitis. Inflammation of a Meckel's diverticulum, pelvic pathology in the female, and idiopathic mesenteric adenitis are the most likely alternative diseases that are seen. If the condition of the appendix does not obviously explain the symptoms the surgeon should carry out a wider exploration involving observation of the female pelvis, withdrawal of the terminal 3 feet of ileum to eliminate the possibility of a Meckel's diverticulum, and examination of the mesentery of the terminal ileum for any enlarged lymph nodes.

Incidental Appendectomy

Incidental appendectomy done at the time of some other major operative procedure is a very common operation. While it is generally tolerated very well, there are times when it introduces additional hazards, and the

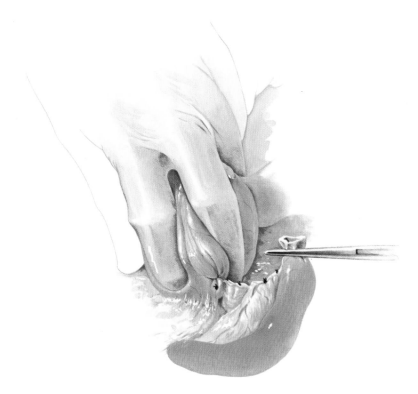

Fig. 26.3. Retrograde appendectomy. The appendix has been divided at its base and the stump has been turned in as shown in the previous figure. The cecum can now be retracted with the fingers and the mesentery divided in a retrograde fashion. Thus the appendix is removed from base to tip.

surgeon must exercise discretion in every instance. The exposure needs to be adequate. The major operative procedure should have been done first in an expeditious competent fashion so that the addition of another procedure will not be disadvantageous for the patient. Since the exposure is sometimes somewhat limited, great care must be taken to prevent any contamination. As a general rule, incidental appendectomy is tolerated extremely well with pelvic operations in the female. Unless an appendix is present in a hernial sac, it is not removed incidental to a herniorrhaphy because there is a risk of sepsis. If an inflamed Meckel's diverticulum is found, it is generally wise to remove the appendix as well even though it is not inflamed. With cholecystectomy, the decision to perform an appendectomy generally depends upon the adequacy of the exposure. If mesenteric adenitis is found or no pathologic process is encountered at the time of an exploratory laparotomy, the appendix is removed. Appendectomy is not advocated in conjunction with operations on the stomach or left colon except in unusual circumstances. If an ileitis suggesting Crohn's disease is found and the cecum appears normal, the appendix is removed even if it appears grossly normal. However, in the presence of an acute colitis involving the cecum that is the result of either idiopathic ulcerative colitis or Crohn's disease, appendectomy is hazardous.

Appendicitis with Complications

Local Perforation and Peritonitis or Appendiceal Abscess
In these instances the perforation has led to a localized accumulation of pus that is usually walled off by intestines and omentum. In early cases it is

263

always possible to remove the appendix, and this certainly should be done whenever it is feasible. Sometimes a smoldering abscess may be encountered many days or even 1–2 weeks after the original perforation. In these cases it may be necessary merely to incise and drain the abscess, and plan to carry out an elective appendectomy 6 weeks later.

Generalized Peritonitis

This situation is encountered more commonly in young children than in adults. Experience has shown that whenever possible it is desirable to explore these patients as soon as the fluid and electrolyte balance can be corrected, antibiotics administered, and fever and pulse rate reduced by cooling. This preparation can be completed in a few hours and the appendectomy can then be done. Today the old fashioned method of treating peritonitis by ochsnerization is no longer applicable. Impressive series without mortality have been reported by Law et al.[4] and Marchildon and Dudgeon.[5] The latter authors used kanamycin, gentamycin, and clindamycin; the peritoneal cultures showed anaerobic *Bacteroides fragilis* in 93% of the cases and *Clostridium* in 43%.

Drainage is not employed for early acute appendicitis. It is used in the operation for appendiceal abscess. One drain is placed down toward the pelvis and the other is placed lateral to the cecum and is brought out through the McBurney incision. With generalized peritonitis, if there is no localized area to drain and no necrotic tissue present, the abdomen is usually closed without drainage. However, there is usually evidence of necrotic material near the appendiceal stump and it is best to insert a drain.

Complications of Appendectomy

The important complications of appendectomy include sepsis, intestinal obstruction, and fecal fistula.

Wound sepsis is a common complication after the treatment of perforated appendicitis. The incidence of sepsis can be reduced by the use of preoperative and intraoperative antibiotics, particularly irrigation of the incision with neomycin prior to closure. Delayed primary closure of the wound has also been very effective.

Sepsis is usually manifested by an infected wound or by a residual abscess. Residual abscesses are more common in the right gutter and in the pelvis than elsewhere, but a right subdiaphragmatic, left subdiaphragmatic, left gutter, or intramesenteric abscess may occur (Fig. 26.4). If primary drainage has been used, right gutter abscesses eventually subside. However, other abscesses, particularly pelvic or subdiaphragmatic, will not drain in this fashion and require a seconday procedure.[1] Helpful diagnostic x-ray examinations include upright films for demonstration of subdiaphragmatic gas, simultaneous liver and lung scans, and gallium scans.

Following operation a rectal examination should be carried out to be certain that there is no accumulation in the pouch of Douglas. If induration and tenderness appear, the possibility of a pelvic abscess is great. A bulge will appear in the pouch of Douglas; drainage should be carried out as soon as this occurs. It is not necessary to wait for the area to become fluctuant or for a spontaneous evacuation to occur because this may lead to a huge intraperitoneal collection.

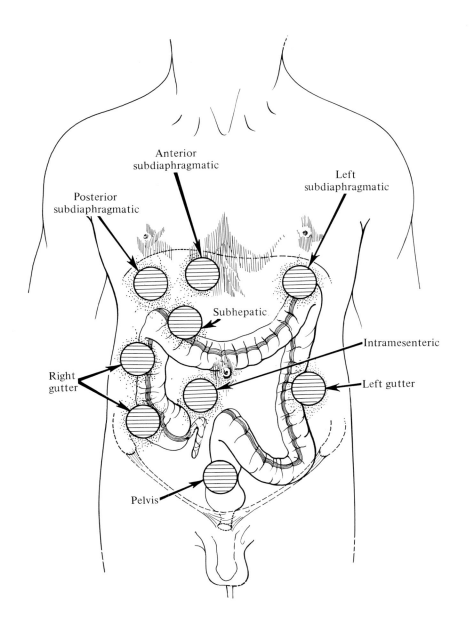

Fig. 26.4. Location of post-appendectomy abscess. Abscesses are most common in the retrocecal area or in the pelvis. However, all of the other areas shown in this diagram may be involved. Gutter, subhepatic, subdiaphragmatic, and intramesenteric abscesses occur.

Drainage of a pelvic abscess is easily accomplished. The patient is placed under full anesthesia in the laparotomy position. The anal sphincter is dilated. The spot of maximum induration or the area of fluctuance, if there is one, is identified. A needle is inserted exactly in the midline anteriorly into the pouch of Douglas (Fig. 26.5a). If pus is encountered the needle is left in place; a Kelly clamp is passed beside it and then spread in order to evacuate the pus. The opening is enlarged in a vertical direction until fingers can be passed into the cavity and loculations can be broken up. A large rubber tube is then sutured in place and brought out through the anus; it is left in place for 5 days, and then removed (Fig. 26.5b).

Subdiaphragmatic abscesses usually occur on the right side. An anterior subcostal incision will allow exploration of both the subhepatic and right subdiaphragmatic spaces through a single incision. If, on the other hand, localization to a posterior location has been ascertained by x-ray studies, the posterior exposure may be employed. The 12th rib may be resected subperiosteally. The peritoneal cavity is entered and a finger is

265

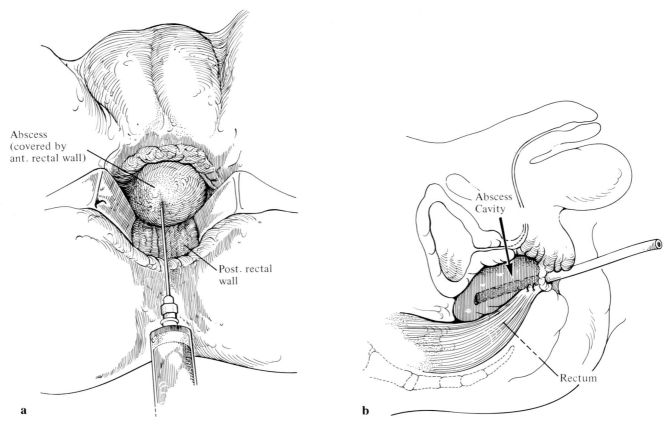

Fig. 26.5a and b. Drainage of pelvic abscess. a. The anal canal has been dilated and a bulge is seen on the anterior wall originating from the pouch of Douglas. An aspirating needle is inserted exactly in the midline; assuming that pus is found, the needle is left in place and the drainage tract is enlarged with a Kelly clamp. A finger is introduced to break up all adhesions. b. A moderately stiff rubber tube is inserted and brought out through the anus.

passed up behind the liver until the abscess is encountered and evacuated. Sumps are placed; they will be withdrawn gradually over a period of 10 days.

Intestinal obstruction following an appendectomy is not as common an occurrence as it was many years ago. It is usually a result of persistent sepsis and is often accompanied by small abscesses located in the right lower quadrant. Plastic adhesions lead to obstruction of the terminal ileum. If the patient does not respond rapidly to nasogastric intubation and intravenous fluids, a secondary operation should be carried out within 10 days. After this period the dissection will become exceedingly difficult and more dangerous. The abdomen is entered through an adequate incision. The bowel is mobilized, adhesions are broken up, and abscesses are evacuated as they are found.

If the surgeon waits for a protracted period, he may find the dissection in the right lower quadrant extremely difficult and may have to be content with a side-to-side ileotransverse colostomy above the point of obstruction.

The use of the long intestinal tubes for the relief of obstruction after appendectomy is much less popular now than it was a few years ago. In our experience they have been far less effective than one would like. Although they may relieve distention, they rarely allow the regression of the obstructing adhesions. As a preoperative method of preparation they are valuable, but they cannot be expected to lead to complete resolution in many cases.

Pylephlebitis is rare, but is manifested by chills and fever and, if untreated, by jaundice and multiple liver abscesses. Antibiotic therapy is essential.

Postoperative fecal fistulas may occur for several reasons. The appendiceal stump may have been closed inadequately and may have opened, particularly if a drain had been left down in apposition with the closure. A fecalith may be free in the peritoneal cavity and lead to continued drainage. In a patient who had Crohn's disease of the terminal ileum, despite the care taken to avoid the ileum during the dissection, a fistula may appear from somewhere in the ileum. If the cecum was involved in inflammatory disease it is also possible that the closure is not satisfactory and perforation could lead not only to peritonitis but also to a fecal fistula.

These fistulas are usually treated conservatively in the absence of any evidence of distal intestinal obstruction. The great majority of them will gradually close spontaneously. There was an old clinical aphorism that if a patient developed a fecal fistula after an appendectomy for ruptured appendititis, he was sure to get well. If, however, the fistula tends to persist over a long period of time, the possibility of Crohn's disease must be entertained. A formal resection of the terminal ileum and right colon is occasionally necessary if the fistula persists. Another cause of a fistula is a retained fecalith, lying free in the peritoneal cavity following a ruptured appendix.

A special type of appendicitis should be mentioned. The appendix becomes acutely inflamed and so inextricably meshed with the terminal ileum and cecum that at the time of operation the surgeon is entirely uncertain as to whether this is appendicitis or some other type of inflammatory disease. In these cases it is far safer to carry out a right colectomy with an ileocolic anastomosis than to attempt to dissect out the appendix. The diagnosis will always be in doubt until the pathologist examines the specimen because this disease can be easily confused with diverticulitis, cancer of the cecum, or Crohn's disease.

Other Diseases of the Appendix

Mucocele

A hugely distended appendix filled with mucus should always raise the suspicion of a low-grade carcinoma of the base of the appendix. These mucoceles may perforate and produce pseudomyxoma peritonei. This appears to be a low-grade type of adenocarcinoma that becomes incurable after perforation has occurred.

Great care should be taken when a mucocele is encountered to be certain that the entire pathologic process is removed intact (Fig. 26.6). This may involve the removal of a section of cecum or right colon.

A greatly distended appendix in the absence of mucus within the lumen may be secondary to an obstructing carcinoma of the colon. The important point is that a distended, noninflamed appendix may point to a much more serious disease than appendicitis.

Carcinoid

About 1 in every 1000 appendixes contains a carcinoid tumor (Fig. 26.7). Usually they are small and are only found by the pathologist on his examination. Appendectomy is considered curative in nearly all cases. However,

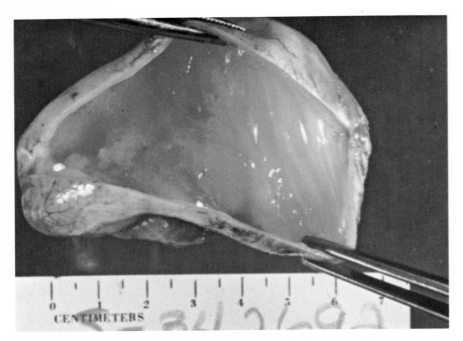

Fig. 26.6. Operative specimen of mucocele of the appendix.

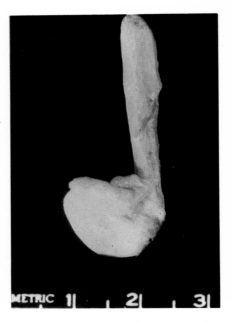

Fig. 26.7. Carcinoid tumor of the appendix. This was an incidental finding during appendectomy (operative specimen).

there are instances in which a right colectomy should be considered either as a primary or secondary procedure. They include those cases in which the appendiceal carcinoid is over 2 cm in diameter, the examination of the specimen shows invasion of the lymphatics by tumor, or carcinoid is demonstrated microscopically at the line of dissection.

The appendix may be the site of numerous other types of pathology. Carcinomas of the appendix should be treated exactly as carcinomas of the right colon, that is, by right colectomy.[2] Villous adenomas of the appendix have been reported. Diverticula of the appendix also occur.[6,7] Special infections of the appendix include infestation with pinworms. The sulfur granules of actinomycosis are occasionally found in excised appendices. Amebae can involve the appendix. In short, the appendix may be involved by any of the diseases observed in the colon.

References

1. Altemeier W.A., Culbertson W.R., Fullen W.D. (1971) Intra-abdominal sepsis. Adv Surg 5: 281
2. Andersson A., Bergdahl L., Boquist L. (1976) Primary carcinoma of the appendix. Ann Surg 183: 53
3. Babaknia A., Hossein P., Woodruff J.D. (1977) Appendicitis during pregnancy. Obstet Gynecol 50: 40
4. Law D., Law R., Eiseman B. (1976) The continuing challenge of acute and perforated appendicitis. Am J Surg 131: 533
5. Marchildon M.B., Dudgeon D.L. (1977) Perforated appendicitis: Current experience in a children's hospital. Ann Surg 185: 84
6. Wolff M., Ahmend N. (1976) Epithelial neoplasms of the vermiform appendix (exclusive of carcinoid). I. Adenocarcinoma of the appendix. Cancer 37: 2493
7. Wolff M., Ahmed N. (1976) Epithelial neoplasms of the vermiform appendix (exclusive of carcinoid). II. Cystadenomas, papillary adenomas, and adenomatous polyps of the appendix. Cancer 37: 2511

Index